Fundamentals of Sports Injury Management

THIRD EDITION

Marcia K. Anderson, PhD, LATC
Professor and Director, Athletic Training Education Program
Department of Movement Arts,
Health Promotion, & Leisure Studies
Bridgewater State University
Bridgewater, Massachusetts

Gail P. Parr, PhD, ATC
Associate Professor
Department of Kinesiology
Towson University
Towson, Maryland

Wolters Kluwer | Lippincott Williams & Wilkins
Health
Philadelphia · Baltimore · New York · London
Buenos Aires · Hong Kong · Sydney · Tokyo

Acquisitions Editor: Emily Lupash
Associate Product Manager: Erin M. Cosyn
Marketing Manager: Allison Powell
Product Director: Tanya M. Martin
Compositor: Aptara, Inc.

Copyright © 2011 Lippincott Williams & Wilkins

351 West Camden Street
Baltimore, Maryland 21201

Two Commerce Square
2001 Market Street
Philadelphia, PA 19103

Printed in the United States of America

First Edition, 1997
Second Edition, 2003

Library of Congress Cataloging-in-Publication Data

Anderson, Marcia K.
  Fundamentals of sports injury management / Marcia K. Anderson,
Gail P. Parr. – 3rd ed.
    p. cm.
  Summary: "The book focusses on establishing a comprehensive content,
'user-friendly' format for a target audience that includes individuals
asked to provide immediate first aid care for physically active
individuals across the lifespan in the absence of a certified athletic
trainer. These individuals may include coaches, exercise science/health
fitness professionals, physical education instructors, supervisors in
recreational sports programs, and directors in YMCA or other community
sports-related programs"– Provided by publisher.
  Includes bibliographical references and index.
  ISBN 978-1-4511-0976-4 (pbk.)
  1. Sports injuries.   I. Parr, Gail P.   II. Title.
  RD97.A527 2011
  617.1'027--dc22

                                           2010043272

The publishers have made every effort to trace the copyright holders for borrowed material. If they have inadvertently overlooked any, they will be pleased to make the necessary arrangements at the first opportunity.

To purchase additional copies of this book, call our customer service department at (800) 638-3030 or fax orders to (301) 824-7390. International customers should call (301) 714-2324.

Visit Lippincott Williams & Wilkins on the Internet: http://www.LWW.com. Lippincott Williams & Wilkins customer service representatives are available from 8:30 am to 6:00 pm, EST.

We are so excited to present the third edition of *Fundamentals of Sports Injury Management* to our many textbook adopters. In this edition, we have focused our attention on establishing a comprehensive content, "user-friendly" format for a target audience that includes individuals asked to provide immediate first aid care for physically active individuals across the life span in the absence of a certified athletic trainer. These individuals may include coaches, exercise science/health fitness professionals, physical education instructors, supervisors in recreational sports programs, and directors in YMCA or other community sports-related programs. In an effort to facilitate ease of reading, the term "coach" is used to collectively identify individuals who may be asked to be responsible for initial assessment and immediate care of an injured patient. This text can be used in an introductory athletic training class or sports first aid class. Because of the content, it is advisable that the student complete parallel coursework and receive current certification in cardiopulmonary resuscitation and airway management.

NEW FEATURES IN THIS EDITION

Fundaments of Sports Injury Management has undergone extensive review from certified athletic trainers, leading to a more reader-friendly text that includes pertinent information that can be easily taught in a one-semester course. As in previous editions, we have expanded illustrations of anatomy, critical information boxes, tables, and application strategies in each chapter to enhance the learning process. We have separated some critical information into new chapters and added a new section with the Injury Prevention chapter on the importance of conditioning to prevent injuries. Many of the highlighted changes and additions include the following:

- Highlighted medical terms are defined within the text and in the glossary.

- Wherever possible, injuries and conditions are organized on the basis of the specific joint or body part affected. The conditions are defined or explained, signs and symptoms are identified, and general immediate management protocols are provided. Guidelines for the coach for referral to an athletic trainer or physician are also provided.

- The end of each chapter includes Application Questions, which allow the student to integrate the information presented in each chapter into practical application. Scenarios are presented from various settings sites and involve individuals of different ages. Open discussion is encouraged on each of these scenarios. There are no "right" answers per se. Rather, the intent is to allow the students and instructor to critically assess the situation and determine the best course of action. In some scenarios, it will be as important to determine actions that should be taken as it is to define actions that should not be taken.

- **Chapter 1,** *Introduction to Injury Care,* introduces the student to the athletic training profession and explains the primary sports medicine team and its responsibilities, and discusses the coach's role in providing basic acute injury care.

- **Chapter 2,** *Legal Issues,* is a new chapter that introduces legal considerations in providing injury care and explains several strategies to prevent litigation.

- **Chapter 3,** *Injury Prevention,* introduces the three most important concepts to prevent injuries: physical conditioning, proper skill techniques, and protective equipment.

- **Chapter 4,** *Injury Mechanism and Classification of Injury,* describes general anatomical terms and concepts; mechanisms of injuries; anatomical properties and classifications of injury to soft-tissue, bone, and nerves; and finally explains basic theories of pain and its management.

- **Chapter 5,** *The Healing Process,* expands on Chapter 4 to introduce the stages of healing in soft-tissue, bones, and nerve, and explains factors that may delay the healing process.

- **Chapter 6**, *Injury Management*, begins by introducing the need for developing and implementing an emergency care plan. This is followed by information on open and closed soft-tissue wound care including current universal precautions and infection control standards. General principles in moving an injured athlete are then explained followed by a discussion on using cold versus heat in the injury process.

- **Chapter 7**, *Injury Assessment*, introduces the student to the HOPS format to assess injuries and discusses the role of the coach in injury assessment.

- **Chapter 8**, *Emergency Conditions*, explains some common emergency conditions, such as airway obstruction, cardiopulmonary emergencies, the unconscious individual, shock, anaphylaxis, and hemorrhage.

- **Chapters 9 to 16** cover specific injuries or conditions organized by body regions. The organization of the chapters has been changed to reflect a better flow through the body, beginning at the head and face; moving down the spine, thorax, and abdomen; then moving to the shoulder, elbow, wrist, and hand; and finally moving to the hip, knee, lower leg, ankle, and foot.

  - Each chapter opens with an expanded coverage of joint anatomy with detailed illustrations drawn by a medical illustrator. Joint motions are demonstrated and the primary muscles responsible for the motions are listed. Injury prevention strategies including protective equipment are then discussed.

  - Chapters are organized to provide information on contusions, sprains, strains, overuse conditions, and fractures. Each condition is defined, signs and symptoms are identified, and management protocols are provided.

  - Assessment highlights the role and responsibility of the coach in assessing each body region with recommendations for disposition of the more severe injuries.

- **Chapter 17**, *Environmental Conditions*, discusses heat- and cold-related injuries and discusses safe sport participation during potential thunderstorms.

- **Chapter 18**, *Systemic Conditions*, highlights several conditions that coaches may encounter in working with physically active individuals, such as bronchial asthma, exercise-induced bronchospasm, diabetes mellitus, seizure disorders, and epilepsy.

PEDAGOGICAL FEATURES

As educators, we have highlighted and summarized information in the text by incorporating several pedagogical features to enhance the text's usefulness as a teaching tool. This is designed to increase readability and retention of relevant and critical information. These in-text features include the following.

Learning Outcomes
Each chapter opens with a series of learning outcomes and important concepts in the chapter that the student should focus on during reading.

Key Terminology
New and difficult medical terminology is listed at the start of each chapter, is bolded and defined in the text, and can be found in the glossary.

Critical Information Boxes
Boxes are interspersed throughout each chapter to list or summarize critical information to supplement material in the text. In the joint chapters, for example, these boxes summarize signs and symptoms of specific conditions.

Tables
Several chapters have tables that expand upon pertinent information discussed in the text. This allows a large amount of knowledge to be organized in an easy-to-read summary of information.

Art and Photography Program
Art plays a major role in facilitating the learning process for visual learners. As such, the art in this edition has been thoroughly updated to provide appropriate, detailed illustrations and

photographs incorporated to supplement material presented in the text. The illustrations provide realistic and accurate figures to depict anatomical structures and to illustrate injury mechanisms.

Chapter Summary
Each chapter has a summary of key concepts discussed in the text. Although provided as a summary, they in no way denote all of the critical information covered in the chapter.

Application Questions
Several injury scenarios are provided to challenge each student to clinically apply the knowledge from the text into a real-life experience. There are no correct answers provided. The intent is to spark classroom discussion, facilitated by the instructor, to encourage students to think creatively and logically in managing each injury.

References
Any valuable teaching tool must include a listing of cited references used to gather information for the text. We have tried to limit the references to a 5-year period, except where the reference is considered to be the original groundbreaking research. The bibliography can be used by the instructor or the student to find additional information on a topic, if needed.

Glossary and Index
An extensive glossary of terms from highlighted words in the individual chapters is provided at the end of the book. Furthermore, the comprehensive index contains cross-referencing information to locate specific information within the text.

ANCILLARY MATERIALS
Online resource centers are available for both the instructor and the student on *thePoint*.

Instructor's Resource Center
The online resource center will be organized by chapters and include the following:

- **PowerPoint Presentations.** The PowerPoint presentations were developed with an understanding that instructors and students adopt various strategies when using PowerPoint. The slides provide detailed rather than general information, recognizing that it is simpler for an educator to delete rather than add information. In addition, given the tendency of many students to take notes verbatim from a slide, an effort was made to condense the actual wording of statements to streamline the note-taking process. The presentations can be downloaded and customized to meet specific needs.

- **Supporting Lecture Notes.** The lecture notes correspond to the individual slides comprising the PowerPoint presentations. The notes are not intended to serve as an actual lecture. Rather, they are designed to provide the instructor with information that supports the material presented on the slides. As such, the notes include additional explanation and background information, as well as examples of concepts.

- **Worksheets.** Utilizing various formats, the exercises in the worksheets require students to demonstrate knowledge and comprehension, as well as apply, analyze, synthesize, and evaluate information. Answer sheets are provided for the worksheets.

- **Image Bank.** A bank of the various illustrations contained in the text is provided for classroom use.

- **Test Bank.** The bank includes more than 1,000 sample test questions composed of multiple choice, true/false, and short answer questions. The program will allow faculty to add/customize their own test questions.

Student Resource Center. The online resource center for students will include:

- **PowerPoint Presentations.** The slides will be the same as those available to the instructor. However, the student will not have access to the supporting lecture notes.

- **Glossary.** The glossary available in the text will also be readily accessible online.

- **Quizzes.** Quizzes containing multiple choice and true/false questions will be available for each chapter.

We hope the new format and level of the material is well received by our colleagues. It is very difficult to please all educators who are looking for that one book that can meet all their needs. We hope this edition of *Fundamentals of Sports Injury Management* will be that book and look forward to your comments.

Marcia K. Anderson, PhD, LATC
Bridgewater State University
Bridgewater, Massachusetts

Gail P. Parr, PhD, ATC
Towson University
Towson, Maryland

ACKNOWLEDGMENTS

We thank several of our colleagues, many of whom assisted in the development of the text through their critical analysis and review of the initial drafts. These individuals include:

Susan J. Hall, Ph.D.
University of Delaware,
Wilmington, Delaware

Patricia L. Ponce, DPT, ATC, CSCS
Towson University
Towson, Maryland

Anonymous Reviewers
We also thank the talented, hardworking individuals at Lippincott Williams and Wilkins: Emily Lupash and Erin Cosyn. Their patience and attention to detail were a strong foundation for producing such an excellent text.

Special thanks must be extended to Dr. Victoria Bacon for her support and encouragement to stick to the project and meet the deadlines, a daunting task for anyone. Thank you to all!

Marcia K. Anderson
Gail P. Parr

CONTENTS IN BRIEF

CONTENTS

APPLICATION STRATEGIES

Foundations of Injury Prevention

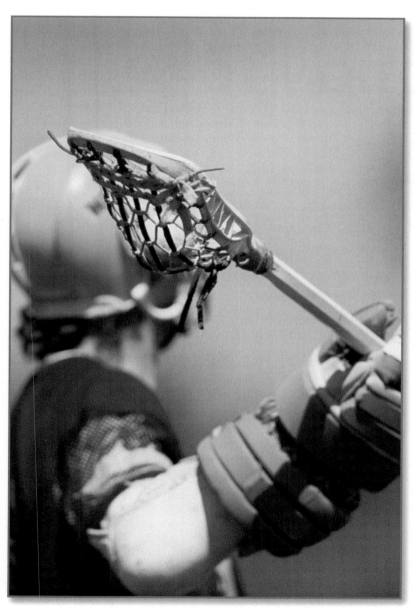

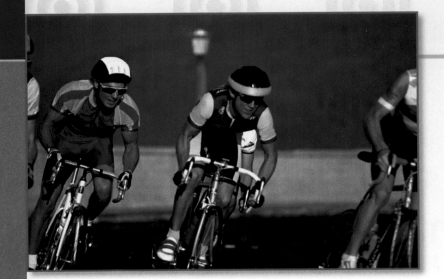

INTRODUCTION TO INJURY CARE

KEY TERMS

athletic training
diagnosis
sports medicine

LEARNING OUTCOMES

1. Differentiate between sports medicine and athletic training.
2. Identify and explain the performance domains of a certified athletic trainer.
3. Describe the team approach to the delivery of healthcare to participants in sport and physical activity programs.
4. Identify responsibilities of the primary care physician, team physician, and athletic trainer in providing care for physically active individuals.
5. Identify responsibilities of the coach, physical educator, fitness specialist, and sport supervisor in injury prevention and management.
6. Identify responsibilities of physically active individuals (participants) in injury prevention and management.

Sport, with the inherent risks involved, leads to injury at one time or another for nearly all participants. In an organized sport setting, such as interscholastic, intercollegiate, and professional level of play, team physicians and athletic trainers are responsible for the daily health and safety of physically active individuals. Furthermore, these professionals serve as a valuable resource to educate and counsel athletes to prevent chronic degenerative injuries and diseases through life-long activity-related fitness and health education. At times, however, these professionals may not be readily accessible at all arenas and venues, where injuries to physically active individuals may occur. Therefore, other professionals, such as physical educators, coaches, sport supervisors, and fitness specialists, find themselves in situations that require them to take steps to reduce the likelihood of injury and to render immediate care to an injured participant. This book is intended to provide physical educators, coaches, sport supervisors, and fitness specialists with information that should be considered when providing care to an injured individual. For the sake of brevity, these professionals will be referred to as coaches.

This chapter will first examine the profession of **athletic training**. In the absence of an athletic trainer, the coach must assume a more active role in providing healthcare to participants. As such, it is essential that the coach understands the responsibilities of the athletic trainer to ensure that the coach acts within their appropriate duty of care in tending to an injured participant. A team approach to the delivery of healthcare will be presented with reference to the responsibilities of the coach, team physician, primary care physician, and the participant.

SPORTS MEDICINE

Sports medicine is a broad and complex branch of healthcare, encompassing several disciplines. Essentially, it is an area of healthcare and special services that applies medical and scientific knowledge to prevent, recognize, assess, manage, and rehabilitate injuries or illnesses related to sports, exercises, or recreational activities, and in doing so, it enhances the health fitness and performance of the participant. No single profession can provide the expertise to carry out this enormous responsibility. Rather, professionals from several disciplines play key roles in providing healthcare for physically active individuals. These professionals may include certified athletic trainers, team physicians and/or primary care physicians, orthopedic physicians, physical therapists, emergency medical technicians, radiologists, dentists, nutritionists, exercise physiologists, biomechanists, sport psychologists, and massage therapists.

ATHLETIC TRAINING

The National Athletic Trainers' Association (NATA) represents over 30,000 members in the athletic training profession.[1] The current mission of the NATA is to enhance the quality of healthcare provided by certified athletic trainers and advance the athletic training profession.[1]

According to the NATA, athletic training is a discipline practiced by athletic trainers. Athletic trainers are allied healthcare professionals, who work in collaboration with physicians to "optimize activity and participation of clients."[1] As medical experts in the prevention, assessment, **diagnosis**, and intervention of emergency, acute, and chronic medical conditions, involving impairment, functional limitations, and disabilities, athletic trainers are uniquely qualified to provide healthcare services to athletes and the physically active. While athletic trainers have a solid presence in the traditional settings of college/university and professional sports, athletic trainers have expanded their medical expertise to include work in clinics (e.g., sports medicine and physical therapy centers), offices (e.g., hospitals), and industrial/occupational settings.

The Board of Certification for the Athletic Trainer is the professional organization responsible for both the certification of athletic trainers and defining the major performance domains of the athletic trainer.[2] These domains include the following.[3]

Prevention

The domain of prevention encompasses a broad spectrum of knowledge and skills that address the risks associated with participation in sports and physical activities. Such risks range in severity from minor to potentially catastrophic injuries or illnesses. In a similar manner, the strategies used to minimize such risks can vary from relatively simple to complex. Examples of injury and illness prevention could involve preparticipation physical examinations; regular safety checks of equipments, facilities, and field areas; designing and implementing year-round conditioning programs to develop and maintain strength, flexibility, agility, and endurance; promoting proper lifting techniques and safety in the weight room; following universal safety precautions to prevent the spread of infectious diseases; applying appropriate taping, wrappings, protective devices, or braces; and monitoring environmental conditions, such as temperature, humidity, or lightning during thunderstorms, and following guidelines for safe participation in adverse weather conditions.

Clinical Evaluation and Diagnosis

The domain of clinical evaluation and diagnosis addresses the responsibilities of the athletic trainer in using standardized clinical practices to make decisions regarding the nature and severity of an injury or illness. Evaluation, or assessment, can involve several scenarios, including on-field (or on-site) primary assessments, off-field initial assessments, and follow-up assessments (FIG. 1.1). In each situation, the evaluation must follow a systematic format that includes a history of the injury or illness; observation and inspection of the condition; palpation of soft tissues and bony structures; and a variety of tests (e.g., range-of-motion, muscle strength, sensory and motor neurologic function, ligamentous/capsular integrity, and functional status). This information is essential in determining the extent and seriousness of an injury or illness, and ultimately, deciding the appropriate management of the condition.

Immediate Care

The immediate-care domain identifies the role of the athletic trainer subsequent to determining the nature and extent of an injury or illness. The athletic trainer must be prepared to care for and prevent further harm for various conditions. As such, immediate care could range from the implementation of standard emergency care for a life-threatening condition (e.g., activating the emergency medical plan) to rendering standard immediate care for a musculoskeletal injury, such as immobilizing a possible fracture and applying cold and compression to a sprain or strain.

Treatment, Rehabilitation, and Reconditioning

The athletic trainer is responsible for the implementation of treatment, rehabilitation, and reconditioning programs appropriate to the diagnosis made during the evaluation and assessment phase (FIG. 1.2). In consultation with a physician, a comprehensive treatment program is developed, including therapeutic goals and objectives, selection of appropriate therapeutic modalities

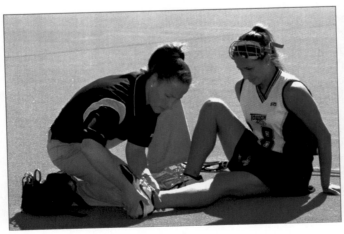

FIGURE 1.1 Injury assessment. Athletic trainers perform assessments in a variety of settings, including on the field.

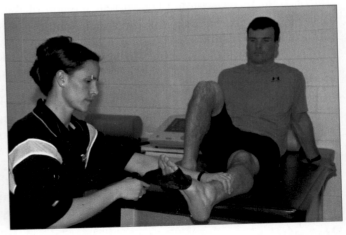

FIGURE 1.2 Injury rehabilitation. A major performance domain of the athletic trainer includes the development and implementation of rehabilitation programs.

and exercise, use of pharmacologic agents, methods to assess and document progress, and criteria for return to participation. Information gathered and documented during rehabilitation assists the physician in determining when the individual may be cleared for participation.

Organization and Administration

The organization and administration domain describes the responsibilities of the athletic trainer in developing and executing a series of plans, policies, and procedures to ensure responsive and efficient operation of the athletic training program. General areas that warrant attention in this domain include documentation and maintenance of the healthcare records, including those pertaining to health services (i.e., preparticipation examinations, injury evaluations, immediate treatment of injuries/illnesses, rehabilitation progress, and medical clearance to participate); other services rendered to an injured party (e.g., counseling, educational programs, referrals to specialists); confidentiality of medical records; financial management; facility management; personnel management; purchase of equipments and supplies; equipment-reconditioning records; compliance with defined safety standards; emergency care protocols; public relations; and normal operating procedures.

Professional Responsibility

The domain of professional responsibility focuses on the expectations of the athletic trainer relative to adhering to ethical, legal, and other professional standards. The knowledge and skills identified in this area are intended to ensure appropriate care in all aspects of healthcare delivery (e.g., patient assessment, care, and treatment; knowledge of current best practices; administrative functions).

TEAM APPROACH TO THE DELIVERY OF HEALTHCARE

The risk of injury is inherent with participation in sports and physical activities. While participation in sports and physical activities can be an important component of a healthy lifestyle for both children and adults, participants can expect to sustain an injury at some point in time.

The team approach to the delivery of healthcare allows for a comprehensive prevention, assessment, and management of an injury or illness, as it taps the expertise of individual specialists working in conjunction with one another and the patient. By having healthcare professionals from different disciplines work collaboratively, a venue is in place for addressing an injury from different perspectives. For example, a 14-year-old adolescent having sustained a serious head injury while participating in interscholastic soccer presents with different concerns than a 30-year-old professional soccer player. Having a pediatrician or a neurologist specializing in pediatrics serve on the healthcare team would benefit the 14-year-old adolescent, but those specialists would not be necessary in treating the 30 year old. In a similar manner, a collaborative care or team approach would best serve the healthcare needs of an older adult participating in a cardiac rehabilitation program. An understanding of the appropriate exercise parameters, impact of medications on exercise participations, and provisions for managing an emergent situation must extend beyond the traditional doctor-to-patient approach to include at a minimum the fitness specialist, the cardiac rehabilitation specialist, and the personnel responsible for onsite management of cardiac-related emergencies.

A majority of professional and college sport programs have access to a team of professionals that oversee the healthcare of their participants relative to injury prevention, assessment, immediate management, and rehabilitation. Unfortunately, the same personnel and provisions are not readily available to the millions of other participants in sport, recreation, exercise, and physical activity programs. In particular, the areas of injury prevention and immediate management are often overlooked or relegated to the coach, physical educator, or fitness specialist, regardless of their background.

While it may not be by choice, the coach is a member of the healthcare delivery team. In many instances, the coach is the first individual to respond to an injured participant. As such, it is essential that the coaches understand their roles and responsibilities to ensure the safety of the participant, as well as to ensure their own protection in a potentially liable situation.

A team approach can provide an effective means for ensuring quality healthcare for physically active individuals. Establishing the responsibilities of the various members of the healthcare team is essential to ensuring appropriate care.

Primary Care Physician

In some settings, particularly outside the traditional athletic setting, the primary care physician or family physician assumes a key role in providing medical care to athletes and physically active individuals of all ages. The services provided by the primary care physician can vary with the background and expertise of the individual. Services performed by a primary care physician can range from completing a preparticipation examination for a young athlete to counseling a middle-aged patient with multiple risk factors for coronary artery diseases on the parameters for safely beginning an exercise program.[4] In some settings, the primary care physician assumes the responsibility of determining the medical eligibility or clearing an individual for participation in an activity.

Team Physician

In organized sports, such as interscholastic, intercollegiate, or professional athletic programs, a team physician may be hired or may volunteer their services to direct the healthcare team. This individual supervises the various aspects of healthcare and is the final authority to determine the mental and physical fitness of athletes in organized programs.

In an athletic program, the team physician should administer and review preseason physical examinations; review preseason conditioning programs; assess the quality, effectiveness, and maintenance of protective equipments; diagnose injuries; dispense medications; direct rehabilitation programs; educate the athletic staff on emergency policies, procedures, healthcare insurance coverage, and legal liability; and review all medical forms, policies, and procedures to ensure compliance with school and athletic association guidelines.[4] This individual may also serve as a valuable resource on current therapeutic techniques, facilitate referrals to other medical specialists, and provide educational counseling to sport participants, parents, athletic trainers, coaches, and sport supervisors.

The Coach, Physical Educator, Fitness Specialist, and Sport Supervisor

These professionals are responsible for teaching various skills and/or strategies related to sports and physical activities. In many cases, these individuals are also responsible for administering and supervising activities or activity areas within an institution or health club facility. In both instances, these specialists are responsible for injury prevention, onsite assessment, and management of injuries, including reducing the potential for further injury or harm.

As such, the coach must encourage appropriate behavior and develop an overall awareness of safety and injury prevention. In general, responsibilities of the coach associated with injury prevention include teaching proper skill development and techniques; providing conditioning programs that are physiologically and developmentally appropriate; checking to ensure that equipments, facilities, and playing fields are safe for participation; evaluating the status of participants prior to permitting them to engage in an activity; and providing appropriate supervision during activities[5] (Box 1.1).

BOX 1.1   Injury Prevention: Responsibilities of the Coach

- **Instructions for proper skill development and techniques**
- **Development and implementation of conditioning programs that are physiologically and developmentally appropriate**
- **Inspection of equipment, facilities, and playing fields/courts to ensure that their use is safe for participation**
- **Evaluation of the status of participants prior to permitting them to engage in activities**
- **Supervision during activities**

BOX 1.2	Injury Assessment and Management: Responsibilities of the Coach in the Absence of an Athletic Trainer

- Assessment of the nature and severity of injury
- Determination of the appropriate course of action in managing an injury
- Implementation of the appropriate course of action (e.g., administering basic first aid and initiating an emergency care plan as necessary)

The role of these specialists as members of the healthcare delivery team will vary based on both the setting and the staff employed (e.g., athletic trainer; school nurse). In the absence of an athletic trainer, the coach must assume a more active role in providing healthcare to participants. As such, the coach must be able to recognize a potentially serious injury and be able to determine the immediate care that should be provided. In general, responsibilities of the coach associated with immediate management of an injury include assessing the nature and severity of an injury; determining the appropriate course of action in managing the injury; providing the appropriate course of action (e.g., emergency first aid); and initiating an emergency care plan as necessary[5] (Box 1.2). As such, coaches, physical educators, fitness specialists, and sport supervisors should complete a basic athletic training class and maintain a current certification in emergency cardiac care (i.e., cardiopulmonary resuscitation [CPR] and automated external defibrillator [AED]) and emergency first aid.

In performing their duties, it is essential that the coach understands the concepts of standards of care and duty of care. In the capacity of being responsible for the medical well-being of participants, a coach is legally responsible for their actions. As such, it is imperative that the coach has an understanding of legal issues pertaining to injury care and management. Chapter 2 of this book addresses legal considerations, legal liabilities, and legal defenses pertaining to a coach.

Sport/Physical Activity Participant

The participant must also play a role in efforts to maximize injury prevention. It is the responsibility of the participant to adhere to prescribed guidelines for their activity. Such responsibilities could include maintaining an appropriate level of fitness; performing within the rules or guidelines of an activity; and maintaining and wearing safety equipments. In the event of an injury, the participant should know the protocol for reporting an injury and seeking immediate healthcare. In some cases, an injury may be apparent to the coach or supervisor, but there will definitely be scenarios in which an injury is not readily apparent to an observer. Participants must understand their responsibility for reporting an injury. If participants understand and practice safety and preventive measures, the number of injuries or illnesses can be reduced significantly.

Additional Professionals Involved in Healthcare of Physically Active Individuals

Physical Therapist

Physical therapists provide a unique and valuable resource in the overall rehabilitation of an individual. Physical therapists often supervise the rehabilitation of injured participants in a hospital setting, an industrial clinic, or a sports medicine clinic.[6]

Exercise Physiologist

An exercise physiologist can provide information pertaining to the physiological mechanisms underlying physical activities. As such, the exercise physiologist can offer theoretical and practical suggestions regarding the analysis, improvement, and maintenance of health and fitness as well as rehabilitation of heart diseases and other chronic diseases and/or disabilities.[7]

Nutritionist

Nutritionists are primarily concerned with the role of proper dietary care in the prevention and treatment of illnesses. However, a nutritionist can provide valuable input regarding the specialized needs of athletes and physically active individuals. Examples of particular needs include diets for enhancing performance and preventing injury; effective weight management strategies (e.g., weight gain, loss, or maintenance); physical activity and diabetes; individual special dietary needs; counseling with regard to disordered eating; and nutrient supplementation.[8]

Biomechanist

Applying basic laws of physics in performing mechanical analyses of human movement, a biomechanist can offer practical insight into improving human performance as well as preventing sport and physical activity related injuries. Information pertaining to kinematics, the study of spatial and temporal aspects of motion, can provide valuable information pertaining to injury prevention, while information regarding kinetics, the study of forces associated with motion, provides a basis for understanding injury mechanisms.[9]

SUMMARY

1. Sports medicine is a branch of medicine that applies medical and scientific knowledge to improve sport performance.

2. The NATA establishes standards for professionalism, education, research, and practice settings for athletic trainers. As medical experts in the prevention, assessment, diagnosis, intervention of emergency, acute, and chronic medical conditions involving impairment, functional limitations, and disabilities, athletic trainers are uniquely qualified to provide healthcare services to athletes and the physically active.

3. The major performance domains of an athletic trainer include (1) prevention, (2) clinical evaluation and diagnosis, (3) immediate care, (4) treatment, rehabilitation, and reconditioning, (5) organization and administration, and (6) professional responsibility.

4. The team approach to the delivery of healthcare allows for a comprehensive prevention, assessment, management, and rehabilitation of injury. The collaborative efforts of various specialists can best serve participants in sport and physical activities.

5. In the absence of an athletic trainer, the coach should be able to:
   - Assess and recognize potentially severe injuries;
   - Provide emergency first aid; and
   - Initiate appropriate referral for advanced medical care, if necessary.

APPLICATION QUESTIONS

1. Should the terms "sports medicine" and "athletic training" be used interchangeably?

2. Injury prevention is one of the major domains of the athletic trainer. A high school with an interscholastic athletic program cannot afford to hire an athletic trainer. What general strategies could the coaches at the school implement in an effort to reduce the incidence and severity of injury (i.e., injury prevention)?

3. You are a fitness specialist at a commercial fitness facility. What instructions would you give to your clients regarding their role in ensuring appropriate and quality healthcare on-site?

4. What are the responsibilities of a physical education teacher in reducing the incidence of injury during class?

5. Why is the team approach to healthcare delivery preferable to a traditional doctor-to-patient approach to ensure quality healthcare for participants in sport and physical activities?

6. Why should the coach of a youth sports team complete a basic athletic training class and maintain current certification in emergency cardiac care (i.e., CPR and AED) and emergency first aid?

REFERENCES

1. National athletic trainers' association. (n.d.). Retrieved from http://www.nata.org/index.htm.
2. Board of certification for the athletic trainer. (n.d.). Retrieved from http://www.bocatc.org/.
3. Fincher L, et al. 2010. Athletic training services: an overview of skills and services performed by certified athletic trainers. Retrieved from http://www.nata.org/about_AT/docs/GuideToAthletic-TrainingServices.pdf.
4. American academy of family physicians. (n.d.). Retrieved from http://www.aafp.org/online/en/home/policy/policies/p/primarycare.html#Parsys0004.
5. National federation of state high school associations. (n.d.). Retrieved from http://www.nfhs.org/.
6. Sports physical therapy section. (n.d.). Retrieved from http://www.spts.org/about-spts/what-is-sports-physical-therapy.
7. Lowery L. (n.d.). American society of exercise physiologists. Retrieved from http://www.asep.org/.
8. National association of sports nutrition. (n.d.). Retrieved from http://www.nasnutrition.com/define.htm.
9. American sports medicine institute. (n.d.). Retrieved from http://www.asmi.org/asmiweb/education/careerInfo.htm.

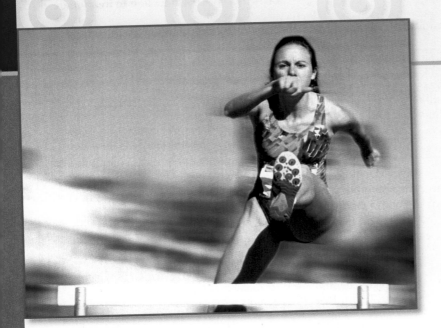

LEGAL ISSUES

KEY TERMS

assumption of risk

battery

commission

comparative negligence

duty of care

exculpatory waiver

expressed warranty

foreseeability of harm

HIPPA

implied warranty

informed consent

malfeasance

misfeasance

negligence

nonfeasance

omission

standard of care

tort

LEARNING OUTCOMES

1. Explain the concepts of standard of care and duty of care with specific reference to the responsibilities of a coach.

2. Identify the factors that must be proved to show legal breach of duty of care (i.e., negligence).

3. Describe measures that can reduce the risk of litigation, including clearance for participation, assumption of risk, informed consent, exculpatory waivers, confidentiality, foreseeability of harm, instruction and supervision, participant responsibility, Good Samaritan laws, and risk management.

Preventing injuries, managing injuries, and reducing the potential for further injury or harm are major responsibilities for individuals involved in the instruction, supervision, or administration of programs involving physical activity. Evidence of the significance of this responsibility can be found in the number and extent of lawsuits filed by individuals who have sustained injuries during participation in sport and physical activity.

By understanding legal issues relating to the provision of injury prevention and management, the coach can take active steps toward reducing the risk of liability. This chapter will begin with an explanation of legal considerations applicable to the coach. It will be followed by strategies that the coach should consider as a means for reducing the risk of litigation.

LEGAL CONSIDERATIONS

In ensuring proper care for the individuals under their care, it is essential that coaches, physical educators, personal trainers, and other specialists responsible for the medical well-being of their players, students, and clients protect themselves with regard to liability, a legal responsibility for one's acts. Failure to attend to that responsibility could result in a lawsuit for damages sustained (Box 2.1).

Standard of Care

In defining **standard of care**, it is important to distinguish between reasonable person standard of care and professional standard of care. Reasonable person standard of care is a minimum standard that requires an individual to act as a reasonably prudent person.[1,2] For example, while riding a bicycle on a city street, a reasonably prudent person would wear an appropriate helmet. In doing so, the individual is taking a precaution to reduce the risk and severity of injury.

In comparison, the professional standard of care requires an individual to use the knowledge, skills, and abilities that conform to the standard of care for their particular specialization.[2] Professional standards of practice are established by professional organizations, such as the National Athletic Trainers' Association, the National Association for Sport and Physical Education, the American College of Sports Medicine, and the National Strength and Conditioning Association. In a liability case, standard of care is measured by what another minimally

---

BOX 2.1   Actions that Can Result in Litigation

- Failing to warn an individual about the risks involved in participation.
- Treating an injured party without their consent.
- Failing to provide medical information concerning alternative treatments or the risks involved with the treatment to a participant.
- Failing to provide safe facilities, fields, and equipments.
- Being aware of a potentially dangerous situation and failing to do anything about it.
- Failing to provide an adequate injury prevention program.
- Allowing an injured or unfit player to participate resulting in further injury or harm.
- Failing to provide quality training, instruction, and supervision.

- Using unsafe equipments.
- Negligently moving an injured athlete before properly immobilizing the injured area.
- Failing to employ qualified medical personnel.
- Failing to have a written emergency action plan.
- Failing to properly recognize an injury or illness, both as immediate acute care and long-term treatment.
- Failing to immediately refer an injured party to the proper physician.
- Failing to keep adequate records.
- Treating an injury that did not occur within the school athletic environment.

competent individual educated and practicing in that profession would have done to protect an individual from harm or further harm. As such, the standard of care differs depending upon the profession. For example, an athletic trainer would be held to the standards of a certified athletic trainer.[2] A coach would not be expected to conform to the standards of an athletic trainer, but rather the national standards for sport coaches. In fact, if an individual performs actions that are outside the parameters of their standard of care, the potential for negligence exists. For example, if a coach dispenses medication to an injured participant, then the coach has rendered a medical service that is outside their standard of care. In that scenario, the coach is liable for an action, which was outside their scope of practice and not consistent with their duty of care.

Duty of Care

Coaches, physical educators, personal trainers, and other specialists have a legal obligation to provide a professional standard of care to protect individuals under their care or supervision from unreasonable risks that could potentially be harmful. This obligation, referred to as **duty of care**, encompasses a variety of responsibilities, such as teaching proper and appropriate techniques for an age group, providing appropriate supervision of activities, providing quality safety equipments, ensuring a safe participation environment, and taking proper actions when an injury is sustained.[2,3]

Negligence

Legal action involving the practice of sport and physical activity injury care is typically tried under tort law. A **tort** is a civil wrong done to an individual, whereby the injured party seeks a remedy for damages suffered. Such wrongs may be attributed to negligence. **Negligence** can occur as a result of an action or lack of an action by a professional who had a legal duty of care.[2,4]

Negligent torts include nonfeasance, malfeasance, and misfeasance (Box 2.2). **Nonfeasance**, also known as an act of **omission**, occurs when an individual fails to perform a legal duty of care. For example, if a coach knows that a player has sustained an injury and permits or persuades the athlete to continue to play, the coach has not exercised reasonable care. **Malfeasance**, also known as an act of **commission**, occurs when an individual commits an act that is not their responsibility to perform. For example, if a physical education teacher suspects that a student has sustained a lower leg fracture due to the visible angulation of the involved bones, the teacher could be liable, if their management of the injury included straightening the leg and immobilizing it in a splint. **Misfeasance** occurs when an individual commits an act that is their responsibility to perform, but uses the wrong procedure or performs the correct procedure in an improper manner.[2,4] For example, if a personal trainer responsible for conducting a pre-activity participant screening fails to perform the screening in a manner consistent with professional guidelines and standards, the personal trainer could be held liable, if the participant later sustains an injury or illness related to their participation in a fitness program.

BOX 2.2   Definition of Negligent Torts

- **Malfeasance** occurs when an individual commits an act that is not their responsibility to perform.
- **Misfeasance** occurs when an individual commits an act that is their responsibility to perform, but uses the wrong procedure, or does the right procedure in an improper manner.
- **Nonfeasance** occurs when an individual fails to perform their legal duty of care.

In cases involving negligence, an individual is potentially entitled to compensation for injury or harm sustained. The burden of proof of negligence lies with the harmed individual. Specifically, the person must prove the four elements of negligence. These include[3,4]:

- There was a duty of care owed to the injured person by the person responsible for the injury.
- There was a breach of that duty.
- There was harm (e.g., pain and suffering, permanent disability, or loss of wages).
- The resulting harm was a direct cause of the breach of duty.

For example, a soccer coach has a duty of care to the participants to check the playing field for hazards. If during a soccer game, a player sustains an injury subsequent to stepping into a hole on the playing field, the coach could be held liable for the harm to the participant. In comparison, if a spectator notices a large hole in the field prior to a soccer game, the spectator has no legal duty to report the potential hazard. The spectator is not liable for any harm sustained by the soccer player.

REDUCING LITIGATION

All individuals responsible for providing healthcare to athletes or physical activity participants should be aware of their duty of care consistent with existing state laws, and complete that duty of care within established policies and standards of practice for their respective professions. In addition, they should actively engage in steps to reduce the risk of litigation (Box 2.3). (Again, for the sake of brevity, coaches, physical educators, and personal trainers will be referred to as coaches.)

Clearance for Participation

The use of a preparticipation examination (PPE) performed by a licensed physician as a requirement for participation in a sports team or in a physical fitness program can be an effective strategy for ensuring an individual's health and safety as it pertains to their participation in physical activity or sport (Box 2.4). A PPE can obtain information on an individual's general health, maturity, and fitness level. The PPE can also identify any underlying or pre-existing conditions that could predispose an individual to injury or illness subsequent to their participation in sport or physical activity.[2–4]

The focus of a PPE is dependent on the specific age group. For example, in the prepubescent child (i.e., 6 to 10 years of age), the focus may be on identifying previously undiagnosed congenital abnormalities. In the pubescent child (i.e., 11 to 15 years of age), the examination should center on maturation and establishing good health practices for safe participation. In the postpubescent or

---

BOX 2.3 Strategies that Coaches Can Take to Avoid Litigation

- Inform the individual about the inherent risks of participation.
- Obtain informed consent from the individual or their guardian prior to participation in the sport/activity and prior to any treatment should an injury occur.
- Provide proper supervision and instruction.
- Foresee the potential for injury and correcting the situation before harm occurs.
- Perform regular inspection of fields, gymnasiums, and activity rooms.
- Use quality products and equipments that do not pose a threat to the individual.

- Post warning signs in plain sight on and around equipments to inform about the risks involved in abuse of equipments and to describe proper use of the equipments.
- Maintain accurate healthcare records; maintaining strict confidentiality of all medical records.
- Establish a well-organized emergency action plan.
- Act as a reasonably prudent professional in caring for all participants.

BOX 2.4	**Goals of the Preparticipation Exam**

- Determine general health and current immunization status.
- Detect medical conditions that are not healed or may predispose the individual to injury or illness so medical treatment can start prior to sport/activity participation.
- Identify health risk behaviors that may be corrected through informed counseling.
- Establish baseline parameters for determining when an injured individual may return to activity.
- Assess physical maturity.
- Evaluate the level of physical fitness.
- Classify the individual as to readiness for participation.
- Recommend appropriate levels of participation for individuals with medical contraindications to exercise.
- Meet legal and insurance requirements related to participation in physical activity or sport.

young adult group (i.e., 16 to 30 years of age), the history of previous injuries and sport-specific examinations are critical. For individuals with cardiovascular or pulmonary diseases, the strenuousness of a physical activity is an additional consideration. Because the adult population (i.e., 30 to 65 years of age) has a high incidence of overuse injuries, these individuals need an examination based on the nature of the activity in which they intend to engage. The final group, those older than 65 years of age, often begins or increases activity to prevent a major medical illness. These individuals need an extensive examination based on individual needs, taking into consideration not only their physical needs, but also medications being taken and their possible side effects.[5]

Subsequent to the conclusion of the PPE, the physician must determine the level of participation based on conditions identified during the examination and knowledge of the physical demands of the physical activity. The physician must ask:

- Will the condition increase the risk of injury to the individual or other participants?
- Can participation be allowed, if medication, rehabilitation, protective bracing, or padding is used? If so, can limited participation be allowed in the interim?
- If clearance is denied for a particular activity, are there other activities in which the individual can participate safely?

Recent interpretations of the Federal Rehabilitation Act and Americans with Disabilities Act have stated that individuals have the legal right to participate in any competitive sport, regardless of a pre-existing medical condition. For this reason, physicians cannot totally exclude an individual from participation, but rather can only recommend the individual not to participate because of a medical condition that increases the risk of further injury and/or death as a result of participation.[6,7] In these situations, an **exculpatory waiver** may be used. An exculpatory waiver is based on the individual's **assumption of risk** and is a release signed by the individual or parent of an individual under the age of 18 that releases the physician from liability of negligence.

In addition to a PPE, a mechanism should be in place for permitting a participant to return to activity following injury or illness. The final authority in measuring an individual's status for participation typically rests with a physician. In settings in which a team physician is employed, it is the team physician who makes the determination. In other settings, policies should be established that identify the conditions under which an individual can return to activity. Such policies should include conditions, which automatically warrant medical clearance before return to activity. For example, if a member of a fitness facility reports a cardiac-related symptom during a workout, it would be advisable to require the individual to obtain clearance from their primary care physician or a cardiologist before permitting the individual to return to the facility. It would not be prudent to permit the individual to self-diagnose, as it could place both the participant and the fitness instructor in compromising positions.[2,3]

A second example can be seen in a scenario in which a middle-school physical education student sustains head trauma. Following an incident in which a student's head strikes the gymnasium floor, the student presents with momentary confusion and a headache, which persisted until the student's parent arrived 45 minutes later. Given the medical consequences associated with concussion and return to play following concussion, it would be advisable to require physician's approval for return to participation in a physical education class.

Another factor to consider is the level of the healthcare provider (e.g., physician; physician assistant; nurse care practitioner; physical therapist; athletic trainer) capable of making acceptable recommendations for return to activity. For example, the physical education student in the previous example may have been seen by a physician assistant in an emergency room setting. In this scenario, the physical education teacher should consider the recommendations of the physician assistant to be legally defensible. In following the recommendations of the physician assistant, the physical education teacher is performing their duty of care to the student.

Assumption of Risk

Coaches should inform potential participants of the risks for injury during sport and physical activity participation. Participants and parents of minor children should understand that the risk for injury exists as well as the nature of that risk, so that informed judgments can be made about participation. Understanding and comprehending the nature of the risk is determined by the participant's age, experience, and knowledge of pertinent information about the risk. An advanced gymnast, for example, knows and appreciates the risk of injury much more than a novice gymnast. Therefore, it is crucial to warn the novice of any inherent dangers in the activity and continually reinforce that information throughout the entire sport season. Warnings may be communicated at the preseason meeting with parents and participants; during prescreening when the client is first introduced into the fitness or health facility; and by posting visible warning signs around equipments, requiring protective equipments, and discouraging dangerous techniques.

Participants and parents of minor children should (1) understand that risk for injury exists, (2) appreciate the nature of the risk, and (3) voluntarily accept the risk. Understanding and comprehending the nature of the risk is determined by the participant's age, experience, and knowledge of pertinent information about the risk.[1,2]

As evidence that a participant has been warned of and understands the risks for injury, it is advisable to have participants sign an expressed assumption of risk form (APPLICATION STRATEGY 2.1) (BOX 2.5). By signing the form, the individual affirms an understanding and appreciation of the risks of their participation in the activity.[1,5,6] In addition, the form acknowledges their voluntary choice to participate and assume the risks inherent in the activity. An assumption of risk form should acknowledge that injury could range in nature from minor to catastrophic, including the potential for traumatic brain injury, paralysis, and even death.[2,4]

An assumption of risk form does not exempt coaches from liability. An individual does not assume the risk that a professional will breach their duty of care. Accordingly, an assumption of risk form does not absolve a coach of liability for inappropriate actions or conduct.[2]

Exculpatory Waiver

It is not unforeseen that an individual will challenge their right to participate, regardless of a physician's recommendation that participation not be permitted. In these situations, several professionals (e.g., physician; athletic trainer; school administrators; facility owners/directors) directly or indirectly involved in the healthcare of the participant may request that the individual sign an exculpatory waiver. An exculpatory waiver is a contract that releases the professional from any liability to the individual executing the release.[8] Similar to an assumption of risk, in signing an exculpatory waiver, the participant acknowledges their understanding of the risks involved in their participation and their voluntary choice to participate in the face of those risks. In addition, an exculpatory waiver states that the participant will not hold the noted professionals liable in the event of injury. Because the validity of this type of waiver varies based on state law, professionals should seek assistance from legal professionals before establishing an exculpatory waiver.

Informed Consent

Authorization to provide treatment for an injury should be obtained in writing prior to the beginning of participation (APPLICATION STRATEGY 2.2). **Informed consent** implies that an injured party has been reasonably informed of the needed treatment for the services that a

APPLICATION STRATEGY 2.1

Assumption of Risk Form–Interscholastic Athletics Sample

I understand that there are certain inherent risks involved in participating in interscholastic athletics. These risks include injuries/illness that may be minor, career-ending, or life-threatening. These injuries/illnesses could result in permanent physical or mental impairment or even death. I understand that these injuries/illnesses may occur in the absence of negligence.

I understand, as does my son/daughter, that he/she has a responsibility to adhere to the established injury management guidelines. These guidelines include (1) reporting any problems related to their physical condition to appropriate school personnel (e.g., athletic trainer; coach), (2) following prescribed conditioning programs, and (3) wearing and inspecting the proper equipment as dictated by the rules of the sport.

I have reviewed this document with my son/daughter. My signature below (1) indicates that my son/daughter and I am aware of the risks of injury inherent in participation in interscholastic athletics and (2) acknowledges my son/daughter's voluntary participation in interscholastic athletics at _____ High School.

_____

Print Name

_____

Parent/Guardian Signature   Date

_____

Signature of Student-Athlete   Date

coach may need to perform, possible alternative treatments, and advantages and disadvantages of each course of action.[1–3] To be valid, consent can only be obtained from one who is competent to grant it, that is, an adult who is physically and mentally competent or the parent in the case of children under the age of 18. For minors, exceptions exist in emergency situations when parents are unavailable. The ideal time to obtain informed consent is during preparticipation meetings as part of the documentation that provides consent to participate in that activity.[1–3,8]

Failure to receive informed consent may constitute **battery**, which is any unpermitted or intentional contact with another individual without their consent. Although many courts require that intent to harm be present in an allegation of battery, a written documentation of the informed consent should be obtained from an individual or parents of minor children prior to treatment to avoid litigation. The consent should be obtained in writing prior to beginning participation in sport or physical activity programs.[6]

BOX 2.5	**Forms Required for Participation**

Preparticipation meetings are opportune times for the coach to distribute and explain the submission of various forms as a requirement prior to participation in an activity. These forms could include:

- **Preparticipation Physical Examination Form (performed by a licensed physician)**
- **Assumption of Risk Form (completed by the participant and/or parent/guardian)**
- **Informed Consent Form (completed by the participant and/or parent/guardian)**
- **Exculpatory Waiver Form (if necessary)**

APPLICATION STRATEGY 2.2

Informed Consent for Medical Care–Fitness Club Sample

The _____ Fitness Club has been designed to provide exercise and physical activity programs without compromising the health and safety of its participants. However, due to the nature of the available programs and the equipments available for use, there is an inherent risk of injury.

If I should sustain an injury or illness while participating in an activity at _____ Fitness Club, I give permission for a member of the professional training staff to assess and provide immediate management for the condition as they deem reasonably necessary to my health and well-being. I understand that the professional training staff at _____ Fitness Club uses only those procedures within their training, credentialing, and scope of professional practice in caring for onsite injuries/conditions.

_____
Print Name

_____
Signature   Date

Although rare, an injured participant may refuse emergency first aid for a variety of reasons, including religious beliefs, cultural differences, avoidance of additional pain or discomfort, or the desire to be evaluated and treated by a more medically qualified individual. Regardless of the reason given to refuse help, the conscious and medically competent individual has the right to refuse treatment.[2,5]

Confidentiality

A major concern affecting all healthcare providers is the individual's right to privacy. Coaches have a duty of care to protect the constitutional rights of their participants by ensuring their right to confidentiality regarding medical information. If a coach releases any information, even accurate information, the coach could be liable for breach of duty of confidentiality to which the participant is entitled. Individuals are entitled to access their medical records as well as make them available to other individuals. If an individual chooses to have their personal records released, regardless of the recipient (e.g., physician, insurance company; college scout), then a written authorization to release the records should be required. If the individual is older than 18 years of age, release of any medical information can be acknowledged by the individual. For individuals younger than 18 years of age, parents or legal guardians must provide consent for the dissemination of this information. This permission should identify what, if any, information should be released.[2,3,5]

The Health Insurance Portability and Accountability Act (**HIPAA**) of 1996 includes laws that are intended to protect the privacy of patients. The component referred to as the Privacy Rule was designed to ensure patient confidentiality by establishing standards for controlling the use and disclosure of an individual's health records. The interpretation of the application of these laws in sport settings has been a source of confusion for professionals in the sports medicine community. Detailed information on HIPAA as it applies to professionals involved in the delivery of healthcare to physically active individuals is beyond the scope of this book. Coaches should meet with the appropriate administration personnel at their institution or facility to ensure understanding of their responsibilities with regard to both oral and written communication as it pertains to HIPPA regulations.[3,5]

Foreseeability of Harm

A duty of care for coaches is to recognize the potential for injury and remove that danger before an injury occurs. **Foreseeability of harm** exists when danger is apparent or should have been apparent, resulting in an unreasonably unsafe condition. This potential for injury can be identified during regular inspections of gymnasiums, field areas, swimming pools, safety equipments, and athletic training facilities.[5] For example, unpadded walls under basketball hoops, glass or potholes on playing fields, slippery floors on a pool deck, exposed wiring, weight training machines that do not operate properly, and failure to follow universal safety precautions against the spread of infectious diseases all pose a threat to safety. Unsafe conditions should be identified, reported in writing to appropriate personnel, restricted from use, and repaired or replaced as soon as possible.

Instruction and Supervision

It is essential that skill techniques, performance tactics, and rules be taught and continually reinforced by coaches in an effort to reduce the potential for injury. Coaches should present information in a manner that is both developmentally and instructionally appropriate. Instruction that is developmentally appropriate takes into consideration characteristics of the participant, such as age, physical maturation, fitness and skill level, previous physical activity experiences, and intellectual capacity.[9,10] For example, it is not developmentally appropriate to teach a 6-year-old soccer player an abstract strategy concept, because it requires intellectual capacity, which exceeds the ability of most 6 year olds. Coaches have a responsibility to recognize individual differences among participants and develop instructional strategies that incorporate those differences to maximize the learning experience, increase the opportunity for skill development, and reduce the susceptibility to injury.

Proper supervision of participants involved in sport and physical activity can help to reduce the rate of injuries. In the capacity of a supervisor, coaches must be alert and attentive. Proper supervision involves active monitoring, not passive observation. In providing supervision, the coach should be positioned such that all participants can be systematically and routinely observed.[9,10] For example, when supervising work-outs in a weight training room, the coach should be positioned on the perimeter of the room and continually scan the room working in a decided direction (e.g., clockwise), so that all participants are viewed on a regular basis (e.g., every 15 to 20 seconds). The coach should also actively listen as part of their supervisory capacity. By engaging in active supervision, coaches are positioned to prevent injuries as well as respond promptly should any injury take place.

Participant's Responsibility

Coaches should advise individuals of their responsibility as participants to use reasonable care to protect their own health. Individual participants play an essential role in working with the professional staff (e.g., athletic trainer; coach; fitness specialist; physical educator) to maximize injury prevention. It is the responsibility of the participant to adhere to prescribed guidelines for their activity.[1-3,8] Such responsibilities could include maintaining an appropriate level of fitness; performing within the rules or guidelines of an activity; and maintaining and wearing safety equipments. In the event of an injury, the individual should know the procedure for seeking immediate healthcare and follow medical advice from the healthcare provider. If participants understand and practice safety and preventive measures, the number of injuries or illnesses can be reduced significantly.

Comparative negligence refers to the relative degree of negligence on the part of the professional (defendant) and the participant (plaintiff), with damages awarded on a basis proportionate to each person's carelessness.[2,3,5] For example, if an athlete was found to be 30 percent at fault for their own injury (contributory negligent) and the coach 70 percent, then on a $100,000 judgment, the coach would be responsible for $70,000 in damages and the athlete would assume an equivalent of $30,000 in damages. The court would also weigh the relative degree of negligence on the part of each defendant and award payment of damages on a basis proportionate to each person's carelessness that lead to the eventual injury.

Product Liability

Participants, parents, and coaches place a high degree of faith in the quality and safety of equipments used in sport and physical activity participation. Manufacturers have a duty of care to design, manufacture, and package equipments that will not cause injury to an individual when used as intended. This is called an **implied warranty**. An **expressed warranty** is a written guarantee that the product is safe for use. Strict liability makes the manufacturer liable for all defective or hazardous equipments that unduly threaten an individual's personal safety.[7,8]

Any alteration or modification to any protective equipment may negate the manufacturer's liability. Coaches should know the dangers involved in using sport equipments and have a duty to properly supervise their fitting and intended use. Furthermore, they should continually warn participants of the inherent dangers, if the equipment is used in a manner for which it was not intended.

Good Samaritan Laws

Beginning in the early 1960s, several states enacted legislation to protect physicians or other recognized medical personnel from litigation that may stem from emergency treatment provided to injured individuals at the scene of an accident. These laws, nicknamed "Good Samaritan Laws," were developed to encourage bystanders to assist others in need of emergency care by granting them immunity from potential litigation. Although the laws vary from state to state, immunity generally applies only when the emergency first aider (1) acts during an emergency, (2) acts in good faith to help the victim, (3) acts without expected compensation, and (4) is not guilty of any malicious misconduct or gross negligence toward the injury party (i.e., does not deviate from acceptable first aid protocol).[2]

While Good Samaritan Laws were intended to protect physicians and medical personnel, several states have expanded the language to include laypersons serving as emergency first aiders. However, these laws are subject to a variety of interpretations. The laws do not automatically protect an emergency care responder from litigation. It is essential that coaches be properly trained in emergency first aid and care of sport/physical activity injuries, if they are expected to supervise athletes/physical activity participants and render immediate first aid should an individual be injured during participation.

Risk Management

The duty of care for a coach includes reducing the risk of injury. As such, the coach is responsible for providing an environment that makes participation in an activity as safe as possible and minimizing opportunities for participants to sustain injury. However, responsibility for risk management cannot be the sole responsibility of the coach. It is essential that institutions, facilities, and organizations that provide sport and physical activity programs develop policies and procedures pertaining to the healthcare of participants, including steps to be taken to prevent injuries and the actions to be taken when an injury is sustained (e.g., emergency plan). Such procedures should be reviewed in advance of implementation by appropriate personnel (e.g., physician; athletic trainer; legal counsel) to ensure their accuracy. In addition, policies and procedures should be reviewed and updated on a regular basis. Accordingly, it is advisable to appoint an individual or a standing committee to coordinate and oversee a risk management program.[2,7,8]

SUMMARY

1. Standard of care is measured by what another minimally competent individual educated and practicing in that profession would have done to protect an individual from harm or further harm.

2. Duty of care refers to the legal obligation to provide a professional standard of care to protect individuals under their care or supervision from unreasonable risks that could potentially be harmful. Duty of care for a coach includes teaching proper and appropriate techniques for an age group; providing appropriate supervision of activities; providing quality safety equipments; ensuring a safe participation environment; and taking proper actions when an injury is sustained.

3. The following elements must be proven with regard to a coach being negligent:
   - A duty of care
   - A breach of that duty
   - Harm directly caused by that breach of duty

4. In the absence of an athletic trainer, the coach should be able to:
   • Assess and recognize potentially severe injuries
   • Provide emergency first aid
   • Initiate appropriate referral for advanced medical care, if necessary

5. The basic objective of the PPE is to determine the general health and fitness level of a physically active individual to ensure safe participation in a particular sport/activity.

6. Coaches have a responsibility to inform participants of the potential for harm associated with participation in physical activity. Coaches should require participants to complete an assumption of risk form confirming their understanding of the risk of injury.

7. Informed consent implies that an injured individual has been reasonably informed of needed treatment and consents to receiving that treatment.

8. Foreseeability of harm exists when danger is apparent or should have been apparent, resulting in an unreasonably unsafe condition.

9. Coaches have a duty of care to provide developmentally appropriate instructions to participants. In addition, they have a responsibility to supervise attentively.

10. Participants have a responsibility to use reasonable care to protect their own health.

11. Manufacturers have a duty of care to design, manufacture, and package equipments that will not cause injury to an individual when used as intended.

12. A coach cannot release any medical information about an injured individual without that person's written consent, if the person is older than 18 years of age. Release of any medical information for individuals younger than 18 years of age must be granted by the child's parent or legal guardian.

13. Although Good Samaritan Laws were developed to encourage bystanders to assist others in need of emergency care by granting the bystanders immunity from potential litigation, these laws do not protect an employee of an institution or fitness facility who renders improper care to a participant. Coaches should complete a basic athletic training class and be certified in standard first aid and cardiopulmonary resuscitation as minimal protection against litigation.

14. The coach should actively engage in actions to reduce the risk of injury and potential litigation.

APPLICATION QUESTIONS

1. You are the coach of a high school athletic team. What standard of care and professional conduct should the parents of the athletes expect from you as the first responder during practices and games? Are you protected by the "Good Samaritan Laws?"

_____

_____

2. A physical education teacher takes his seventh grade class to an outdoor field for a class on soccer. During play, one of the students inadvertently falls, lands on a broken bottle, and sustains a significant laceration to the forearm. In responding to the student, the teacher notices several broken bottles in the area. Is the teacher liable for the injury sustained by the student? Why?

_____

_____

3. A member of your high school basketball team was seen by their family physician for an injury sustained during practice. The physician determined that the athlete should not participate in activity for 1 week. After 3 days, the athlete's parent calls you to give approval for their child to play. How would you respond to this situation?

_____

_____

4. You are the coach of a high school soccer team. Following a game, a college coach comes to your office expressing interest in one of the players on the team. What (if any) medical information would you give the individual?

_____

_____

5. You are self-employed as a fitness/exercise specialist. Before working with a new client, what information would you provide to, and request from, the individual to reduce the risk of litigation related to injury?

6. A high school physical education teacher decides to supplement his income by offering summer sport camps. The camp is open to boys and girls aged 8 to 14 years. The activities will include basketball, soccer, and swimming. What strategies should the teacher implement to avoid the risk of litigation due to a participant sustaining an injury?

7. A 50-year-old member of a fitness club advises his personal trainer that he had a "bit of a scare" 2 days earlier. He reports that while doing some yard work, he began to experience tightness in his chest, labored breathing, and dizziness. He went to the emergency room, but after waiting for 2 hours, he found himself feeling better and opted to leave before being seen by a physician. How should the personal trainer respond to the client? Why?

8. An elementary school physical education teacher has the gymnasium set up with a variety of learning stations that include balance beams, climbing apparatus, ropes, floor scooters, etc. Because the set-up is complex and the unit lasts for 2 weeks, the stations must be left in place throughout the school day. What strategies should the physical education teacher use to reduce the risk of injury during class? What strategies should the physical education teacher use to reduce the risk of injury between class periods and when the gymnasium is not in use by classes?

REFERENCES

1. American Medical Association. (n.d.). Informed consent. Retrieved from http://www. ama-assn. org/ama/pub/physician-resources/legal-topics/patient-physician-relationship-topics/informed-consent.shtml
2. Chen S, and Esposito R. 2004. Practical and critical legal concerns for sports medicine physicians and athletic trainers. Sport J, 7:1–7.
3. Fuller C, and Drawer S. 2004. The application of risk management in sport. Sports Med, 34(6): 349–356.
4. Johnson MVM, and Easter BA. 2007. Legal liability for cheerleading injuries: implications for universities and coaches. J Legal Aspects Sport, 17(2):213–252.
5. Mazur D. 2003. Influence of the law on risk and informed consent. BMJ, 327(7417):731–734.

Retrieved from Academic Search Premier database. DOI:10.1136/bmj.327.7417.731.
6. Mitten MJ. 2002. Legal issues in sports medicine. St Johns Law Rev, 76(5):7–86.
7. Steven K, Richard W. 2009. Medical malpractice and the sports medicine clinician. Clin Orthop Relat Res, 467(2):412–419. Retrieved from Academic Search Premier database. DOI: 10.1007/s11999-008-0589-5
8. National Association for Sport and Physical Education. (n.d.). Position statements. Retrieved from http://www.aahperd.org/naspe/standards/.
9. Nohr K. *Managing risk in sport and recreation: the essential guide for loss prevention.* Champaign, IL: Human Kinetics, 2009.
10. Northern Arizona University. General liability. (2001). Retrieved from http://www.prm.nau.edu/prm383/liability.htm.

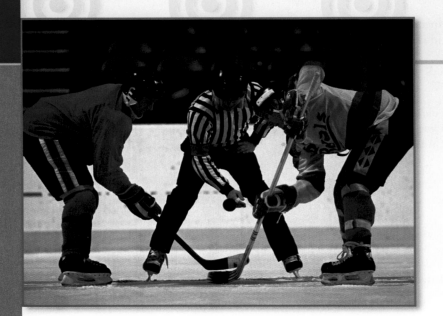

INJURY PREVENTION

KEY TERMS

active inhibition
ballistic stretching
Golgi tendon organs
individuality
muscle spindles
overload
proprioceptors
reciprocal inhibition
SAID principle
static stretching

LEARNING OUTCOMES

1. Explain the basic principles of conditioning (i.e., specificity; overload; individuality; progression).

2. Define flexibility, muscular strength, muscular endurance, and cardiovascular endurance; explain the physiological principles for each component and their role in the prevention of injury during sport and physical activity.

3. Explain the principle of overload as it applies to flexibility, muscular strength, muscular endurance, and cardiovascular endurance.

4. Explain the importance of using proper techniques in executing physical/sport skills as a factor in the prevention of injury.

5. Describe the use of protective equipments as a means for reducing the incidence and severity of injuries sustained during sport and physical activity.

6. Explain the need for the coach to be informed of, and understand, their responsibilities with regard to the use of protective equipments.

7. Identify and describe common protective equipments for the head and face, torso, and the upper and lower body.

While injury is inherent to participation in sport and physical activity, strategies to reduce the incidence and severity of injury must be implemented. Regardless of the setting or the age of the participants, active steps must be taken to promote a healthy and safe environment. In particular, three areas that should be addressed include physical conditioning, proper skill techniques, and use of protective equipments.

In this chapter, basic principles of conditioning will be discussed. The principles will be applied to the areas of flexibility, muscular strength, muscular endurance, and cardiorespiratory endurance. The importance of proper techniques, which is both age and developmentally appropriate, will then be presented. Finally, the use of protective equipments will be discussed with reference to liability issues and specific equipments for various body areas.

CONDITIONING AND INJURY PREVENTION

An effective, physiologically appropriate physical conditioning program can not only improve performance, but it can also minimize the risk of injury and illness. The coach should be familiar with the basic principles of conditioning as a way to ensure a program is safe and effective and void of practices that could predispose the participant to injury.

Note: It is not within the scope of this book to provide detailed information pertaining to fitness assessment and exercise prescription. Rather, the intent is to provide basic information that should be considered by the coach in an effort to prevent injury attributed to improper conditioning techniques.

Basic Principles of Conditioning

In developing a physical conditioning program, several basic principles must be addressed. In efforts to develop a specific component of fitness (e.g., flexibility; strength; endurance; particular skill), the **Specific Adaptation to Imposed Demands (SAID)** principle or specificity must be followed. The SAID principle states that the body responds to a given demand with a specific and predictable adaptation. An exercise program must address the specific needs of the individual with regard to their fitness and skill goals as well as to the various body parts. For example, an individual who possesses adequate flexibility in the upper extremities, but lacks flexibility in the lower extremities, will require specific exercises to increase lower extremity flexibility. In a similar manner, if an individual wants to improve muscular endurance in the lower extremities, the individual must perform endurance training exercises for the lower extremities. If the focus of a program is muscular endurance, then an expectation of improvement in muscular strength is inappropriate. Consistent with the principle of specificity, a goal of improved muscular endurance requires different criteria from that of a program focused on the development of muscular strength. Specificity also applies to the development of particular skills. For example, exercises that mimic the throwing action will benefit a baseball pitcher, but are not applicable to a football lineman.

The principle of **overload** states that physiologic improvements occur only when an individual physically demands more of the body than is normally required. If the demands are within appropriate physiological limits, the body will adapt and improve its function. As such, if the demands are insufficient (e.g., too little exercise), improvement will not take place. If the demands are too strenuous, there is a risk for injury. A common error in carrying out a conditioning program is doing "too much too soon." The body must be stressed at tolerable physiological limits. Exceeding those parameters by performing at an inappropriate intensity, for too long a duration, or for too many consecutive days, can lead to injury and setbacks, rather than improvement. As such, a program based on progression is essential to ensure that the individual does not overuse any structure(s) (e.g., joints; muscles; tendons).

Overload is achieved by manipulating frequency, intensity, and duration in the exercise program.

Frequency

Frequency refers to the number of exercise sessions per day or week. The number of days in which an individual should engage in a conditioning program will vary depending on various factors (e.g., goals; current fitness level). In determining the number of days of a specific exercise/activity, progression must be considered. Specifically, the overload principle should be implemented on a gradual and systematic basis over a period of time. In doing so, the individual will have time to adapt physiologically to the demands. In some cases, recognizing the need for recovery time is the key. For example, an individual focusing on the development of muscular strength should not work the same muscle groups on successive days, in order to allow recovery from fatigue and muscle soreness. If daily bouts are planned, strength and power exercises may be alternated with cardiovascular conditioning, or exercises for the lower extremity may alternate with exercises for the upper extremity.

It is also important to ensure that an individual maintains an appropriate frequency. For example, if a training program is based on participation in an activity 3 days a week without participation in back-to-back days, a lack of adherence on the part of the participant will require adjustments to the program. Both the participant and the coach must understand that failure to adhere to a defined schedule can result in lack of improvement and increased susceptibility to injury. Developing the various components of fitness (e.g., flexibility; strength; endurance) takes time and requires adherence to an established training routine.

Intensity

Intensity reflects both the caloric cost of the work and the specific energy systems activated. It refers to the amount of work being done during an exercise. The level of intensity for any given activity should be based on the component being developed, the current performance level, and desired goals.

Duration

Duration refers to the length of a single exercise session. The recommended duration may be stated in terms of minutes (e.g., walking 45 minutes) or the number of repetitions and sets (e.g., muscular endurance training three sets of 12 to 15 repetitions).

Another principle that warrants attention is **individuality**. From various perspectives, it is important to recognize that each participant is potentially different. As such, individual participants will have different responses to a conditioning program. Several factors can influence differences, including age, gender, body type, heredity, lifestyle, fitness level, illness/chronic conditions, and previous experience. Accordingly, an effective conditioning program is designed based on the individual. Developing and implementing a conditioning program for a group of participants (e.g., physical education class; members of a high school athletic team) is not an easy task, but it is a manageable and necessary one.

Finally, in developing the conditioning program, it is important to design a program that addresses total body fitness. A program based entirely on strengthening muscles is not sufficient. Rather, the program should also include flexibility, muscular endurance, cardiovascular conditioning, and sport-specific conditioning as appropriate. In a similar manner, a program that focuses on the upper and lower extremities, but does not address the body's core muscles, is not an optimal program.

Flexibility

Flexibility is the total range of motion (ROM) at a joint that occurs pain-free in each of the planes of motion. Joint flexibility is a combination of normal joint mechanics, mobility of soft tissues, and muscle extensibility. For example, the hip joint may have full passive ROM, but when doing active hip flexion from a seated position, as in touching one's toes, resistance from tight hamstrings may limit full hip flexion. This type of resistance may be generated from tension in muscle fibers or connective tissue. In a similar manner, flexibility in one body part (e.g., the hip joint) does not guarantee normal ROM in another body part (e.g., the ankle).

Flexibility can influence performance in physical activity. An absence of flexibility or excessive flexibility can potentially reduce the ability to effectively perform an action or skill and, in doing so, improve or hinder performance of a particular action or skill.

Physiological Principles

Muscles contain two primary **proprioceptors** that can be stimulated during stretching, namely the **muscle spindles** and **Golgi tendon organs**. Because muscle spindles lie parallel to muscle fibers, they stretch with the muscle. When stimulated, the spindle sensory fibers discharge and through reflex action in the spinal cord initiate impulses to cause the muscle to contract reflexively and, in doing so, inhibit the stretch. Muscles that perform the desired movement are called agonists. Muscles that oppose or reverse a particular movement are referred to as antagonists.

Unlike muscle spindles, Golgi tendon organs are connected in a series of fibers located in tendons and joint ligaments, and respond to muscle tension rather than length. If the stretch continues for an extended time (i.e., over 6 to 8 seconds), the Golgi tendons are stimulated. This stimulus, unlike the stimulus from muscle spindles, causes a reflex inhibition in the antagonist muscles. This sensory mechanism protects the musculotendinous unit from excessive tensile forces that could damage muscle fibers.

Stretching Techniques

Flexibility can be increased through **ballistic** or **static** stretching techniques. Ballistic stretching uses repetitive bouncing motions at the end of the available ROM. Muscle spindles are repetitively stretched, but because the bouncing motions are of short duration, the Golgi tendon organs do not fire. As such, the muscles resist relaxation. Because generated momentum may carry the body part beyond normal ROM, the muscles being stretched often remain contracted to prevent overstretching, leading to microscopic tears in the musculotendinous unit. In a static stretch, movement is slow and deliberate. Golgi tendon organs are able to override impulses from the muscle spindles, leading to a safer, more effective muscle stretch. A stretch must be held for a minimum of 8 seconds for the Golgi tendon organ to activate. Box 3.1 outlines guidelines for static stretching to improve flexibility.

Proprioceptive neuromuscular facilitation (PNF) promotes and hastens the response of the neuromuscular system through stimulation of the proprioceptors. These exercises increase flexibility in one muscle group (i.e., agonist), and simultaneously improve strength in another muscle group (i.e., antagonist). While PNF exercises can be very effective in increasing flexibility, the coach should only perform PNF exercises having been appropriately trained by a qualified professional to do so.

BOX 3.1 | **Guidelines for Static Stretching to Improve Flexibility**

1. Stretching is facilitated by warm body tissues; therefore, a brief warm-up period is recommended. If it is not possible to jog lightly, stretching could be performed after a superficial heat treatment.
2. In the designated stretch position, the individual should move to a position in which a sensation of tension is felt.
3. There should be no bouncing associated with the stretch. The stretch position should be held for 10 to 30 s until a sense of relaxation occurs. The individual should be aware of the feeling of relaxation, or "letting go." A stretch should be repeated six to eight times.
4. Breathing should be performed rhythmically and slowly. The individual should exhale during the actual stretch.

5. It is important to avoid being overly aggressive in stretching. Increased flexibility may not be noticed for 4 to 6 weeks.
6. If an area is particularly resistant to stretching, partner stretching or PNF may be used.
7. Vigorous stretching of tissues should be avoided in the following conditions:
   • After a recent fracture
   • After prolonged immobilization
   • With acute inflammation or infection in or around the joint
   • With a bony block that limits motion
   • With muscle contractures or when joint adhesions limit motion
   • With acute pain during stretching

> ## BOX 3.2   Active Inhibition Techniques
>
> To stretch the hamstring group on a single leg using the three separate PNF techniques, the following guidelines should be followed:
>
> 1. CONTRACT – RELAX
>   - The thigh is stabilized and the hip passively flexed into the agonist pattern, until limitation is felt in the hamstrings.
>   - The individual then performs an isotonic contraction with the hamstrings through the antagonist pattern.
>   - A passive stretch is then applied into the agonist pattern, until limitation is felt; the sequence is repeated.
>
> 2. HOLD-RELAX
>   - The leg is passively moved into the agonist pattern, until resistance is felt in the hamstrings.
>   - The individual performs an isometric contraction to "hold" the position for about 10 s.
>
> - The individual should then relax for about 5 s.
> - A passive stretch is then applied into the agonist pattern, until limitation is felt; the sequence is repeated.
>
> 3. SLOW REVERSAL – HOLD-RELAX
>   - The individual consciously relaxes the hamstring muscles, while doing a concentric contraction of the quadriceps muscles into the agonist pattern.
>   - The individual then performs an isometric contraction, against resistance, into the antagonist pattern for 10 s.
>   - The individual should then relax for about 10 s.
>   - The individual then actively moves the body part further into the agonist pattern; the sequence is repeated.

Proprioceptive neuromuscular facilitation technique recruits muscle contractions in a coordinated pattern as agonists and antagonists move through a ROM. One technique utilizes **active inhibition,** whereby the muscle group reflexively relaxes prior to the stretching maneuver. Common methods include contract–relax, hold–relax, and slow reversal–hold–relax (Box 3.2). The coach or a teammate stabilizes the limb to be exercised. Alternating contractions and passive stretching of a group of muscles are then performed. Contractions may be held for 3, 6, or 10 seconds, with similar results obtained.[1]

A second technique, known as **reciprocal inhibition,** uses active agonist contractions to relax a tight antagonist muscle. In this technique, the individual contracts the muscle opposite the tight muscle, against resistance. This causes a reciprocal inhibition of the tight muscle, leading to muscle lengthening.

Application Principles: Flexibility

Achieving or maintaining normal flexibility can be achieved by following the overload principle.

- Frequency: The American College of Sports Medicine recommends that stretching exercises be performed a minimum of 2 to 3 days per week, but more optimally, 5 to 7 days a week.[2] Muscles should be stretched when warm, so the best time for stretching is following exercise (e.g., after a cardiovascular endurance activity; after a weight training session; the end of a practice session). It is contraindicated to stretch muscles that are "cold" (i.e., prior to activity), as it can increase the risk of injury (i.e., tearing) of the muscles.
- Intensity: Movement to the desired stretch position should be initialed slowly and continue until to a feeling of slight tension or burn is felt.
- Duration: The final position should be held for 15 to 30 seconds, and repeated—two to four times with a 30 to 60 second rest period between repetitions.

Muscular Strength and Endurance

Strength is the ability of a muscle or group of muscles to produce force in one maximal effort. Muscular strength influences the ability to execute normal activities of daily living and aids in reducing or preventing postural deformities.

Muscular endurance is the ability of muscle tissue to exert repetitive tension over an extended period. The rate of muscle fatigue is related to the endurance level of the muscle (i.e., the more rapid the muscle fatigues, the less muscle endurance). A direct relationship exists between muscle strength and endurance. As muscle endurance is developed, density in the capillary beds increases, providing a greater blood supply, and thus a greater oxygen supply, to the working muscle. Increases in muscle endurance may influence strength gains; however, strength development has not been shown to increase muscle endurance.

Performance in most physical activities and sport skills/activities requires or is enhanced by muscular strength and/or muscular endurance. By strengthening the muscles involved in throwing a baseball, a shortstop will be able to throw the ball with greater speed and, as such, increase the potential for throwing out the base runner. A basketball player can enhance performance by following a training program that increases both the strength and endurance of the muscles in the lower extremities. The increased muscular endurance will enable the basketball player to sustain activity for longer periods of time, while the increased muscle strength will enable the individual to generate more force in executing a variety of skills (e.g., jumping; throwing)

An appropriate level of muscular strength and endurance is necessary to prevent injury during participation in sport and physical activity. The muscles must be prepared to withstand the forces associated with the demands of a particular sport or activity. It is essential that the demands of the sport or activity be identified, so that an appropriate training program can be developed. Some activities may require a focus on endurance, while others warrant a focus on muscular strength.

In the role of providing stability for any given joint, the basic principle is that the stronger the muscle, the better the protection for the joint. In developing muscular strength, the concept of muscle imbalance should not be overlooked. The major muscle groups function in a complex manner that requires balanced symmetry. Imbalances in muscle strength can lead to musculoskeletal dysfunction and pain.

Physiological Principles

The development of muscular strength and endurance depends on several factors. These factors include, but are not limited to, the number and size of muscle fibers, the type of muscle fiber, neuromuscular coordination, and gender.

The strength of a skeletal muscle is determined by the cross-sectional diameter of the muscle fibers. The size of the muscle fiber will increase in response to progressive resistance exercise (i.e., overload). An exercise program cannot increase the numbers of fibers. Rather, it increases the size of the fibers present. Muscle hypertrophy refers to the increase in the size of muscle fibers in response to physical activity. In comparison, atrophy is a decrease in size or a wasting away of muscle fiber. Atrophy can be attributed to some common diseases (e.g., cancer; pulmonary disease), but it can also be due to a lack of physical activity. Muscle atrophy results in muscle weakness. The actual number of muscle fibers is an inherited trait.

Gender differences exist with regard to the absolute strength of males and females. While the muscle properties of males and females are the same, the size of the muscle fibers and, as such, the cross-sectional diameter of a muscle is greater for males than for females. The difference in size is attributed to the presence of the hormone testosterone.

For both males and females, the initial 3 to 4 weeks of a strength training program are characterized by a rapid increase in strength. This phenomenon is attributed to an improvement in neuromuscular coordination. During the initial stage of a strength training program, the nervous system begins to innervate an increased number of motor units and there is an increased rate in the firing of motor units. As a result, the muscle is capable of generating increased force. The training effect results in improved coordination of the motor unit that allows for more efficient and effective functioning.

Skeletal muscles are composed of two primary types of fibers, namely slow twitch (Type I) and fast twitch (Type II). Slow-twitch fibers have a slow contraction time and they yield relatively low levels of force production. Slow-twitch muscles are more resistant to fatigue and are best suited for aerobic activities that require relatively low levels of force production (e.g., walking; distance running; posture maintenance).

Fast twitch fibers have a faster contraction rate than slow twitch fibers. They are able to generate higher levels of force production in a short period of time, but they are more prone to fatigue. Fast-twitch fibers are further categorized as Type IIa and Type IIb. The Type IIa fiber has a relatively high force production and moderate resistance to fatigue. As such, they are used for both aerobic and anaerobic activities. The Type IIb fibers have the fastest rate of contraction, but they are the most sensitive to fatigue. They are recruited for anaerobic activities that require quick, powerful force production. From a functional perspective, a track athlete specializing in the 1-mile race would benefit from a larger percentage of Type IIa fibers as it is an intense activity that lasts for 4 to 5 minutes. A track athlete specializing in the 100-m sprint would be better served by a higher proportion of Type IIb fibers.

Because of the unique properties of the three types of muscle fibers, each responds differently to training and physical activity. If a strength training program is characterized by low-intensity, high-duration exercises, the slow-twitch muscles will be recruited and subsequently developed. A strength training program that focuses on high-intensity, short-duration exercises will neglect the slow-twitch fibers, but develop the fast-twitch fibers.

Static Strength Versus Dynamic Strength

Strength can be described as static or dynamic. Static strength involves an isometric contraction. Tension is produced by the muscle, but there is no change in muscle length. Dynamic strengthening involves an isotonic contraction.

In an isotonic contraction, two types of contractions occur, namely concentric and eccentric. A concentric contraction involves a shortening of muscle fibers, which decreases the angle of the associated joint. In an eccentric contraction, the muscle resists its own lengthening, so that the joint angle increases during the contraction. Concentric and eccentric may also be referred to as positive and negative work, respectively. Concentric contractions work to accelerate a limb. For example, the gluteus maximus and quadriceps muscles concentrically contract to accelerate the body upward from a crouched position. In contrast, eccentric contractions work to decelerate a limb and provide shock absorption, especially during high-velocity dynamic activities. For example, the shoulder external rotators decelerate the shoulder during the follow-through phase of the overhead throw.

Eccentric contractions generate greater force than isometric contractions, and isometric contractions generate greater force than concentric contractions. In addition, less tension is required in an eccentric contraction. However, one major disadvantage of eccentric training is delayed-onset muscle soreness (DOMS). Delayed-onset muscle soreness is defined as muscular pain or discomfort 1 to 5 days following unusual muscular exertion. Delayed-onset muscle soreness is associated with joint swelling and weakness, which may last after the cessation of pain. This differs from acute-onset muscle soreness, where pain during exercise ceases after the exercise bout is completed. To prevent the onset of DOMS, eccentric exercises should progress gradually. Dynamic muscle strength is gained through isotonic or isokinetic exercise.

Isotonic Training (Variable Speed/Fixed Resistance)

A common method of strength training is isotonic exercise, or progressive resistive exercise , as it is sometimes called. In this technique, a muscle contraction generates a force to move a constant load throughout the ROM at a variable speed. Both concentric and eccentric contractions are possible with free weights, elastic or rubber tubing, and weight machines.

- Free weights are inexpensive and can be used in diagonal patterns for sport or activity-specific skills, but adding or removing weights from the bars can be troublesome. In addition, a spotter may be required for safety purposes to avoid dropping heavy weights.
- Thera-Band, or surgical tubing, is inexpensive and easy to set up, can be used in diagonal patterns for sport or activity-specific skills, and can be adjusted to the individual's strength level by using bands of different tension.
- Weights on commercial machines can be changed quickly and easily. Utilizing several stations of free weights and commercial machines, an individual can perform circuit

training to strengthen multiple muscle groups in a single exercise session. However, the machines are typically large and expensive, work only in a single plane of motion, and may not match the biomechanical makeup or body size of the individual.

Isotonic training permits exercise of multiple joints simultaneously, allows for both eccentric and concentric contractions, and permits weight-bearing, closed kinetic chain exercises. A disadvantage is that when a load is applied, the muscle can only move that load through the ROM with as much force as the muscle provides at its weakest point. Nautilus and Eagle equipments are examples of variable resistance machines with an elliptical cam. The cam system provides minimal resistance, where the ability to produce force is comparatively lower (i.e., early and late in the ROM), and greatest resistance, where the muscle is at its optimal length-tension and mechanical advantage (i.e., usually the midrange). The axis of rotation generates an isokinetic-like effect, but angular velocity cannot be controlled.

Isokinetic Training (Fixed Speed/Variable Resistance)

Isokinetic training, or accommodating resistance, allows an individual to provide muscular overload and angular movement to rotate a lever arm at a controlled velocity or fixed speed. Theoretically, isokinetic training should activate the maximum number of motor units, which consistently overloads muscles and achieves maximum tension-developing or force output capacity at every point in the ROM, even at the relatively "weaker" joint angles. Cybex, Biodex, and Kin Com are examples of equipments that use this strength training method.

Two advantages of isokinetic training are that a muscle group can be exercised to its maximum potential throughout the full ROM. However, as the muscles fatigue, isokinetic resistance decreases. In contrast, with an isotonic contraction, because the resistance is constant, as the muscle fatigues, it must either recruit additional motor units, requiring an increase in muscle force, or fail to perform the complete repetition.

Application Principles: Muscular Strength

Strength gains depend primarily on the intensity of the overload, more so than the specific training method used to improve strength.

- Frequency: A strength-development program requires a minimum of 2 days per week. The 2 days should not be back to back, as the muscles must be given time to rest between exercise sessions. The absence of a rest period can lead to injury as well as an inability of the muscle to sustain sufficient intensity to create the necessary overload. However, it is acceptable to engage in strength-development exercises on a daily basis, if the muscle groups are stressed on alternate days. For example, the lower body training could take place one day and the upper body exercises the next.

- Intensity: The intensity of the overload should be a weight that is at least 80% of the individual's maximum capacity (1 RM). The maximum capacity is the amount of weight that can be lifted as a single repetition.

- Duration: In developing strength, high intensity is combined with low repetitions (i.e., one to five). The number of sets can vary from one to three with a period of rest from 3 to 5 minutes between sets.

In general, the individual can determine whether the intensity was sufficient by assessing their response to the work. If the goal is to complete five repetitions of a particular weight, the individual should feel fatigue and the inability to complete another repetition (i.e., is not able to complete the sixth repetition). If after the five repetitions, the individual feels comfortable with completing additional repetitions, the weight is too low (i.e., insufficient intensity). If the individual is unable to complete five repetitions (i.e., completes four or less), the weight is too high. The weight should be adjusted as necessary, rather than continuing with an inappropriate intensity. In completing each repetition, it is essential that the individual focuses on the proper technique and avoids compensating due to fatigue. In both scenarios, there is an increased risk for injury and decreased probability of strengthening the targeted muscles.

Application Principles: Muscular Endurance

Similar to the development of strength, it is the intensity and duration of exercises that will determine improvement in muscular endurance. Muscular endurance is gained by lifting low weights at a faster contractile velocity with more repetitions in the exercise session.

- Frequency: A muscular endurance program requires a minimum of 2 to 3 days per week. Similar to strength training, training days should not be back to back as the muscles must be given time to rest between exercise sessions.
- Intensity: The intensity of the overload should be a weight that is 40 to 60% of the individual's maximum capacity (1 RM).
- Duration: The development of muscular endurance requires 12 to 20 repetitions per set. The number of sets can vary from one to three with a period of rest from 3 to 5 minutes between sets.

Again, it is important to determine the appropriate amount of weight (i.e., intensity) that should be used. The initial goal should be to complete 12 repetitions of an exercise. If 12 repetitions cannot be performed, the weight is too high; if completion of 12 repetitions is relatively easy, the weight is too low. When the individual becomes comfortable with or adapts to the ability to complete 12 repetitions, the next step is to increase the number of repetitions performed, rather increasing the amount of weight. The goal is to increase gradually the repetitions until having reached 20 repetitions per set. When that goal is achieved, the next step is to return the number of repetitions to 12 and increase the amount of weight. The process continues in the same manner (i.e., work toward the ability to complete 20 repetitions of an exercise for two to three sets).

Cardiorespiratory Endurance

Cardiorespiratory exercise can be aerobic or anaerobic depending upon the energy system being utilized. An aerobic exercise requires oxygen to produce energy. The aerobic energy system is utilized for activities that last longer than several minutes. In comparison, anaerobic exercise does not require oxygen for energy, but rather it uses lactic acid to convert nutrients to energy. Anaerobic exercises are short, intense bursts of activity that last for less than several minutes. While both aerobic and anaerobic cardiovascular training is beneficial, regular participation in activities, which require utilization of aerobic energy (e.g., cardiovascular endurance activities), is associated with numerous physiological benefits (Box 3.3).

BOX 3.3   **Physiological Benefits of Cardiovascular Endurance**

- **Increase in the size (i.e., volume and weight) of the heart that improves the strength and pumping efficiency of the heart**
- **Increase in cardiac output**
  - Decrease in heart rate results in less stress on the heart during exercise and at rest
  - Increase in stroke volume results in the heart being able to pump more blood per beat
- **Increase in the number of red blood cells in the body enabling a more efficient transport of oxygen throughout the body**
- **Improved circulatory efficiency that results in the working muscles requiring less blood due to an improvement in the delivery, extraction, and utilization of oxygen**
- **Reduced blood pressure resulting in a more efficient cardiovascular system as well as decreased susceptibility to hypertension**
- **Decrease in total cholesterol with an increase in the level of high-density lipoprotein cholesterol (i.e., "good cholesterol")**
- **Increase in the strength of the muscles involved in respiration that results in more efficient pulmonary function (i.e., flow of air in and out of the lungs)**

Cardiorespiratory endurance refers to the ability to sustain prolonged exercise. It involves activities that use the large muscle groups to engage in dynamic exercise at moderate or higher levels of intensity for an extended period of time.[2] Examples of these activities include running, fast-paced walking, swimming, and cycling. Cardiovascular endurance is generally considered the most important component of any fitness program. This recognition is attributed to the numerous benefits associated with participation in a cardiovascular conditioning program. It also reflects the relationship between poor cardiovascular fitness and a variety of health risks (e.g., cardiac disease; diabetes; stress; cancer).

Cardiovascular endurance is also required for participation in many sports. In the absence of appropriate levels of cardiovascular endurance, an individual can become fatigued. Fatigue can result in making abnormal movements or mistakes that can lead to both poor performance and increased susceptibility to injury. In some physical activities and sports, it is also important to engage in anaerobic training. Based on the specific demands of the sport, aerobic and anaerobic cardiovascular conditioning should be incorporated as part of the training regimen.

Physiological Principles

The cardiovascular and respiratory systems are two distinct systems, but they work together (i.e., cardiorespiratory system) for transporting oxygen to the various organs and muscles of the body and removing waste products from those structures. The cardiovascular system includes the heart, blood vessels, and the blood. The respiratory system includes the nasal cavity, the pharynx, the larynx, the trachea, and the lungs.

The functioning of the cardiorespiratory system occurs at predictable rates. During rest or light activities, the normal heart rate for adults is 60 to 100 beats per minute; for children, the normal resting range is from 120 to 140 beats per minute. Respiration rate ranges from 10 to 20 breaths per minute for adults and 20 to 25 breaths per minute for children. Normal healthy rates for blood pressure are 120/70 to 120/80 mm Hg for adults and 125 to 140/80 to 90 mm Hg for children aged 10 to 18 years. In response to the demands of exercise or strenuous activities, changes in the resting rates occur, including:

* Increased heart rate
* Increased systolic blood pressure
* Increased respirations

In general, these changes result in an increase in the amount of blood pumped per beat (i.e., stroke volume), an increase in the rate at which blood circulates, and an increase in the amount of blood and oxygen delivered to the working muscles.

Aerobic capacity refers to the maximum amount of oxygen that the body can use during a period of high-intensity exercise. It depends on the efficiency of the pulmonary and cardiovascular systems to supply oxygen to working muscles and the ability of those muscles to use the oxygen to produce energy. As the intensity of an exercise or physical activity increases, there is an increase in oxygen consumption that continues until the individual reaches his/her maximal aerobic capacity. When maximal capacity is attained, the oxygen consumption no longer increases, rather it plateaus.

The measurement of an individual's maximal aerobic capacity is their VO_2 max. It reflects the highest rate of oxygen consumed by an individual when exercising as hard as possible. VO_2 max, which is measured as milliliters of oxygen used in one minute per kilogram of body weight, is considered the best measure of cardiovascular endurance.

VO_2 max appears to be a genetic trait. An individual inherits a range of maximum aerobic capacity. While the average individual has a range of 50 to 60 mL/kg/minute, elite runners typically have a high VO_2 max range (i.e., 70 to 80 mL/kg/minute). Regardless of their inherited range, an individual can reach the higher level of their range through participation in an appropriate cardiovascular endurance training program. In a similar manner, regardless of their inherited range, improvements in cardiovascular endurance yield physiological benefits.

Application Principles: Cardiovascular Endurance

Maintaining and improving cardiovascular endurance is influenced by an interaction of frequency, duration, and intensity. The American College of Sports Medicine recommends that aerobic training includes activity 3 to 5 days per week lasting for 20 to 60 minutes more than twice weekly at an intensity of 55 to 60 to 90% of maximal heart rate (HRmax) (lower number for unfit, elderly, or sedentary persons).[2,3] Targeted heart rate can be calculated in the following two manners:

1. An estimated HRmax for both men and women is about 220 beats/minute. Heart rate is related to age, with maximal heart rate decreasing as an individual ages. A relatively simple calculation is

$$HRmax = 220 - Age.$$

(With a 20-year-old individual working at 80% maximum, the calculation is $0.8 \times (220 - 20)$ or 160 beats per minute.)

2. Another commonly used formula (Karvonen formula) assumes that the targeted heart rate range is between 60 and 90%. The calculation is

$$Target\ HR\ range = [(HRmax - HRrest) \times 0.60\ and\ 0.90] + HRrest.$$

(If an individual's HRmax is 180 beats/minute and the HRrest is 60 beats/minute, this method yields a target HR range of between 132 and 168 beats/minute.)

When an individual is unable to continue or chooses to stop aerobic training, detraining occurs within 1 to 2 weeks.[3] As such, when the individual returns to cardiovascular endurance training, it will be necessary to recalculate the appropriate intensity, rather having the individual continue at the same level, which he/she had previously achieved. If the individual returns to activity without an appropriate cardiovascular endurance level, fatigue can set in quickly and place the individual at risk for injury.

PROPER TECHNIQUE AND INJURY PREVENTION

Proper technique is important with regard to efficient and effective skill performance. It is also an important factor in the prevention of injury. Use of improper techniques in executing sport-specific skills has been identified as a factor that can contribute to injury.[4] Subsequently, it has been suggested that poor coaching can result in increased injuries.[5]

One of the responsibilities of the coach is to teach proper skill techniques and to continually reinforce the use of proper techniques. Unfortunately, many coaches lack the proper knowledge for the correct instruction of sport skills.[6] In many cases, coaches rely on the information they collected while playing the sport or information obtained from anecdotal sources (e.g., other coaches; sport magazines); information is not always based on sound principles.

Instruction of proper techniques requires knowledge of basic biomechanical principles (e.g., kinetics; kinematics) to ensure that structures within the body are not sustaining forces that will cause soft or bony tissues to fail (i.e., rupture of soft tissue; fracture of bone). For example, a poor overhead throwing technique could place adverse stress on the elbow, leading to trauma to the ligaments, tendons, or muscles encompassing the elbow. In a similar manner, poor execution of a swimming stroke could produce forces within the shoulder that tissues are simply not able or designed to sustain. In the lower extremities, poor posture or improper running techniques could lead to a range of injuries (e.g., stress fracture of a metatarsal; stress fracture of the tibia; patella–femoral pathology; lumbar sprain or strain). In some cases, too much repetition of a particular skill or motion, in and of itself, can lead to injury. However, if the motion or skill is not being performed using proper techniques, injury can occur, regardless of the extent of repetition. For example, a football player executing a tackle by leading with the head could sustain a catastrophic injury (e.g., head trauma; spinal paralysis) on a single hit. In addition to teaching the correct technique, the coach should be able to recognize improper techniques and provide instruction for correcting them.

While the use of proper techniques is essential for physically active individuals of all ages, it is especially important for youth and adolescent participants. If an individual learns the correct technique for performing a skill on their initial exposure to the skill and continues to practice the skill correctly, neuromuscular communication and proprioceptive feedback will enable the continued appropriate execution of the skill. In the same manner, if the individual learns an improper technique and continues to practice with that technique, the internal feedback will result in continued poor technique. Correcting poor technique is not necessarily an easy task. It is a process that takes time as the body needs to learn a new pattern. Initially, the new pattern often feels awkward and does not produce the desired performance results. Unfortunately, those results often lead to frustration and a return to the more comfortable but incorrect technique. The coach should constantly reinforce the need to continue to practice the proper technique and educate the individual about potential injury susceptibility, if there is a return to improper techniques.

Consideration must also be given to ensure that the instruction and expectation of performance of any given skill is age and developmentally appropriate. While a 10-year-old baseball player may demonstrate excellent throwing techniques, it is not developmentally appropriate to provide instructions in some pitching techniques (e.g., throwing a curve ball; throwing at high speeds) to a 10 year old. Prior to and during puberty, the body experiences numerous physical and physiological stresses as part of the normal growth process. Compounding those stresses with performing developmentally inappropriate physical skills can increase the potential for injury. In some cases, the resultant injuries can result in permanent deformities or alteration of normal growth. Such conditions can potentially lead to various additional injuries or problems that can have long-term or life-long consequences. As such, the coach must be familiar with the age and developmentally appropriate skill level in providing instructions of proper techniques.

PROTECTIVE EQUIPMENTS AND INJURY PREVENTION

Specialized equipments, when properly used, can protect a participant from accidental or routine injuries associated with a particular sport or physical activity. However, there are limitations to the effectiveness of protective equipments. A natural outcome of wearing protective equipments is to feel more secure. Unfortunately, this often leads to more aggressive play, which can result in injury to the participant or an opponent. In many cases, it is the shared or sole responsibility of the coach to ensure that protective equipments meet minimum standards of protection, are in good condition, clean, properly fitted, used routinely, and used as these were intended.

In events involving impact and collisions, the participant must be protected from high-velocity, low-mass forces, and low-velocity, high-mass forces. High-velocity, low-mass forces occur, for example, when an individual is struck by a ball, puck, bat, or hockey stick. The low-mass and high speed of impact can lead to forces concentrated in a smaller area, causing focal injuries (i.e., injuries concentrated in a small area, such as a contusion). An example of low-velocity, high-mass forces is an individual falling on the ground or ice, or checked into the side-boards of an ice hockey rink, thereby absorbing the forces over a larger area, and leading to diffuse injuries (i.e., injuries spread over a larger area, such as a concussion).

Potential means by which equipments can protect an area from accidental or routine injuries associated with a particular activity are listed in BOX 3.4. Equipment design extends

---

| BOX 3.4 | **Equipment Design Factors That Can Reduce Potential Injury** |

- **Increase the impact area**
- **Transfer or disperse the impact area to another body part**
- **Limit the relative motion of a body part**
- **Add mass to the body part to limit deformation and displacement**
- **Reduce friction between contacting surfaces**
- **Absorb energy**
- **Resist the absorption of bacteria, fungus, and viruses**

beyond the physical protective properties to include size, comfort, style, tradition, and initial and long-term maintenance costs. Individuals responsible for the selection and purchase of equipments should be less concerned about appearance, style, and cost, and most concerned about the ability of equipments to prevent injury.

Liability and Equipment Standards

Legal issues concerning protective equipments are a major concern for every organized sport or physical activity program. An organization's duty to ensure the proper use of protective equipments is usually a shared responsibility among the members of the athletic staff. For example, the head coach may be responsible for recommending specific equipments for their sport. The athletic director may be responsible for purchasing these recommended equipments. The equipment manager or athletic trainer then may be responsible for properly fitting the equipment based on the manufacturer's guidelines, instructing and warning the individual about the proper use of the equipment, regularly inspecting the protective equipment, and keeping accurate records of any repair or reconditioning of the equipment.

It is essential that the coach is informed of, and understands, their role in ensuring the proper use of protective equipments. For example, in some settings, it may be determined that the coach is legally responsible for:

- Selecting the most appropriate equipment.
- Properly fitting the equipment to the individual.
- Instructing the individual in proper care for the equipment.
- Warning the individual of any danger in using the equipment inappropriately.
- Supervising and monitoring the proper use of all protective equipments.

In an effort to protect the participant from ineffective and poorly constructed equipments, several agencies have developed standards of quality to ensure that equipments do not fail under normal athletic circumstances or contribute to injury. The National Operating Committee on Standards for Athletic Equipment (NOCSAE) sets the standards for football helmets to tolerate certain forces when applied to different areas of the helmet. Currently, baseball, softball, and lacrosse helmets and face masks must also be NOCSAE certified. Other testing agencies for protective equipments include the American Society for Testing and Materials (ASTM) and the Hockey Equipment Certification Council (HECC) of the Canadian Standards Association (CSA). These agencies have established material standards for equipments, such as protective eye wear, ice hockey helmets, and face masks.

In addition to agencies that establish standards for the manufacture of equipments, athletic governing bodies establish rules for the mandatory use of specific protective equipments and determine rules governing special protective equipments. These governing bodies include the National Federation of State High School Associations (NFSHSA), the National Association of Intercollegiate Athletics (NAIA), the National Collegiate Athletic Association (NCAA), and the United States Olympic Committee (USOC). For example, the NCAA requires football players to use a face mask and helmet with a secured, four-point chin strap. All players must wear helmets that carry a warning label regarding the risk of injury and a manufacturer's or reconditioner's certification indicating that the equipment meets the NOCSAE test standards.[7]

After equipments have been purchased, the manufacturer's information materials, such as brochures and warranties used in the selection process, should be cataloged for reference in the event an injury occurs. This information can document the selection process and particular attributes of the equipment ultimately chosen. When an individual provides his/her own protective equipment, the responsibilities of the coach do not automatically change. The coach must ensure that the equipment meets safety standards and is fitted correctly, properly maintained and cleaned, and used appropriately. Coaches should know the dangers involved in using sport equipments and have a duty to properly supervise its fitting and intended use. Athletes should not be allowed to wear any equipment or alter any equipment that may endanger the individual or other team members.

Protective Equipments: Head and Face

Many head and facial injuries can be prevented with regular use of properly fitted helmets and facial protective devices, such as face guards, eye wear, ear wear, mouthguards, and throat protectors. Helmets, in particular, are required in football, ice hockey, men's lacrosse, baseball, softball, and bicycling, and must be fitted properly to disperse impact forces.

Football Helmets

Footballs helmets consist of an outer shell constructed of plastic or a polycarbonate alloy, a material that is lightweight and impact-resistant. The inside of the helmet contains a single or double air bladder, closed-cell pads, or a combination of the two. The football helmet is designed to reduce the incidence and severity of head trauma. While a football helmet will not prevent concussion, it has been found to reduce the incidence of cerebral concussions in high school football players.[8] The helmet also features increased side and facial protection to lessen the impact in these areas.

The NOCSAE mark should be on every football helmet. It indicates that the helmet meets minimum impact standards and can tolerate forces applied to several different areas of the helmet. The NOCSAE also includes a warning label regarding risk of injury on each helmet that states:

Warning: Do not strike an opponent with any part of this helmet or face mask. This is a violation of football rules and may cause you to suffer severe brain or neck injury, including paralysis or death. Severe brain or neck injury may also occur accidentally while playing football. NO HELMET CAN PREVENT ALL SUCH INJURIES. USE THIS HELMET AT YOUR OWN RISK.

This warning label must be clearly visible on the exterior shell of all new and reconditioned helmets. In addition, the coach should continually warn athletes of the risks involved in football and ensure that the helmet is properly used within the guidelines and rules of the game.

Manufacturer's guidelines should always be followed when fitting a football helmet. Prior to fitting, the individual should have a haircut in the style that will be worn during the athletic season, and wet their heads to simulate game conditions. Once fitted, the helmet should be checked daily for proper fit, which can be altered by hair length, deterioration of internal padding, loss of air from cells, and spread of the face mask.

Each helmet should have the purchase date and tracking number engraved on the inside. Detailed records should be kept that identify the purchase date, use, reconditioning history, and certification seals. Each individual should also be instructed on the proper use, fit, and care of the helmet. In addition, each individual should sign a statement that confirms having read the NOCSAE seal and been informed of the risks of injury through improper use of the helmet or face mask when striking an opponent. This statement should be signed, dated, and kept as part of the individual's medical files.

Ice Hockey Helmets

As with football helmets, ice hockey helmets reduce head injuries; however, they do not prevent neck injuries caused by axial loading. The use of head protection with a face mask seems to have given many players a sense of invulnerability to injury. Studies have shown that the risk of spinal cord injury, and in particular, quadriplegia, may be three times greater in hockey than in American football.[9] The major mechanism for this injury is head-first contact with the boards secondary to a push, or a check from behind.

Ice hockey helmet standards are monitored by the ASTM and the HECC and are required to carry the stamp of approval from the CSA. Helmets should be fitted and maintained in accordance with manufacturer's guidelines.

Batting Helmets

Batting helmets are now compulsory in baseball and softball and require the NOCSAE mark.[1] Most batting helmets are open-faced with a double ear-flap design and can protect the majority of the superolateral cranium, but not the jaw or facial area. Although some studies claim that batting helmets fitted with face shields may prevent or reduce severity of facial injuries to children, there are no rigorous data to support such a claim.[10] The helmet should be snug enough so that it does not move or fall off during batting and running bases.

Other Helmets

Lacrosse helmets are mandatory in the men's game, optional in the women's game, and are also worn by field hockey goalies. The helmet is made of a high-resistant plastic or fiberglass shell, and must meet NOCSAE standards. The helmet, wire face guard, and chin pad are secured with a four-point chin strap.

An effective bicycle helmet has a plastic or fiberglass rigid shell with a chin strap and an energy-absorbing foam liner. Regardless of the type, the helmet can provide substantial protection against head injuries and injuries to the upper and midface region. Improved designs have produced helmets that are lightweight and aerodynamic with an increase in the number of ventilation ports. Wearing a cycling helmet does not increase thermal discomfort to the head or body and has no additional impact on the core temperature, head skin temperature, thermal sensation, heart rate, sweat rate, and overall perceived exertion.[11]

Although the rate of bicycle helmet usage has increased in the United States, at least one study has found that the overwhelming majority of children, adolescents, and their parents cannot properly fit a bicycle helmet. This increases the potential for exposure of the head's frontal region, which is the most common site of impact in bicycle head injuries.[12]

Bicycle helmet fitting should first begin with a properly conditioned helmet (i.e., being certified by the Consumer Product Safety Commission, American Society for Testing and Materials, American National Standards Institute, or Canadian Standards Association). The manufacturer's guidelines should be followed to ensure proper fit. Common fitting errors include having the helmet rest too high on the forehead, improper strap position (failure of strap to make a "V" around the ear, and excessive front-to-back movement of the helmet).[12,13]

Face Guards

Face guards, which vary in size and style, protect and shield the facial region from flying projectiles. The NOCSAE has set standards for strength and deflection for football face guards worn at the high school and college levels. Football face guards are made of heavy-gauge, plastic-coated steel rod, designed to withstand impacts from blunt surfaces, such as the turf or another player's knee or elbow. The effectiveness of a football face guard depends on the strength of the guard itself, the helmet attachments, and the four-point chin strap on the helmet.

Ice hockey face guards are made of clear plastic (polycarbonate), steel wire, or a combination of the two, and must meet the HECC and ASTM standards. Hockey face guards primarily prevent penetration of the hockey stick, but are also effective against flying pucks and collisions with helmets, elbows, side boards, and the ice. The use of full-coverage face masks in amateur ice hockey has greatly reduced facial trauma. The use of a single chin strap, however, still allows the helmet to ride back on the head when a force is directed to the frontal region, and, in doing so, exposes the chin to lacerations.

Lacrosse face guards must meet NOCSAE standards. The wire mesh guard stands away from the face, but the four-point chin strap has a padded chin region in case the guard is driven back during a collision with another player. Face masks used by catchers and the home plate umpire in baseball and softball should fit snugly to the cheeks and forehead, but should not impair vision. These devices can be used by players in the field and must meet ASTM standards.

Eye Wear

Eye injuries are relatively common and almost always preventable, if proper protective wear is worn. There are three types of protective eyewear: goggles, face shields, and spectacles. The type of eyewear will vary depending upon the sport or physical activity. A qualified specialist (e.g., athletic trainer; coach) or healthcare practitioner should be consulted regarding the use of protective eyewear.

Mouthguards

An intraoral readily visible mouthguard is required in all interscholastic and intercollegiate football, ice hockey, field hockey, and men's and women's lacrosse. The American Dental Association has recommended requiring a mouthguard in acrobatics, basketball, bicycling, boxing, equestrian events, extreme sports, field hockey, football, gymnastics, handball, ice hockey, inline skating, lacrosse, martial arts, racquetball, rugby, skateboarding, skiing, skydiving, soccer, softball, squash, surfing, volleyball, water polo, weightlifting, and wrestling.[14]

Properly fitted across the upper teeth, a mouthguard can absorb energy, disperse impact, cushion contact between the upper and lower teeth, and keep the upper lip away from the incisal edges of the teeth. This action significantly reduces dental and oral soft-tissue injuries, and to a lesser extent jaw fractures, cerebral concussions, and temporomandibular joint injuries. The practice of cutting down mouthguards to cover only the front four teeth invalidates the manufacturer's warranty, cannot prevent many dental injuries, and can lead to airway obstruction, should the mouthguard become dislodged. Although some individuals may complain that use of a mouthguard adversely effects speech and breathing, a properly fitted mouthguard should not interfere with either function. The benefits of preventing oral injuries through the use of mouthguards far outweigh any disadvantages.

Throat and Neck Protectors

Blows to the anterior throat can cause serious airway compromise as a result of a crushed larynx and/or upper trachea, edema of the glottic structures, vocal cord disarticulation, hemorrhage, or laryngospasm. The NCAA requires that catchers in baseball and softball wear a built-in or attachable throat guard on their mask.[1] Helmets used in field hockey, lacrosse, and ice hockey also provide anterior neck protectors to protect this vulnerable area.

Cervical neck rolls and collars are designed to limit excessive motion of the cervical spine and can be effective in protecting players with a history of repetitive burners or stingers. However, properly fitted shoulder pads are perhaps the most critical factor in preventing brachial plexus injuries.

Protective Equipments: Upper Body

In the upper body, special pads and braces are often used to protect the shoulder region, ribs, thorax, breasts, arms, elbows, wrists, and hands. Depending on the activity, special design modifications are needed to allow maximum protection, while providing maximal performance.

Shoulder Protection

Shoulder pads should protect the soft- and bony-tissue structures in the shoulder, upper back, and chest. The external shell is generally made of a lightweight, yet hard plastic. The inner lining may be composed of closed- or open-cell padding to absorb and disperse the shock; however, use of open-cell padding reduces peak impact forces when compared with closed-cell pads.

Football shoulder pads should be selected based on the player's position, body type, and medical history. Linemen need more protection against constant contact and use larger cantilevers. Quarterbacks, offensive backs, and receivers require smaller shoulder cups and flaps to allow greater ROM in passing and catching.

Elbow, Forearm, Wrist, and Hand Protection

The entire arm is subjected to compressive and shearing forces in a variety of sports, such as those seen in blocking and tackling an opponent, deflecting projectiles, pushing opponents away to prevent collisions, or breaking a fall. Goalies and field players in many sports are required to have arm, elbow, wrist, and hand protection. However, in high school and collegiate play, no rigid material can be worn at the elbow or below, unless covered on all sides by closed-cell foam padding.[1]

The use of a counterforce forearm brace may provide some relief for individuals with lateral and medial epicondylitis. These braces are designed to reduce tensile forces in the wrist flexors and extensors, particularly the extensor carpi radialis brevis. Although these braces may relieve pain on return to activity, debate continues about the effectiveness of counterforce forearm braces. These braces should not be used for other causes of elbow pain, such as growth plate problems in children and adolescents or medial elbow instability in adults.

The forearm, wrist, and hand are especially vulnerable to external forces and often neglected when considering protective equipments. In collision and contact sports, this area should be protected with specialized gloves and pads.

Thorax, Rib, and Abdominal Protection

Many collision and contact sports require special protection of the thorax, rib, and abdominal areas. Catchers in baseball and softball wear full thoracic and abdominal protectors to prevent high-speed blows from a bat or ball. Individuals in fencing, and goalies in many sports, also wear full thoracic protectors. Quarterbacks and wide receivers in football often wear rib protectors composed of air-inflated, interconnected cylinders to absorb impact forces caused during tackling. These protectors should be fitted according to the manufacturer's instructions.

Lumbar/Sacral Protection

Lumbar/sacral protection includes weight-training belts used during heavy weight lifting, abdominal binders, and other similar supportive devices. Each should support the abdominal contents, stabilize the trunk, and prevent spinal deformity or injury during heavy lifting. Use of belts or binders can significantly increase proprioception and intra-abdominal pressure to reduce compressive forces in the vertebral bodies and, in doing so, potentially lessens the risk of low back trauma. The use of back belts to prevent occupational low-back pain or to reduce lost work time due to occupational low-back pain is not supported by the Canadian Centre for Occupational Health and Safety and the United States National Institute for Occupational Safety and Health.[15,16] In contrast, the United State Occupational Safety and Health Administration's recent ergonomics regulation classified lumbar supports as personal protective equipments and suggested that they may prevent back injuries in certain industrial settings.[16]

Protective Equipments: Lower Body

In the lower body, commercial braces are commonly used to protect the knee and ankle. In addition, special pads are used to protect bony and soft-tissue structures in the hip and thigh region. Depending on the sport/activity, special design modifications are needed to allow maximum protection, while providing maximal performance.

Hip and Buttock Protection

In collision and contact sports, the hip and buttock regions require special pads typically composed of hard polyethylene covered with layers of Ensolite™ to protect the iliac crest, sacrum, coccyx, and genital region. A girdle with special pockets can effectively hold the pads in place. The male genital region is best protected by a protective cup placed in an athletic supporter.

Thigh Protection

Thigh and upper leg pads slip into readymade pockets in the girdle to prevent injury to the quadriceps area. Thigh pads should be placed over the quadriceps muscle group, approximately 6 to 7 inches proximal to the patella. When using asymmetrical thigh pads, the larger flare should be placed on the lateral aspect of the thigh to avoid injury to the genitalia. In addition to thigh pads, neoprene sleeves can provide uniform compression, therapeutic warmth, and support for a quadriceps or hamstring strain.

Knee and Patella Protection

The knee is second only to the ankle and foot in incidence of injury. Knee pads can protect the area from impact during a collision or fall, and in wrestling, can protect the prepatellar and infrapatellar bursa from friction injuries. In football, knee pads reduce contusion and abrasions when falling on artificial turf.

Knee braces fall into three broad functional categories: prophylactic, functional, and rehabilitative. Prophylactic knee braces are designed to protect the medial collateral ligament by redirecting a lateral valgus force away from the joint itself to points more distal on the tibia and femur. Functional knee braces are widely used to provide proprioceptive feedback and to protect unstable anterior cruciate ligament (ACL) injuries, or in postsurgical ACL ligament repair or reconstruction cases. Rehabilitative braces provide immobilization at a selected angle after injury or surgery, permit controlled ROM through predetermined arcs, and prevent accidental loading in non–weight-bearing patients. Knee braces should only be worn based on the recommendation of a qualified healthcare practitioner.

Patellofemoral Protection

Patella braces are designed to dissipate force, maintain patellar alignment, and improve patellar tracking. A horseshoe-type silicone or felt pad is sewn into an elastic or neoprene sleeve to relieve tension in recurring patellofemoral subluxation or dislocations. These braces relieve anterior knee pain syndrome.[17]

Lower Leg Protection

Pads for the anterior tibia area should consist of a hard, deflective outer layer, and an inner layer of thin foam. Velcro straps and stirrups help stabilize the pad inside the sock. Many styles also incorporate padding or plastic shells over the ankle malleoli, which are often subject to repeated contusions. Several commercial designs are available.

Ankle and Foot Protection

Commercial ankle braces can be used to prevent or support a postinjury ankle sprain and come in three categories: lace-up brace, semirigid orthosis, or air bladder brace. A lace-up brace can limit all ankle motions, whereas a semirigid orthosis and air bladder brace limit only inversion and eversion. Ankle braces have been compared with ankle taping. It is fairly well accepted that maximal loss in taping restriction for both inversion and eversion occurs after 20 min or more of exercise. Ankle braces are more effective in reducing ankle injuries, are easier for the wearer to apply independently, do not produce some of the skin irritation associated with adhesive tape, provide better comfort and fit, and are more cost-effective and comfortable to wear.[18–20]

Selection and fit of shoes may also affect injuries to the lower extremity. Shoes should adequately cushion impact forces and support and guide the foot during the stance and final push-off phase of running. In activities requiring repeated heel impact, additional heel cushioning should be present. Length should be sufficient to allow all toes to be fully extended. Individuals with toe abnormalities or bunions also may require a wider toe box. APPLICATION STRATEGY 3.1 identifies factors to keep in mind when selecting and fitting athletic shoes.

In field sports, shoes may have a flat-sole, long cleat, short cleat, or a multicleated design. The cleats should be properly positioned under the major weight-bearing joints of the foot and should not be felt through the sole of the shoe. Shoes with the longer irregular cleats placed at the peripheral margin of the sole with a number of smaller pointed cleats positioned in the middle of the sole produce significantly higher torsional resistance and are associated with a significantly higher anterior cruciate ligament injury rate when compared with shoe models with flat cleats, screw-in cleats, or pivot disc models.[21] When increased temperature is a factor, such as when playing on turf, only the flat-soled basketball-style turf shoes are reported to have low-release coefficients at varying elevated temperatures.[22] This may lead to a lower incidence of lower leg injuries. In individuals with arch problems, the shoe should include adequate forefoot, arch, and heel support. In all cases, individuals should select shoes based on the demands of the activity.

Foot Orthotics

Orthotics are devices used in the treatment and prevention of foot and gait abnormalities and related conditions, such as plantar fasciitis, heel pain, shin splints, patellofemoral pain, and low back pain. By changing the angle at which the foot strikes the surface, orthotics can make standing, walking, and running more comfortable and efficient. Orthotics are available in several forms and are constructed of various materials. Foot orthotics fall into three broad categories: orthotics to change foot function, protective orthotics, and those that combine functional control and protection. Foot orthotics should be measured and fitted by a qualified medical professional.

APPLICATION STRATEGY 3.1

Factors in the Selection and Fit of Athletic Shoes

- Shoes should be fitted toward late afternoon or evening, preferably after a workout, and with the socks typically worn during sport participation.
- Shoes should be fitted to the longest toe of the largest foot, providing one thumb's width to the end of the toe box.
- The widest part of the shoe should coincide with the widest part of the foot. Eyelets should be at least 1 inch apart with normal lacing. Women with big or wide feet should consider purchasing boy's or men's shoes.
- The sole of the shoe should provide moderate support, but should not be too rigid. Sole tread typically comes in a horizontal bar (commonly used on asphalt or concrete) or a waffle design (used on off-road terrain).
- The midsole may be composed of ethylene vinyl acetate, polyurethane, or preferably, a combination of the two. Ethylene vinyl acetate provides good cushioning, but will break down over time. Polyurethane has minimal compressibility and provides good durability and stability.
- A thermoplastic heel counter maintains its shape and firmness even in adverse weather conditions.
- Running shoes should position the heel at least a half inch above the outsole to minimize stretch on the Achilles tendon.

- While wearing the shoes, athletic skills should be approximated (walking, running, jumping, and changing directions).
- Individuals with specific conditions need special shoes, such as:
  - Runners with normal feet—more forefoot and toe flexibility
  - Overpronation—greater control on the medial side
  - Achilles tendonitis— a heel wedge of at least 15 mm
  - Court sports—added side-to-side stability
  - High, rigid arches—soft midsoles, curved lasts, and low or moderate hindfoot stability
  - Normal arches—firm midsole, semicurved lasts, and moderate hindfoot stability
  - Flexible low arch—very firm midsole, straight last, and strong hindfoot stability
- The newly purchased shoes should be walked in for 2 to 3 days to allow them to adapt to the feet. Next, begin running or practicing in the shoes for approximately 25 to 30% of the workout. In order to prevent blisters, there should be a gradual extension in the length of time that the shoes are worn.
- Avid runners should replace shoes every 3 months and recreational runners every 6 months.

SUMMARY

1. In developing a conditioning program, consideration must be given to the principles of specificity, overload, individuality, and progression.

2. Overload is achieved by manipulating frequency, intensity, and duration in the exercise program.

3. Flexibility is the total ROM at a joint that occurs pain-free in each of the planes of motion.

4. Strength is the ability of a muscle or group of muscles to produce force in one maximal effort. Muscular endurance is the ability of muscle tissue to exert repetitive tension over an extended period.

5. An appropriate level of muscle strength and muscular endurance is necessary to prevent injury. The muscles must be prepared to withstand the forces associated with the demands of a particular sport or activity.

6. Cardiorespiratory endurance refers to the ability to sustain prolonged exercise. It involves activities, which use the large muscle groups to engage in dynamic exercise at moderate or higher levels of intensity for an extended period of time.

7. In the absence of appropriate levels of cardiovascular endurance, an individual can become fatigued. Fatigue can result in making abnormal movements or mistakes that can lead to increased susceptibility to injury.

8. Improper technique has been identified as a factor that contributes to injury.

9. Instruction of proper techniques should be based on sound physiological principles. Instruction of techniques based on personal experiences or anecdotal experiences and absent of a substantiated physiological premise should be avoided.

10. Instruction of proper techniques must be age and developmentally appropriate.

11. The sport participant must be protected from high-velocity, low-mass forces to prevent focal injuries, and low-velocity, high-mass forces to prevent diffuse injuries.

12. The coach must be informed of and understand their responsibilities with regard to the use of protective equipments.

13. Several agencies have developed standards of quality to ensure that the equipment does not fail under normal athletic circumstances or contribute to injury (e.g., NOCSAE; HECC; ASTM).

14. Protective equipment is only effective when it is properly fitted and maintained, periodically cleaned and disinfected, and used as intended.

APPLICATION QUESTIONS

1. A high school basketball coach is concerned about various oral injuries that have occurred on the school's basketball teams. What rationale can be used to convince the administration to purchase mouthguards for the teams?

2. A middle-age female client at the fitness facility requests advice concerning the purchase of running shoes. She reveals that her orthopedic physician has diagnosed her with high arches. What guidelines should be suggested to this individual regarding shoe fit and construction (i.e., sole, midsole, heel, toebox)?

3. A high school physical education curriculum includes a course in cycling. The students are responsible for providing their own helmets. Prior to the start of the course, the instructor approved the helmet style and fit for each student. One day, having left his/her helmet at home, a student borrowed a helmet from a classmate in order to be able to participate in class. The teacher observes that while secured to the student's head, it does not fit properly. The student is an excellent cyclist. Should the instructor permit the student to participate in the class activity? Explain your response.

4. A high school varsity baseball coach is also a volunteer coach for an 8 to 10 year old little league baseball team. Is it advisable for the coach to use the same training and instructional techniques for the boys that play the position of pitcher? Explain your response.

5. A mandate from the Board of Education requires the physical education teachers in middle schools to incorporate 10 min of cardiorespiratory exercise into every physical education class. Would you recommend that the physical educator focus on aerobic or anaerobic cardiorespiratory exercise? Why?

6. A high school football coach has 50 sets of uniforms. The last student selected for the team is also the last student to receive his/her uniform. The available pants and shoulder pads are slightly large for the student. In addition, the helmet does not fit snugly. The coach does not anticipate that the student will see much playing time, rather he kept him on the team roster because the student is enthusiastic and a hard-worker. Is it acceptable for the student to practice in the uniform that is available? Explain your response.

_____

_____

7. When is the best time to incorporate flexibility exercises into a high school basketball practice? Why?

_____

_____

REFERENCES

1. Nelson KC, Cornelius WL. 1991. The relationship between isometric contraction durations and improvement in shoulder joint ROM. J Sports Med Phys Fitness, 31(3):385–388.
2. American College of Sports Medicine. *ACSM's guidelines for exercise, testing and prescription.* Baltimore: Lippincott Williams & Wilkins, 2005.
3. McArdle WD, Katch FI, Katch VL. *Exercise physiology: energy, nutrition, and human performance.* Baltimore: Lippincott Williams & Wilkins, 2007.
4. Koester MC. 2000. Youth sports: a pediatrician's perspective on coaching and injury prevention. J Ath Train, 35(4):466–470.
5. Murphy P. 1985. Youth sport coaches: using hunches to fill a blank page. Phys Sportsmed, 13(4):136–142.
6. Quain RJ. 1989. An overview of youth coaching certification programs. Adolescence, 24: 541–547.
7. *2008-09 NCAA sports medicine handbook.* Overland Park, KS: The National Collegiate Athletic Association, 2008.
8. Collins M, et al. 2006. Examining concussion rates and return to play in high school football players wearing newer helmet technology: A three-year prospective cohort study. Neurosurgery, 58(2):275–286.
9. Reynan PD, Clancy WG Jr. 1994. Cervical spine injury, hockey helmets, and face masks. Am J Sports Med, 22(2):167–170.
10. Nicholls RL, Elliott BC, Miller K. 2004. Impact injuries in baseball: prevalence, aetiology and the role of equipment performance. Sports Med, 34(1):17–25.
11. Sheffield-Moore M, et al. 1997. Thermoregulatory responses to cycling with and without a helmet. Med Sci Sports Exerc, 29(6):755–761.
12. Parkinson GW, Hike KE. 2003. Bicycle helmet assessment during well visits reveals severe shortcomings in condition and fit. Pediatrics, 112(2):320–323.
13. Wellbery C. 2004. Proper bicycle helmet fit reduces head injuries. Am Fam Phys, 69(5): 1271.
14. American Dental Association Division of Communications. 2004. The importance of using mouthguards: tips for keeping you smile safe. J Am Dent Assoc, 135(7):1061.
15. Canadian Task Force on Preventive Health Care. 2003. Use of back belts to prevent occupational low-back pain. Can Med Assoc J, 169(3):213–214.
16. Occupational Safety and Health Administration. 2000. Ergonomic program: final rule. Fed Regist, 65(220):68261–68870.
17. BenGal S, et al. 1997. The role of the knee brace in the prevention of anterior knee pain syndrome. Am J Sports Med, 25(1): 118–122.
18. Osborne MD, Rizzo TD Jr. 2003. Prevention and treatment of ankle sprain in athletes. Sports Med, 33(15):1145–1150.
19. Hume PA, Gerrad DF. 1998. Effectiveness of external ankle support: bracing and taping in rugby union. Sports Med, 25(5):285–312.
20. Thacker SB, Stroup DF, Brance CM, et al. 1999. The prevention of ankle sprains in sports: a systematic review of the literature. Am J Sport Med, 27(6):753–760.
21. Lambson RB, Barnhill BS, Higgins RW. 1996. Football cleat design and its effect on anterior cruciate ligament injuries: a three year prospective study. Am J Sports Med, 24(2): 155–159.
22. Torg JS, Stilwell G, Rogers K. 1996. The effect of ambient temperature on the shoe-surface interface release coefficient. Am J Sports Med, 24(1):79–82.

Injury Pathology, Assessment and Management

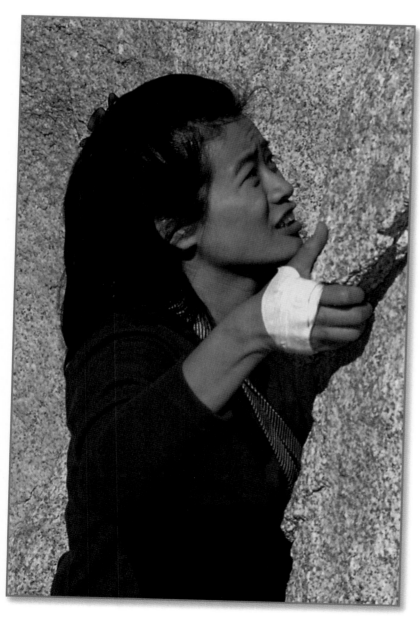

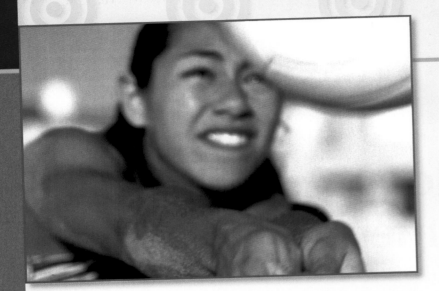

INJURY MECHANISM AND CLASSIFICATION OF INJURY

KEY TERMS

acute injury
anatomic position
anisotropic
axial force
axonotmesis
bending
bursitis
chronic injury
collagen
compressive force

(continued)

LEARNING OUTCOMES

1. Define terminology used to identify body segments, anatomic position, and directional terms used to communicate with the medical community.

2. Describe the major mechanical forces that produce injury to biological tissues, namely, compression, tension, shear, stress, strain, bending, and torsion.

3. Explain the effect of the material constituents and structural organization of skin, tendon, ligament, muscle, bone, and nerve on their ability to withstand the mechanical loads to which each is subjected.

4. List common injuries of skin, muscles and tendons, joints, bone, and nerve.

5. Explain the neurologic basis of pain, including factors that mediate pain.

KEY TERMS (CONTINUED)

coronal plane	irritability	shear force
cramp	mechanism of injury	somatic pain
dislocation	musculotendinous unit	spasm
ecchymosis	myositis ossificans	sprain
elastin	neurapraxia	stress
elasticity	neurotmesis	subluxation
epiphyseal plates	nociceptors	tendinitis
extensibility	osteoarthritis	tenosynovitis
extrinsic	osteochondrosis	tensile force
force	psychogenic pain	torsion
frontal plane	referred pain	visceral pain
hematoma	sagittal plane	yield point
intrinsic		

Injuries sustained as a result of participation in sport and physical activity can be caused by various mechanisms and may be acute or chronic (overuse) in nature. Understanding the different ways in which forces act on the various tissues in the body is necessary in comprehending techniques to prevent injuries. Likewise, knowing the material and structural properties of skin, tendon, muscle, ligament, bone, and nerve can lay a foundation for understanding the response of these tissues to applied forces and the potential resultant injury.

This chapter begins with information pertaining to the terminology used to identify body segments, anatomic positions, and directional terminology. This is followed by a general discussion of the mechanics of injuries to the human body. Finally, information is presented pertaining to the structural properties of soft, bone, and nerve tissue and classification of injuries to these tissues.

ANATOMIC FOUNDATIONS

Using correct terminology is crucial when communicating with members of the medical community. Anatomic terms, such as superior and inferior, medial and lateral, or thoracic and abdominal, help pinpoint the exact location on which to focus. Combined with basic medical terms, one can describe the site and what motions are affected by an injury. Anatomic considerations of skin, muscle, ligaments and joint structures, and bones are discussed in specific sections of this chapter.

Anatomic Position

The human body is separated into two main segments: axial and appendicular. The axial segment relates to the head and trunk and includes the chest and abdomen. The appendicular segment relates to the extremities. Direction or position on the body is based on **anatomic position** (FIG. 4.1). In this position the body is erect, facing forward, with the arms at the side of the body, palms facing forward.

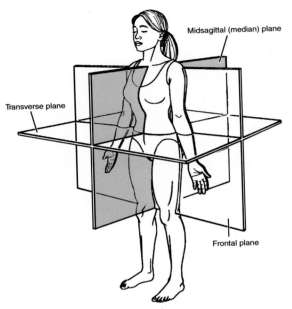

FIGURE 4.1 Anatomic position. All directional terms are based on anatomic position. Movement is described in directional terms—the planes of space along which the movement occurs.

Directional Terms

Directional terms are used to describe the location of one body part relative to another. For example, the elbow is superior to the wrist, the chest is on the anterior thorax, and the big toe is on the medial side of the foot. These terms are always used relative to anatomic position, regardless of the body's actual position. In speaking with the school's athletic trainer, a coach might report that one of the basketball players has pain on the lateral side of the ankle. In this manner, the athletic trainer can better visualize where the pain is located. Common directional terms used in injury assessment are defined in TABLE 4.1.

Movement is described in directional terms relative to the lines, or axes, around which the body part moves and the planes of space along which the movement occurs (TABLE 4.2; FIG. 4.2). Planes are a flat surface that sections the body into two parts. The most frequently used body planes are the **sagittal** or median **plane**, which divides the body vertically into right and left parts; the **frontal** or **coronal plane**, which divides the body vertically into anterior and posterior parts; and the **transverse plane**, which divides the body horizontally into superior and inferior parts.

MECHANISMS OF INJURY

The process by which an injury occurs is referred to as the **mechanism of injury**. Analyzing the mechanics of injuries to the human body is complicated by several factors. First, forces are applied to the body at different angles, over different surface areas, and over different periods of time. Second, the human body is composed of many different types of tissue that respond differently to applied forces. Finally, injury to the human body is not an all-or-none phenomenon. That is, injuries range from mild to moderate to severe.

Injury is caused by an abnormal force. **Force** is a push or pull acting on a body. A multitude of forces act on our bodies routinely during the day. The forces of gravity and friction enable us to move about in predictable ways when muscles produce internal forces.

TABLE 4.1	**Directional Terms**	
TERM	DEFINITION	EXAMPLE
Superior (cranial)	Toward the head or cranium	The heart is superior to the abdomen.
Inferior (caudal)	Toward the lower part of the body	The pelvic cavity is inferior to the thoracic cavity.
Anterior	Toward the front of the body	The quadriceps muscles lie anterior to the femur.
Posterior	Toward the back of the body	The buttock muscles lie posterior to the pelvis.
Proximal	Closest to a reference point	The shoulder is proximal to the elbow.
Distal	Farthest from a reference point	The wrist is distal to the elbow.
Medial	Toward or at the midline of the body	The little finger is medial to the thumb.
Lateral	Away from the midline of the body	The thumb is lateral to the little finger.
Bilateral	Pertaining to both sides of the outer body	The ears are bilateral on the skull body.
Superficial	Toward or at the body surface	The skin is superficial to the muscles.
Deep	Away from the body surface	The femur is deep to the skin.

TABLE 4.2	Joint Movements
Flexion	Movement along the **sagittal plane** that decreases the angle of the joint, e.g., bending the knee.
Extension	Movement along the sagittal plane that increases the angle of the joint, e.g., straightening a flexed knee.
Dorsiflexion and plantar flexion	Because the foot joins the leg at a right angle, both up and down motions of the foot technically decrease the angle and could both be called flexion. To avoid confusion, special terms are used. Lifting the foot toward the shin is called dorsiflexion; depressing the foot away from the shin is called plantar flexion.
Abduction	Movement along the **frontal plane** whereby the limb moves away from the midline of the body, e.g., raising the arm.
Adduction	Movement along the frontal plane whereby the limb moves toward the midline of the body, e.g., lowering a raised arm to the side of the body. Note: abduction and adduction of the fingers relate to movement away from the midline of the body part. In this instance, the midline is the longest digit—the third finger or the second toe.
Circumduction	Movement that involves flexion, abduction, extension, and adduction in succession. While the distal end of the limb moves in a circle, the point of the cone (the shoulder or hip) remains less stationary.
Rotation	Turning of a bone around its own long axis, e.g., movement between the first two cervical vertebrae.
Supination and pronation	Used at the wrist, supination refers to rotating the forearm laterally so that the palm faces anteriorly or superiorly (i.e., you can hold a cup of soup in your hand). In pronation, the forearm rotates medially and the palm faces posteriorly or inferiorly (i.e., palm lying down on a table). Inversion and eversion. Used at the foot, inversion implies that the sole of the foot turns medially. In eversion, the sole faces laterally.
Protraction and retraction	Movement in the transverse plane. For example, the mandible is protracted when you jut out the jaw and is retracted when you move it back into its original position.
Elevation and depression	Elevation means lifting a body part superiorly, such as when you shrug your shoulders. Depression is the opposite; or, moving the elevated part inferiorly.
Opposition	Movement at the joint between the first metacarpal and carpals of the wrist, which involves touching the thumb to the tips of the other fingers of the same hand.

When a force acts, there are two potential effects on the target object. The first is acceleration, or change in velocity, and the second is deformation, or change in shape. For example, when a racquetball is struck with a racquet, the ball is both accelerated (i.e., put in motion in the direction of the racquet swing) and deformed (i.e., flattened on the side struck). The greater the stiffness of the material to which a force is applied, the greater the likelihood that the deformation will be too small to be easily seen. The more elastic the material to which a force is applied, the greater the likelihood that the deformation will be temporary, with the material springing back to regain its original shape.

When tissues sustain a force, two primary factors dictate whether injury occurs, namely, the size, or magnitude, of the force and the material properties of the involved tissues. If the magnitude (or load) is relatively small, the response of the structure is elastic. As such, when the load is removed, the material will return to its original size and shape. However, if the load exceeds the material's **yield point**, or elastic limit, some amount of deformation will remain when the load is removed. Loads exceeding the ultimate failure point result in mechanical failure of the structure, which translates to fracturing of bone or tearing of soft tissues.

The direction of the applied force also has important implications for injury potential. Many tissues are **anisotropic**, meaning that the structure is stronger in resisting force from

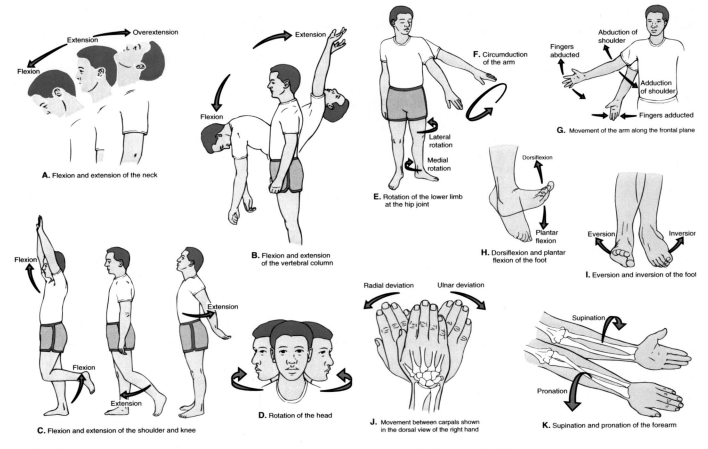

FIGURE 4.2 Joint motions. Movements permitted at the more common freely movable joints.

certain directions than from others. The anatomic makeup of many of the joints of the human body also makes them more susceptible to injury from a given direction. For example, lateral ankle sprains are much more common than medial ankle sprains because the ligamentous support of the ankle is much stronger on the medial side. Consequently, in discussing injury mechanisms, force is commonly categorized according to the direction from which the force acts on the affected structure (FIG. 4.3).

Force acting along the long axis of a structure is termed **axial force**. When the human body is in an upright standing position, body weight creates axial loads on the femur and the tibia.

Axial loading that produces a squeezing or crushing effect is called **compressive force** or compression. The weight of the human body constantly produces compression on the bones that support it. The fifth lumbar vertebra must support the weight of the head, trunk, and arms when the body is erect, producing compression on the intervertebral disk below it. When a football player is sandwiched between two opposing players, the force acting on that

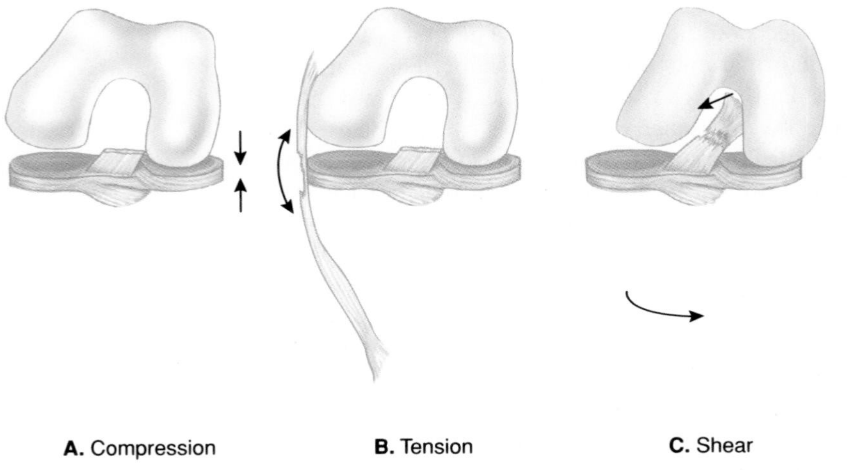

A. Compression   **B.** Tension   **C.** Shear

FIGURE 4.3 Mechanisms of injury. Compression (**A**) and tension (**B**) are directed along the longitudinal axis of a structure, whereas shear (**C**) acts parallel to a surface.

player is compressive. When a lacrosse player receives a blow to the upper arm from an opponent's stick, the force acting on the player is compressive. In the absence of sufficient padding, compressive forces sustained during contact activities often result in bruises or contusions.

Axial loading in the direction opposite to that of compression is called **tensile force**, or tension. Tension is a pulling force that stretches the object to which it is applied. Muscle contraction produces tensile force on the attached bone, enabling movement of that bone. When the foot and ankle are inverted or rotated excessively, the tensile forces applied to the ligaments may result in an ankle **sprain**.

Whereas compressive and tensile forces are directed, respectively, toward and away from an object, a third category of force, termed **shear**, acts parallel or tangent to a plane passing through the object. **Shear force** tends to cause one part of the object to slide against, displace, or shear with another part of the object. In performing a squat exercise, during knee flexion, the shear component of the joint force increases as the joint reaches 90°. Shearing at the knee, which results in a tendency for the femur

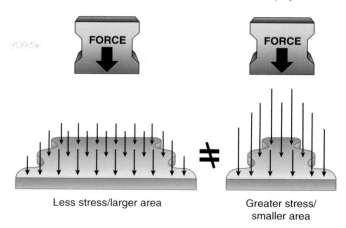

Less stress/larger area   Greater stress/ smaller area

FIGURE 4.4 Stress. The stress produced by a force depends on the area over which the force is spread. For example, the stress sustained by the superficial tissues of the arm would be lower than that with the force distributed directly over a small, bony landmark. The risk of injury increases when force is sustained over smaller areas.

to displace anteriorly on the tibia, is resisted primarily by the anterior and posterior cruciate ligaments. Because of the potential for injury to the cruciate ligaments resulting from shearing, it is recommended that squats be limited to 90° of flexion.

When force is sustained by the human body, the likelihood of injury depends on the magnitude of the **stress** produced by that force. When a given force is distributed over a large area, the resulting stress is less than if the force were distributed over a smaller area (FIG. 4.4). Alternatively, if a force is concentrated over a small area, the stress is relatively high. A high magnitude of stress, rather than a high magnitude of force, usually results in injury to biological tissues. One of the reasons that football and ice hockey players wear pads is that a pad distributes any force sustained across the entire pad, thereby reducing the stress acting on the player.

Injuries can result from a single traumatic force of relatively large magnitude or repeated forces of relatively small magnitude. When a single force produces an injury, the injury is called an **acute injury**. An acute injury, such as a ruptured anterior cruciate ligament or a fractured humerus, is characterized by a definitive moment of onset followed by a relatively predictable process of healing. When repeated or chronic loading over time produces an injury, the injury is called a **chronic injury** or a stress injury. A chronic injury, such as a stress fracture, develops and worsens gradually over time, typically culminating in a threshold episode in which pain and inflammation become evident. Chronic injuries can persist for months or years.

SOFT TISSUE INJURIES

Skin, tendon, muscle, and ligament are soft (nonbony) tissues that behave in characteristic ways when subjected to different forms of loading. The material composition of the anatomic structure influences the mechanical behavior of each tissue.

Anatomic Properties of Soft Tissue

Skin, muscles, tendon, ligaments, and other soft tissue structures are composed of connective tissue. The major building block of connective tissue is **collagen**. Collagen is a protein that is strong in resisting tension. Collagen fibers have a wavy configuration in a tissue that is not under tension (FIG. 4.5). This enables collagenous tissues, which are inelastic, to stretch slightly under tensile loading as these fibers straighten. As such, even though they are relatively inelastic, collagen fibers provide both strength and flexibility to tissues.

Elastin is another protein substance found in connective tissue. It provides added **elasticity** to some connective tissue structures and, in doing so, enables the tissues to return to normal length following stretching or contraction.

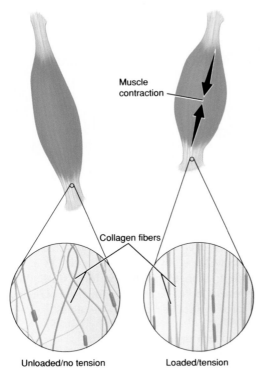

FIGURE 4.5 Collagen fibers. Collagen fibers have a wavy configuration when unloaded and a straightened configuration when loaded in tension.

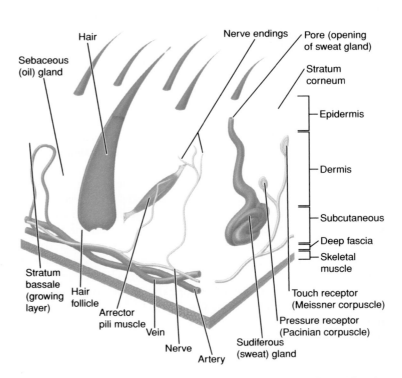

FIGURE 4.6 Skin. The two major regions of the skin are the epidermis and the dermis.

Skin

Anatomic Considerations

The integumentary system comprises the skin, hair, nails, and glands of the skin and is the largest organ in the body. It provides protection and sensation, regulates fluid balance and temperature, and produces vitamins (vitamin D) and immune system components.

The skin is composed of two major regions. The outer region, known as the epidermis, has multiple layers containing the pigment melanin, along with the hair, nails, sebaceous glands, and sweat glands (FIG. 4.6). Beneath the epidermis is the dermis, which contains blood vessels, nerve endings, hair follicles, sebaceous glands, and sweat glands. The dermis is composed of dense, irregular connective tissue, characterized by a loose, multidirectional arrangement of collagen fibers. This fiber arrangement enables resistance to multidirectional loads, including compression, tension, and shear. The skin dermis also contains elastic fibers that provide the skin with some elasticity.

Skin Injury Classification

Because skin is the body's first layer of defense against injury, it is the most frequently injured body tissue. There are five common open wounds seen in sport and physical activity: abrasions, incisions, lacerations, avulsions, and punctures.

Abrasions are caused by shear when the skin is scraped with sufficient force, usually in one direction, against a rough surface such as the floor or the artificial playing surface. The greater the applied force, the more layers of skin that are scraped away. Blood may ooze from the wound, but bleeding is usually not severe. Regardless of size, abrasions are extremely painful because of the number of nerve endings exposed. If the dermis is exposed, a primary concern is that dirt and foreign materials scraped over the wound may penetrate the exposed blood vessels, which increases the risk for infection unless the wound is properly cleansed and debrided.

Incisions are caused by a sharp, cutting object, such as broken glass. They are also caused when the impact causes the skin to be split over an underlying bone (e.g., a basketball player's elbow comes into contact with the supraorbital ridge of another player after pulling down a rebound and leading with the elbow as they turn into position). The wound has sharp, even cuts with smooth edges that tend to bleed freely. If the incision is caused by impact over a bone, an associated contusion usually occurs. These wounds tend to heal better than lacerations because the edges of the wound are smooth and can be approximated more easily during treatment.

A laceration is an irregular tear in the skin that typically results from a combination of tension and shear. As such, the edges are often jagged, leading to significant bleeding, especially if an artery is cut. Skin and tissue may be torn away, increasing the risk of infection.

An avulsion is a severe laceration that results in complete separation of the skin from the underlying tissues. A flap of skin may remain hanging or be torn off completely. Bleeding is profuse, and scarring is often extensive. If the avulsed skin is still attached by a flap of skin, circulation may be compromised. A primary concern with this injury is to make sure that the flap is lying flat and that it is aligned in its normal position before securing a dressing.

A puncture wound is formed when a sharp object, such as a shoe spike or nail, penetrates the skin and underlying tissues with tensile loading. Although the opening in the skin may appear small, the wound may be extremely deep, posing a serious threat for infection. A puncture wound usually does not cause a bleeding problem; however, the object that caused the injury may remain embedded in the wound.

Although not associated with an open skin wound, two other wounds do affect the skin—blisters and skin bruises. Blisters are minor skin injuries caused by repeated application of shear in one or more directions, as happens when a shoe rubs back and forth against the foot. The result is a pocket of fluid between the multiple layers of the epidermis as fluid migrates to the site of injury. If the movement is between the epidermis and the dermis, there may be blood in the pocket of fluid. These wounds are generally closed unless the blister should break, so infection is not the norm. The primary concern with this injury is to prevent further irritation to the area. If the blister should break, it should be treated as an abrasion.

Skin bruises are injuries resulting from compression sustained during a blow. Damage to the underlying capillaries causes the accumulation of blood within the skin. As a closed injury, the primary concern is to control superficial bleeding within the skin and underlying tissues by applying ice and compression.

Muscles and Tendons
Anatomic Considerations

Skeletal muscle is a highly organized structure that functions to produce skeletal movement and maintain postural alignment. A sheath known as the endomysium surrounds each muscle cell, or fiber. Small numbers of fibers are bound up into fascicles by a dense connective tissue sheath called the perimysium. A muscle is composed of several fascicles surrounded by the epimysium (FIG. 4.7).

The structure and composition of muscle enable it to function in a viscoelastic fashion, that is, with both elasticity and time-dependent extensibility. **Extensibility** is the ability to be stretched or increase in length, whereas elasticity is the ability to return to normal length after either lengthening or shortening has taken place. The viscoelastic aspect of muscle extensibility enables muscle to stretch to greater lengths over time in response to a sustained tensile force. This means that a static stretch maintained for 30 seconds is more effective in increasing muscle length than a series of short, ballistic stretches.

Another of muscle's characteristic properties, **irritability**, is the ability to respond to a stimulus. Stimuli affecting muscles can be either electrochemical, such as an action potential from the attaching nerve, or mechanical, as with an external blow to the

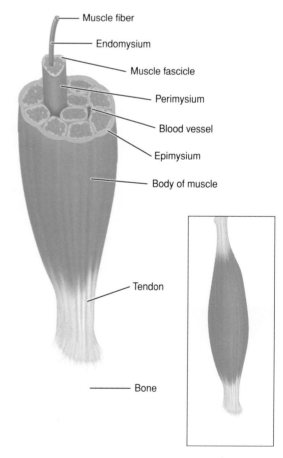

Muscle fiber

Endomysium

Muscle fascicle

Perimysium

Blood vessel

Epimysium

Body of muscle

Tendon

Bone

FIGURE 4.7 Muscle tissue. Skeletal muscle is composed of muscle cells, connective tissue, blood vessels, and nerves.

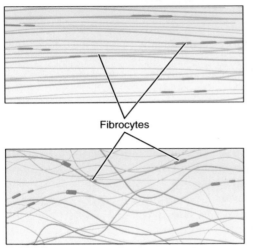

Tendon
Parallel bundles of collagen fibers

Fibrocytes

Ligament
Irregular wavy bundles of collagen fibers

FIGURE 4.8 Collagen arrangements in tendon and ligament tissue. The arrangement of collagen in tendons and ligaments differs, producing differences in their ability to resist tensile loads.

muscle. If the stimulus is of sufficient magnitude, muscle responds by developing tension.

The ability to develop tension is a property unique to muscle. A muscle may or may not shorten when tension is developed. Specifically, isometric contraction involves no joint movement and no change in muscle length; concentric contraction involves a shortening of the muscle developing tension; and eccentric contraction actually involves lengthening of the muscle developing tension. When a stimulated muscle develops tension, the amount of tension present is the same throughout the muscle and the tendon, and at the site of the tendon attachment to bone.

Tendons connect muscle to bone. They are composed of dense, regular connective tissue, consisting of tightly packed bundles of unidirectional collagen fibers (FIG. 4.8). The collagen fibers are arranged in a parallel pattern, enabling resistance to high, unidirectional tensile loads when the attached muscle contracts. By virtue of their collagenous composition, tendons are about twice as strong as the muscles to which they attach. Collectively, the muscle and tendon are referred to as the **musculotendinous unit.**

Muscle/Tendon Injury Classification

Injuries to muscles and tendons are dependent upon the nature of the causative force, the location of the force, and the properties of the involved musculotendinous unit (e.g., cross-sectional area; training state). Injuries can be acute or chronic.

Muscle contusions or bruises result from a direct compressive force sustained from a heavy blow. Such injuries vary in severity in accordance with the area and depth over which blood vessels are ruptured. **Ecchymosis,** or tissue discoloration, may be present if the hemorrhage is superficial. As blood and lymph flow into the damaged area, swelling occurs, often resulting in the formation of a hard mass composed of blood and dead tissue called a **hematoma.** This mass may restrict joint motion. Nerve compression usually accompanies such injuries, leading to pain and sometimes temporary paralysis.

Muscle contusions are rated in accordance with the extent to which the associated joint range of motion is impaired (TABLE 4.3). A first-degree contusion causes little or no range of movement restriction, a second-degree contusion causes a noticeable reduction in range of motion, and a third-degree contusion causes severe restriction of motion. With a third-degree contusion, the fascia surrounding the muscle may be ruptured, causing swollen muscle tissues to protrude.

Traumatic injury to muscles and tendons, termed strains, are caused by indirect forces (i.e., abnormally high tensile forces) that produce rupturing of the tissue and subsequent hemorrhage and swelling. The likelihood of strains depends on the magnitude of the force and the structure's cross-sectional area. The greater the cross-sectional area of a muscle, the greater its strength, meaning it can produce more force and translate that force to the attached tendon. In a similar manner, the larger the cross-sectional area of the tendon, the greater the force it can withstand. The increased cross-sectional area translates to reduced stress.

TABLE 4.3	**Classification of Contusions**		
	FIRST DEGREE	SECOND DEGREE	THIRD DEGREE
Damage to tissue	Superficial tissues are crushed	Superficial and some deep tissues are crushed	Deeper tissues are crushed (fascia surrounding muscle may rupture, allowing swollen tissues to protrude)
Weakness	Mild, if any	Mild to moderate	Moderate to severe
Loss of function	Mild	Moderate	Severe
Range of motion	No restriction	Decreased	Significantly decreased because of swelling

TABLE 4.4	**Classification of Strains**		
	FIRST DEGREE	SECOND DEGREE	THIRD DEGREE
Damage to muscle	Few fibers of muscle are torn	Nearly half of muscle fibers are torn	All muscle fibers are torn (rupture)
Weakness	Mild	Moderate to severe	Moderate to severe
Muscle spasm	Mild	Moderate to severe	Moderate to severe
Loss of function	Mild	Moderate to severe	Severe
Swelling	Mild	Moderate to severe	Moderate to severe
Palpable defect	No	No	Yes (if early)
Pain on contraction	Mild	Moderate to severe	None to mild
Pain with stretching	Yes	Yes	No
Range of motion	Decreased	Decreased	May increase or decrease depending on swelling

Because tendons are stronger than their attached muscle, the muscle portion of the musculotendinous unit almost always ruptures first. Muscle strains tend to be located near the musculotendinous junction, where muscle cross-sectional area is smallest. A tendon begins to develop tears when it is stretched to approximately 5 to 8% beyond normal length.[1]

Strains are categorized as first, second, and third degree (TABLE 4.4). First-degree strains involve only microtearing of the collagen fibers. They are characterized by mild pain and local tenderness, but they may present with no readily observable symptoms. In a first degree strain, there is no loss of function in activities of daily living. Second-degree injuries involve an extensive rupturing of the tissue. They are characterized by moderate pain, muscle weakness, and loss of function. Third-degree injuries produce a major loss of tissue continuity that results in a significant loss of function or movement. Severe pain followed by decreased pain attributed to nerve separation is typical in a third-degree strain. The tearing of muscle tissue can damage small blood vessels, which results in bleeding that may present as swelling and ecchymosis, particularly if the damage is superficial rather than deep.

Although typically not associated with injury, muscle cramps and spasms are painful, involuntary muscle contractions common to participation in sport and physical activity. A **cramp** is a painful involuntary contraction that may be clonic, with alternating contraction and relaxation, or tonic, with continued contraction over a period of time. Cramps appear to be brought on by a biochemical imbalance, sometimes associated with muscle fatigue. A muscle **spasm** is an involuntary contraction of short duration caused by reflex action that can be biochemically derived or initiated by a mechanical blow to a nerve or muscle.

Myositis and fasciitis refer, respectively, to inflammation of a muscle's connective tissues and inflammation of the sheaths of fascia surrounding portions of muscle. These are chronic conditions that develop over time as the result of repeated body movements that irritate these tissues.

Tendinitis and tenosynovitis involve inflammation within the tendon itself, or of the tendon sheath, respectively. **Tendinitis** is closely related to the process of normal aging and degenerative changes within tendons (tendinosis) and is characterized by pain and swelling with tendon movement (BOX 4.1). **Tenosynovitis** may be acute or chronic. Acute tenosynovitis is characterized by a grating sound (crepitus) with movement, inflammation, and local swelling. Chronic tenosynovitis has the additional symptom of nodule formation in the tendon sheath.

Prolonged chronic inflammation of a muscle or tendon can result in the accumulation of mineral deposits resembling bone in the affected tissues, a process known as ectopic calcification. Accumulation of mineral deposits in muscle is known as **myositis ossificans**. A common site for this condition is the quadriceps region. The muscle typically is very tender, and as the

BOX 4.1	**Signs and Symptoms of Tendinitis**

- **History of chronic onset**
- **Mechanism of injury is caused by overuse, or repetitive overstretch or overload**
- **Pain exists throughout the length of the tendon and increases during palpation**
- **Swelling may be minor to major and thickening of the tendon may be present**
- **Crepitus may be present**
- **Pain occurs at the extremes of motion during passive range of motion (PROM) and active range of motion (AROM)**
- **Pain increases during stretching and resisted range of motion (RROM); strength decreases with pain**

ossificans develops, a hardened mass can be palpated within the muscle mass. In tendons, the condition is called calcific tendinitis.

Overuse injuries may result from **intrinsic** factors (e.g., malalignment of limbs, muscular imbalances, and other anatomic factors) or **extrinsic** factors (e.g., training errors, faulty technique, incorrect surfaces and equipment, and poor environmental conditions). Typically, overuse injuries are classified into four stages based on pain and dysfunction:

- Stage 1: Pain after activity only
- Stage 2: Pain during activity, does not restrict performance
- Stage 3: Pain during activity, restricts performance
- Stage 4: Chronic, unremitting pain, even at rest

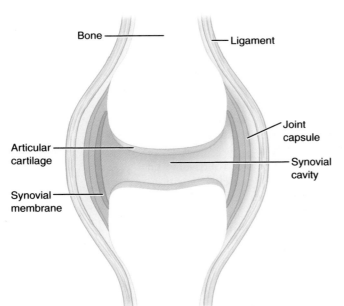

FIGURE 4.9 Joint components. Synovial joints have articular cartilage, a joint (synovial) cavity, an articular capsule, synovial membrane, synovial fluid, and reinforcing ligaments.

Joints
Anatomic Considerations

A joint is the site at which two bones connect. Joints are classified by their structure or function. Structurally, they are grouped as fibrous, cartilaginous, or synovial joints. Fibrous joints occur when the bone ends are united by collagenic fibers, and tend to be immobile (sutures of the skull or joints around the teeth) or slightly mobile (syndesmosis at the distal tibiofibular joint). Cartilaginous joints exist when bone ends/parts are united by cartilage, such as the pubic symphysis (fibrocartilage). Synovial joints occur when the bone ends/parts are covered with articular cartilage and enclosed within an articular capsule lined with synovial membrane. Synovial joints are freely movable, depending on the design of the joint. All joints of the limbs fall into this class.

The functional classification is based on the amount of movement allowed at the joint. Synarthroses are immovable joints, amphiarthroses are slightly movable joints, and diarthroses are freely movable joints. Since many of the joints of the body are freely movable synovial joints, discussion on joint structures will focus on this type of joint.

Diarthrodial joints are distinguished by five features (FIG. 4.9):

1. Articular cartilage. Glassy-smooth hyaline cartilage covers the ends of the bony surfaces. These cushions absorb compression placed on the joint and thereby protect the bone ends from being crushed. The

cartilage has no nerves or blood vessels; it is nourished by the synovial fluid covering its free surface. The nutrients in the synovial fluid come from the capillaries in the synovial membrane.

2. Joint (synovial) cavity. Unique to synovial joints, the joint cavity is filled with synovial fluid.

3. Articular capsule. The joint cavity is enclosed by a double-layered capsule. The external layer is a tough, flexible fibrous capsule that is continuous with the periosteum of the articulating bones. The capsule functions to help hold the bones of the joint in place. The inner layer is a synovial membrane composed of loose connective tissue, which covers all internal joint surfaces that are not hyaline cartilage. The synovial membrane produces synovial fluid that lubricates the joint.

4. Synovial fluid. A small amount of synovial fluid occupies all free spaces within the joint capsule. This fluid is derived largely by filtration from blood flowing through the capillaries in the synovial membrane. Synovial fluid has a viscous, egg-white consistency due to its content of hyaluronic acid secreted by cells in the synovial membrane, but it thins and becomes less viscous as it warms during joint activity. Synovial fluid is also found within the articular cartilages, providing a slippery weight-bearing film that reduces friction between the cartilages. In a weeping action, the fluid is forced from the cartilages when a joint is compressed. As pressure on the joint is relieved, the synovial fluid seeps back into the articular cartilages like water into a sponge. Synovial fluid also contains phagocytic cells that clear the joint cavity of microbes or cellular debris.

5. Reinforcing ligaments. Synovial joints are reinforced by a number of ligaments. More commonly, the ligaments are intrinsic, or capsular; that is, they are thickened parts of the fibrous capsule. In some cases, ligaments may remain distinct and are found outside the capsule (extrinsic or extracapsular) or deep into it (intracapsular). Since intracapsular ligaments are covered with synovial membrane, they do not actually lie within the joint cavity (extrasynovial).

Diarthrodial joints are classified according to their shape, which dictates the type and range of motion permitted. The classification is as follows:

- Plane: The articulating surfaces are nearly flat, and the only movement permitted is nonaxial gliding or short slipping movement. Examples include the intermetatarsal, intercarpal, and facet joints of the vertebrae.

- Hinge: One articulating bone surface is concave and the other convex. Strong collateral ligaments restrict motion to a single plane (uniaxial). Hinge joints permit flexion and extension only and can be seen at the elbow and interphalangeal joints.

- Pivot: A rounded or conical end of one bone rotates within a sleeve or ring composed of bone (and possibly ligaments), allowing for uniaxial rotation of one bone around its own long axis or against another. The atlantoaxial joint and both the proximal and distal radioulnar joints are examples of this type of joint.

- Condyloid: The oval (ellipsoidal) articular surface of one bone fits reciprocally into the concavity of another. These biaxial joints permit all angular motions, namely, flexion, extension, abduction, adduction, and circumduction. The key characteristic of these joints is that both articulating surfaces are oval. The radiocarpal (wrist) joint and the metacarpophalangeal (knuckle) joints are typical condyloid joints.

- Saddle: These biaxial joints resemble a condyloid joint; however, saddle joints allow greater freedom of movement. Each articular surface has both concave and convex areas; that is, it is shaped like a saddle. The carpometacarpal joint of the thumb is an example of this type of joint.

- Ball-and-socket: The spherical or hemispherical head of one bone articulates with the cuplike socket of another. These joints are multiaxial and the most freely moving synovial joints in that they permit universal movement in all axes and planes, including rotation. Examples include the shoulder and hip joints.

TABLE 4.5	**Classification of Sprains**		
	FIRST DEGREE	SECOND DEGREE	THIRD DEGREE
Damage to ligament	Few fibers of ligament are torn	Nearly half of fibers are torn	All ligament fibers are torn (rupture)
Distraction with stress tests	<5 mm distraction	5–10 mm distraction	>10 mm distraction
Weakness	Mild	Mild to moderate	Mild to moderate
Muscle spasm	None	None to minor	None to minor
Loss of function	Mild	Moderate to severe	Severe (instability)
Swelling	Mild	Moderate	Moderate to severe
Pain on contraction	None	None	None
Pain with stretching	Yes	Yes	No
Range of motion	Decreased	Decreased	May increase or decrease depending on swelling; dislocation or subluxation possible

Joint Injury Classification

Sprains are traumatic injury to ligaments. Abnormally high tensile forces produce a stretching or tearing of tissues that compromises the ability of the ligament to stabilize the joint. The tissue tearing also results in the flow of blood and lymph into the damaged area, producing swelling and restricting the range of motion. An example of a sprain is the motion that occurs when a basketball player lands on another player's foot after coming down from an attempted rebound. The action typically results in plantar flexion and inversion that produces tension on the lateral ligaments of the ankle.

Sprains are categorized as first, second, and third degree (TABLE 4.5). First-degree sprains involve only microtearing of the collagen fibers. Signs and symptoms include mild discomfort, mild point tenderness, minimal or no swelling, but minimal or no loss of function. Second-degree sprains involve tearing of nearly half the ligament fibers that result in a moderate loss of function and detectable joint instability. They are characterized by moderate pain, moderate swelling, and ecchymosis. Third-degree sprains produce a major loss of tissue continuity that results in a significant loss of function, severe instability, and severe pain.

A **dislocation** is a traumatic injury that occurs when the bones that comprise a joint are forced beyond their normal position, resulting in the displacement of one joint surface on another. A partial or incomplete dislocation is called a **subluxation**. The resultant damage includes rupturing of the joint capsule and ligaments as well as potential tearing of surrounding muscle-tendon units. In addition, many acute dislocations have an associated fracture or nerve injury. Signs and symptoms associated with a dislocation include pain, swelling, point tenderness, deformity, and loss of limb function.

Because of extensive stretching of the connective tissues surrounding a joint associated with a traumatic dislocation, there is increased susceptibility for chronic or recurrent dislocations. Less force is required to sustain a recurrent dislocation. While recurrent dislocations may be less painful, the subsequent damage to joint structures can be extensive and lead to chronic joint problems. The most common sites for dislocations are the fingers and the glenohumeral joint of the shoulder.

Osteoarthritis is a type of arthritis attributed to degeneration of the articular cartilage in a joint. Individuals with osteoarthritis experience pain and limited movement at the involved joint. While there is no definitive cause of osteoarthritis, it is attributed to a combination of factors, including stresses sustained during certain types of physical activity, joint trauma, and the aging process. It is one of the leading causes of disability among American adults. However, it should be noted that physical activity is being promoted as a potential strategy for managing arthritis.[2]

Bursitis involves irritation of one or more bursae. It may be acute or chronic, depending on whether it is brought on by a single traumatic compression or repeated compressions associated with overuse of the joint. Local swelling of a bursa can be very pronounced, particularly at the olecranon bursa of the elbow and the prepatellar bursa of the knee. An inflamed bursa is point tender and can be warm to the touch.

BONE INJURIES

In keeping with its material constituents and structural organization, bone behaves predictably in response to stress. The composition and structure of bone make it strong for its relatively light weight.

Anatomic Properties of Bone

The primary constituents of bone are calcium carbonate, calcium phosphate, collagen, and water. The minerals, making up 60 to 70% of bone weight, provide stiffness and strength in resisting compression. Collagen provides bone with some degree of flexibility and strength in resisting tension. Aging causes a progressive loss of collagen and increase in bone brittleness. As such, children's bones are more pliable than adults' bones.

Longitudinal bone growth continues only as long as the bone's **epiphyseal plates**, or growth plates, continue to exist (FIG. 4.10). Epiphyseal plates are cartilaginous discs found near the ends of the long bones. Longitudinal bone growth takes place on the diaphysis (central) side of the plates. During or shortly after adolescence, the plate disappears and the bone fuses, terminating longitudinal growth. Most epiphyses close by age 18, but some may be present until about age 25.

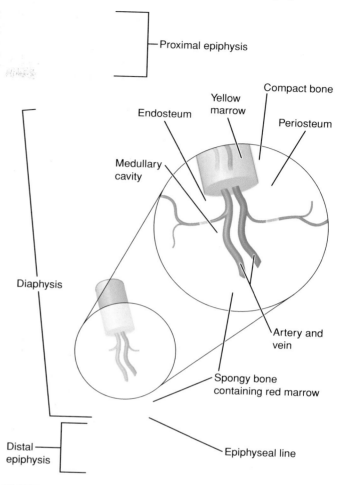

FIGURE 4.10 Bone macrostructure. Epiphyseal growth lines are found at both ends of the bone. Cortical bone surrounds the cancellous bone and the medullary cavity. Cancellous bone is more porous than cortical bone.

Although the most rapid bone growth occurs prior to adulthood, bones continue to grow in diameter throughout most of the life span. The internal layer of the periosteum builds new concentric layers of bone tissue on top of the existing ones. At the same time, bone is reabsorbed or eliminated around the sides of the medullary cavity, so that the diameter of the cavity is continually enlarged. The bone cells that form new bone tissue are called osteoblasts, and those that resorb bone are known as osteoclasts. In healthy adult bone, the activity of osteoblasts and osteoclasts, referred to as bone turnover, is largely balanced. The total amount of bone remains approximately constant until women reach 40 years of age and men reach 60 years of age, when a gradual decline in bone mass begins. As such, physically active individuals past these ages may be at increased risk for bone fractures. However, regular participation in weight-bearing exercise has been shown to be effective in reducing age-related bone loss.

Regardless of age, some bones are more susceptible to fracture as a result of their internal composition. Bone tissue is categorized as either cortical, if the porosity is low (with 5 to 30% nonmineralized tissue), or cancellous, if the porosity is high (with 30% to more than 90% of nonmineralized tissue). Most human bones have outer shells of cortical bone, with cancellous bone underneath. Cortical bone is stiffer, which means that it can withstand greater stress but less strain than cancellous bone. However, cancellous bone has the advantage of being spongier than cortical bone, which means that it can undergo more strain before fracturing. The mineralization of cancellous bone varies with the individual's age and location of the bone in the body.

Both cortical and cancellous bone is anisotropic. As such, they exhibit different strengths and stiffness in response to forces applied from different directions. Bone is strongest in resisting compressive stress and weakest in resisting shear stress.

Bone size and shape also influence the likelihood of fracture. The direction and magnitude of the forces to which they are habitually subjected largely determine the shape and size of the bone. The direction in which new bone tissue forms is in response to adaption required in resisting encountered loads, particularly in regions of high stress such as the femoral neck. Mineralization and girth of the bone increases in response to increased stress levels. For example, the bones of the dominant arm of professional tennis players and professional baseball players have been found to be larger and stronger than the bones of their nondominant arms.[3,4]

Bone Injury Classification

A fracture is a disruption in the continuity of a bone. Signs of fracture include rapid swelling, ecchymosis, deformity or shortening of the limb, precise point tenderness, grating or crepitus, and guarding or disability. See FIGURE 4.11 and BOX 4.2 for the most common types of fractures.

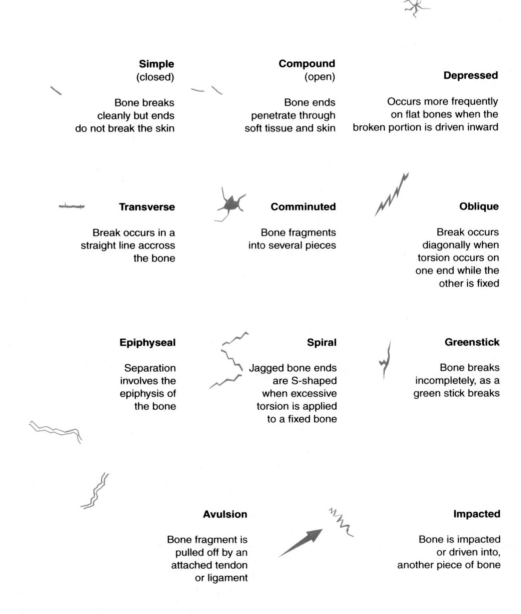

Simple
(closed)

Bone breaks cleanly but ends do not break the skin

Compound
(open)

Bone ends penetrate through soft tissue and skin

Depressed

Occurs more frequently on flat bones when the broken portion is driven inward

Transverse

Break occurs in a straight line accross the bone

Comminuted

Bone fragments into several pieces

Oblique

Break occurs diagonally when torsion occurs on one end while the other is fixed

Epiphyseal

Separation involves the epiphysis of the bone

Spiral

Jagged bone ends are S-shaped when excessive torsion is applied to a fixed bone

Greenstick

Bone breaks incompletely, as a green stick breaks

Avulsion

Bone fragment is pulled off by an attached tendon or ligament

Impacted

Bone is impacted or driven into, another piece of bone

FIGURE 4.11 Types of fractures. The type of fracture sustained is dependent on the type of mechanical load that causes the injury.

BOX 4.2   Common Types of Fractures

- **Simple (closed).** The bone clearly fractures, but the bone ends do not break the skin.
- **Compound (open).** One or both of the bone ends penetrates through the soft tissues and the skin.
- **Depressed.** This fracture occurs more frequently on flat bones when the broken bone portion is driven inward.
- **Transverse.** The fracture occurs on a straight line across the bone.
- **Comminuted.** The bone fragments into several pieces.
- **Oblique.** The fracture occurs diagonally when torsion occurs on one end while the other end is fixed.

- **Epiphyseal.** The separation involves the epiphysis of the bone.
- **Spiral.** Jagged bone ends are S-shaped because excessive torsion is applied to a fixed bone.
- **Greenstick.** The fracture is incomplete (e.g., as a green stick breaks). This fracture is more common in children than in adults.
- **Stress.** The fracture is incomplete, resulting from repeated low-magnitude forces that worsen over time.
- **Avulsion.** A bone fragment is pulled off by an attached tendon or ligament.
- **Impacted.** Bone is impacted, or driven into, another piece of bone.

The type of fracture sustained depends on the type of mechanical loading that caused it, as well as the health and maturity of the bone at the time of injury. In addition to compression, tension, and shearing mechanisms, bone is susceptible to **bending** and **torsion**. The simultaneous application of forces from opposite directions at different points along a structure, such as a long bone, can cause bending and ultimately fracture of the bone. If a football player's leg is anchored to the ground and the player is tackled on that leg from the front while being pushed into the tackle from behind, a bending force is created on the leg. When bending is present, the structure is loaded in tension on one side and in compression on the opposite side (FIG. 4.12A). Because bone is stronger in resisting compression than tension, the side of the bone loaded in tension will fracture if the bending moment is sufficiently large.

The application of a rotational force about the long axis of a structure, such as a long bone, can cause torsion, or twisting of the structure (FIG. 4.12B). Torsion results in the creation of shear stress throughout the structure. This mechanism can be seen in skiing accidents in which one boot and ski are firmly planted as the skier rotates during a fall. The result is a torsion load that can cause a spiral fracture of the tibia.

Fractures are considered to be closed when the bone ends remain intact within the surrounding soft tissues and open or compound when one or both bone ends protrude from the skin.

Excessive torsional and bending loads, as exemplified by tibial fractures resulting from skiing accidents, often produce spiral fractures of the long bones. Such fractures are the result of a combined loading pattern of shear and tension, producing failure at an oblique angle to the long axis of the bone.

Because bone is stronger in resisting compression than tension and shear, acute compression fractures of bone are rare. However, under combined loading a fracture resulting from a torsional load may be affected by the presence of a compressive load. An impacted fracture is one in which the

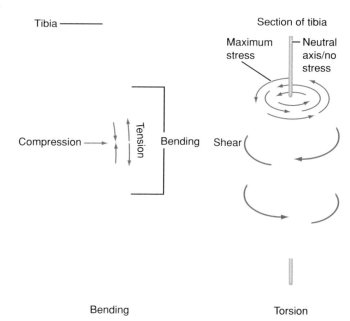

FIGURE 4.12 Bone injury mechanisms. **A.** Bones loaded in bending are subject to compression on one side and tension on the other. **B.** Bones loaded in torsion develop internal shear stress, with maximal stress at the periphery.

opposite sides of the bone are compressed together. Fractures that result in depression of bone fragments into the underlying tissues are termed depressed.

Because the bones of children contain relatively larger amounts of collagen than do adult bones, they are more flexible and more resistant to fracture under day-to-day loading than adult bones. Consequently, greenstick fractures, or incomplete fractures, are more common in children than in adults. A greenstick fracture is an incomplete fracture typically caused by bending or torsional loads.

Avulsions are another type of fracture caused by tensile loading that involve a tendon or ligament pulling a small chip of bone away from the rest of the bone. Explosive throwing and jumping movements may result in avulsion fractures. When loading is very rapid, a fracture is more likely to be comminuted, meaning it contains multiple fragments.

Stress fractures, also known as fatigue fractures, result from repeated low-magnitude forces. Stress fractures differ from acute fractures in that they can worsen over time, beginning as a small disruption in the continuity of the outer layers of cortical bone and ending as complete cortical fracture with possible displacement of the bone ends. Stress fractures of the metatarsals, femoral neck, and pubis have been reported among runners who have apparently overtrained. Stress fractures of the pars interarticularis region of the lumbar vertebrae occur in higher-than-normal frequencies among football linemen and female gymnasts.

Osteopenia, a condition of reduced bone mineral density, predisposes an individual to all types of fractures, but particularly to stress fractures. The condition is primarily found among adolescent female athletes, especially distance runners, who are amenorrheic. Although amenorrhea among this group is not well understood, it appears to be related to a low percentage of body fat and/or high training mileage. The link between cessation of menses and osteopenia is also not well understood. Possible contributing factors include hyperactivity of osteoclasts, hypoactivity of osteoblasts, hormonal factors, and insufficiencies of dietary calcium or other minerals or nutrients.

Epiphyseal Injury Classification

The bones of children and adolescents are vulnerable to epiphyseal injuries, including injuries to the cartilaginous epiphyseal plate, articular cartilage, and apophysis. The apophyses are sites of tendon attachments to bone, where bone shape is influenced by the tensile loads to which these sites are subjected. Both acute and repetitive loading can injure the growth plate, potentially resulting in premature closure of the epiphyseal junction and termination of bone growth. "Little League elbow," for example, is a stress injury to the medial epicondylar epiphysis of the humerus. Salter[5] has categorized acute epiphyseal injuries into five distinct types (FIG. 4.13):

- Type I: Complete separation of the epiphysis from the metaphysis with no fracture to the bone
- Type II: Separation of the epiphysis and a small portion of the metaphysis
- Type III: Fracture of the epiphysis
- Type IV: Fracture of a part of the epiphysis and the metaphysis
- Type V: Compression of the epiphysis without fracture, resulting in compromised epiphyseal function

Another category of epiphyseal injuries is referred to collectively as **osteochondrosis**. Osteochondrosis results from disruption of blood supply to an epiphysis, with associated tissue necrosis and potential deformation of the epiphysis. Because the cause of the condition is poorly understood, it is typically termed idiopathic osteochondrosis.

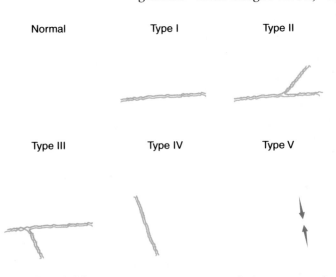

Normal   Type I   Type II

Type III   Type IV   Type V

FIGURE 4.13 Epiphyseal injuries. Five distinct types of injuries involve the epiphysis.

Osteochondrosis occurs more commonly between the ages of 3 and 10, and is more prevalent among boys than among girls.[5] Specific disease names have been given to sites where osteochondrosis is common, such as Legg-Calvé-Perthes disease, which is osteochondrosis of the femoral head.

The apophyses are also subject to osteochondrosis, particularly among children and adolescents. These conditions, referred to as apophysitis, may be idiopathic. However, they can be associated with traumatic avulsion-type fractures. Common sites for apophysitis are the calcaneus (i.e., Sever's disease) and the tibial tubercle at the site of the patellar tendon attachment (i.e., Osgood-Schlatter's disease).

NERVE INJURIES

The nervous system is divided into the central nervous system, consisting of the brain and the spinal cord, and the peripheral nervous system, which includes 12 pairs of cranial nerves and 31 pairs of spinal nerves, along with their branches (FIG. 4.14). There are 8 pairs of cervical spinal nerves (C_1-C_8), 12 pairs of thoracic nerves (T_1-T_{12}), 5 pairs of lumbar nerves (L_1-L_5), 5 pairs of sacral nerves (S_1-S_5), and 1 pair of tiny coccygeal nerves (designated C_0). Injuries to any of these nerves can be devastating to the individual, potentially resulting in temporary or permanent disability.

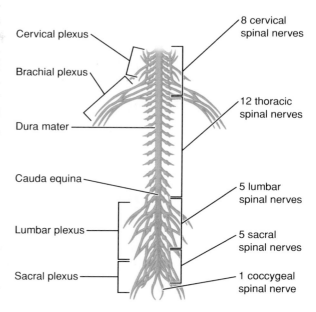

FIGURE 4.14 Spinal nerves. Each spinal nerve is formed from anterior and posterior roots on the spinal cord. The posterior branches are afferent nerves; the anterior branches are efferent nerves.

Anatomic Properties of Nerves

Each spinal nerve is formed from anterior and posterior roots on the spinal cord that unite at the intervertebral foramen. The posterior branches are the afferent (sensory) nerves that transmit information from sensory receptors in the skin, tendons, ligaments, and muscles to the central nervous system. The anterior branches are the efferent (motor) nerves that transmit control signals to the muscles. The nerve fibers are heavily vascularized and encased in a multilayered, segmental protective sheath called the myelin sheath. Myelin protects and electrically insulates fibers from one another, and it increases the speed of transmission of nerve impulses. Myelinated fibers (axons bearing a myelin sheath) conduct nerve impulses rapidly, whereas unmyelinated fibers tend to conduct impulses quite slowly.

Nerve Injury Classification

Tensile or compressive forces most commonly injure nerves. Tensile injuries are more likely to occur during severe high-speed accidents, such as automobile accidents or impact collisions in contact sports. When a nerve is loaded in tension, the nerve fibers tend to rupture prior to the rupturing of the surrounding connective tissue sheath. Because the nerve roots on the spinal cord are not protected by connective tissue, they are particularly susceptible to tensile injury, especially in response to stretching of the brachial plexus or cervical nerve roots.

Nerve injuries caused by tensile forces are typically graded in three levels. Grade I injuries represent **neurapraxia**, the mildest lesion. A neurapraxia is a localized conduction block that causes temporary loss of sensation and/or motor function from selective demyelination of the axon sheath without true axonal disruption. Recovery usually occurs within days to a few weeks. Grade II injuries are called **axonotmesis** injuries that produce significant motor and mild sensory deficits that last at least 2 weeks. Axonotmesis disrupts the axon and myelin sheath but leaves the epineurium intact. The epineurium is the connective tissue that encapsulates the nerve trunk and binds the fascicles together. Axonal regrowth occurs at a rate of 1 to 2 mm per day; full or normal function is usually restored. Grade III injuries represent **neurotmesis** injuries, which disrupt the endoneurium. These severe injuries have a poor prognosis, with motor and sensory deficit persisting for up to 1 year. Surgical intervention often is necessary to avoid poor or imperfect regeneration.

Compressive injuries of nerves are more complex because their severity depends on the magnitude and duration of loading and on whether the applied pressure is direct or indirect. Because nerve function is highly dependent on oxygen provided by the associated blood vessels, damage to the blood supply caused by a compressive injury results in damage to the nerve.

Nerve injuries can result in a range of afferent symptoms, from severe pain through complete loss of sensation. Terms used to describe altered sensation include hypoesthesia, a reduction in sensation; hyperesthesia, heightened sensation; and paresthesia, a sense of numbness, prickling, or tingling. Pinching of a nerve can result in a sharp wave of pain that is transmitted through a body segment. Irritation or inflammation of a nerve can result in chronic pain along the nerve's course, known as neuralgia.

PAIN

Pain is a negative sensory and emotional experience associated with actual or potential tissue damage. It is also a universal symptom common to most injuries. An individual's perception of pain is influenced by various physical, chemical, social, and psychological factors.

The Neurological Basis of Pain

Pain can originate from somatic, visceral, and psychogenic sources. **Somatic pain** originates in the skin as well as internal structures in the musculoskeletal system. **Visceral pain**, which is often diffuse or referred rather than localized to the problem site, originates from the internal organs. Psychogenic pain involves no apparent physical cause of the pain, although the sensation of pain is felt.

Stimulation of specialized afferent nerve endings called **nociceptors** produces the pain sensation. The name nociceptor is derived from the word noxious, meaning physically harmful or destructive. Nociceptors are prevalent in the skin, meninges, periosteum, teeth, and some internal organs.

In most acute injuries, pain is initiated by mechanosensitive nociceptors responding to the traumatic force that caused the injury. In chronic injuries and during the early stages of healing of acute injuries, pain persists because of the activation of chemosensitive nociceptors. Bradykinin, serotonin, histamines, and prostaglandins are all chemicals transported to the injury site during inflammation that activate the chemosensitive nociceptors. Thermal extremes can also stimulate other specialized nociceptors to produce pain.

Two types of afferent nerves transmit the sensation of pain to the spinal cord. Small-diameter, slow-transmission, unmyelinated C fibers transmit low-level pain that might be described as dull or aching. Larger, faster, thinly myelinated A fibers transmit sharp, piercing types of pain. Pain can be transmitted along both types of afferent nerves from somatic and visceral sources. Activity involving A and C fibers from the visceral organs can also provoke autonomic responses, such as changes in blood pressure, heart rate, and respiration.

Afferent nerves carrying pain impulses, along with those transporting sensations such as touch, temperature, and proprioception, articulate with the spinal cord through the substantia gelatinosa of the cord's dorsal horn. Specialized T cells then transmit impulses from all of the afferent fibers up the spinal cord to the brain, with each T cell carrying a single impulse. Within the brain, the pain impulses are transmitted to the thalamus, primarily its ventral posterior lateral nucleus, as well as to the somatosensory cortex, where pain is perceived.

According to the gate control theory of pain proposed by Melzack and Wall[6], the substantia gelatinosa acts as a gatekeeper by allowing either a pain response or one of the other afferent sensations to be transported by each T cell. The theory is substantiated by the observation that increased sensory input can reduce the sensation of pain. For example, extreme cold can often numb pain. Because hundreds or thousands of "gates" are in operation, however, it is more common that added sensory input reduces rather than eliminates the feeling of pain because pain impulses get through to some of the T cells.

Factors That Mediate Pain

Some brain cells have the ability to produce narcotic-like, pain-killing compounds known as opioid peptides, including beta-endorphin and methionine enkephalin. Both work by blocking neural receptor sites that transmit pain. Several different sites in the brain produce endorphins. Stressors, such as physical exercise, mental stress, and electrical stimulation, provoke the release of endorphins into the cerebrospinal fluid. A phenomenon called "runner's high," which is a feeling of euphoria that occurs among long distance runners, has been attributed to endorphin release. The brain stem and pituitary gland produce enkephalins. Enkephalins block pain neurotransmitters in the dorsal horn of the spinal cord.

The central nervous system also imposes a set of cognitive (i.e., quality of knowing or perceiving) and affective (i.e., pertaining to feelings or a mental state) filters on both the perception of pain and the subsequent expression of perceived pain. Social and cultural factors can be powerful influences on pain tolerance level. For example, in American society, it is much more acceptable for females than males to express feelings of pain. Individual personality and a state of mental preoccupation can also be significant modifiers of pain.

Referred Pain and Radiating Pain

Referred pain is perceived at a location remote from the site of the tissues actually causing the pain. A proposed explanation for referred pain begins with the fact that neurons carrying pain impulses split into several branches within the spinal cord. Although some of these branches connect with other pain-transmitting fibers, some also connect with afferent nerve pathways from the skin. This cross-branching can cause the brain to misinterpret the true location of the pain. In some instances, referred pain behaves in a logical and predictable fashion. Pain from the internal organs is typically projected outward to corresponding dermatomes of the skin. For example, heart attacks can produce a sensation of pain in the superior thoracic wall and the medial aspect of the left arm. In most cases, the affected internal organ and the corresponding dermatome receive innervation from the same spinal nerve roots.

Referred pain should not be confused with radiating pain, which is pain that is felt both at its source and along a nerve. Pinching of the sciatic nerve at its root may cause pain that radiates along the nerve's course down the posterior aspect of the leg.

SUMMARY

1. When a force acts, two effects occur on the target tissue: acceleration, or change in velocity, and deformation, or change in shape.

2. Two factors determine whether injury occurs to a tissue: the magnitude of the force and the material properties of the involved tissues.

3. Biological tissues are strongest in resisting the form of loading to which they are most commonly subjected.

4. Force exceeding a structure's yield point causes tearing or fracture.

5. The common mechanisms of injury include compressive force from axial loading, which compresses or crushes an object; tensile force from tension or traction on an object; and shearing force, which acts parallel or tangent to a plane passing through the object.

6. Injury to soft tissue and joints can be acute (results from a single traumatic force) or chronic/stress related (resulting from repeated loading over time).

7. Skin is able to resist multidirectional loads, including compression, tension, and shear. Open skin injuries include abrasions, incisions, lacerations, avulsions, and puncture wounds.

8. A unique property of muscle is the ability to develop tension. Isometric contraction involves no joint movement and no change in muscle length; concentric contraction involves a shortening of the muscle developing tension; and eccentric contraction actually involves lengthening of the muscle developing tension.

9. The viscoelastic aspect of muscle extensibility enables muscles to stretch to greater lengths over time in response to a sustained tensile force.

10. In tendons, the collagen fibers are arranged in a parallel pattern, enabling resistance to high, unidirectional tensile loads when the attached muscle contracts.

11. Contusions and strains are common acute injuries to muscles and tendons. Chronic or stress injuries to the muscles and tendons include myositis, fasciitis, tendinitis, tenosynovitis, and myositis ossificans.

12. Diarthrodial joints are freely moveable joints with distinct features. They are classified according to their shape, which determines the type and range of movement permitted.

13. In ligaments, the collagen fibers are largely parallel, but also interwoven, providing resistance to large tensile loads along the long axis of the ligament, and to smaller tensile loads from other directions.

14. Sprains and dislocations are common acute joint injuries. Chronic or stress injuries to joints include osteoarthritis and bursitis.

15. Because bone is stronger in resisting compressive forces than both tension and shear forces, acute compression fractures are rare. Most fractures occur on the side of the bone placed in tension.

16. Longitudinal bone growth occurs until the epiphysis closes. Bones continue to grow in diameter throughout most of the life span.

17. The type of fracture that occurs depends on the type of mechanical loading that caused the trauma.

18. Bones of children are susceptible to epiphyseal injuries. Damage to the epiphysis can alter normal bone growth.

19. Spinal nerves are formed from anterior and posterior roots on the spinal cord. The posterior branches are the afferent (sensory) nerves that transmit information from sensory receptors in the skin, tendons, ligaments, and muscles to the central nervous system. The anterior branches are the efferent (motor) nerves that transmit control signals to the muscles.

20. Nerve injuries caused by tensile forces are graded in three levels: neurapraxia injury, with temporary loss of sensation or motor function; axonotmesis injury, with significant motor and sensory deficits that last at least 2 weeks; and neurotmesis injury, with significant motor and sensory deficits persisting for up to 1 year.

21. Pain associated with injury is transmitted by specialized afferent nerve endings called nociceptors. Mechanosensitive nociceptors respond to traumatic forces that cause the injury. Chemosensitive nociceptors respond to chronic injuries and are activated during the early stages of healing in acute injuries.

22. Stressors, such as physical exercise, mental stress, and electrical stimulation, provoke the release of endorphins into the cerebrospinal fluid and can mediate pain perception.

APPLIED QUESTIONS

1. When the human body sustains force, there is the potential to strengthen body tissues or injure them. A previously sedentary middle age adult wants to initiate a running program as a way to improve his cardiovascular fitness. As a fitness specialist/personal trainer what advice should you provide to the individual to reduce the risk of sustaining a mechanical stress-related injury? Why?

_____

_____

2. A member of your high school volleyball team reports localized pain along the fifth metatarsal that increases after practice sessions. The pain has been present for over a month and is progressively getting worse. What injury should be suspected? What implications does this injury have for the volleyball player's continued training?

_____

_____

3. While sprinting to the end of the basketball court, a student in your high school physical education class suddenly pulls up limping, grabbing his posterior thigh, and unable to finish the sprint. How would you distinguish the signs and symptoms of a grade I and grade II muscle strain?

_____

_____

4. You are the coach of a boy's high school soccer team. For the past 2 weeks, preseason practice has included practices twice a day (i.e., 2 hours in the morning and 2 hours in the late afternoon). Prior to the start of morning practice on day 14, a player reports that he had a muscle spasm in his calf during the night. The pain was severe enough that it actually woke him from sleep. To date, the player has not sustained any injuries during preseason. Is it likely that the player experienced a muscle spasm? Explain your response.

_____

_____

5. During her junior year, a high school softball player dislocates her shoulder (glenohumeral joint) while sliding into second base. During the offseason, she follows a workout program designed to strengthen the muscles that govern the joint. Even with the offseason workouts, is she susceptible to another dislocation? Explain your response.

_____

_____

6. One of your clients at a fitness club is a middle age runner training for his or her first marathon. The individual asks for an explanation of a "runner's high." How would you respond?

_____

_____

7. You are the coach of a 14- to 16-year age group recreational swim team. A swimmer reports radiating pain down the posterior aspect of the left leg. What condition might be suspected because of the radiating pain? What type of structure may be injured?

_____

_____

8. You are the coach of a high school cheerleading squad. What factors could potentially contribute to a female squad member developing osteopenia?

_____

_____

REFERENCES

1. Standish WB, Curwin S, and Madel S. Tendinitis: its etiolgoy and treatment. New York: Oxford University Press, 2000.
2. National Center for Chronic Disease Prevention and Health Promotion. Physical activity: The arthritis pain reliever. Retrieved July 18, 2005, from http://www.cdc.gov/arthritis/campaigns/physical_activity/download_general.htm.
3. Jones HH, et al. 1977. Humeral hypertrophy in response to exercise. J Bone Joint Surg Am, 59: 204–208.
4. Watson RC. Bone growth and physical activity. In *International conference on bone measurements*, edited by RB Mazess. Washington, DC: Department of Health, Education, & Welfare, 1973. DHEW Pub No. NIH 75-683.
5. Salter RB. *Textbook of disorders and injuries of the musculoskeletal system.* Baltimore: Lippincott Williams & Wilkins, 1999.
6. Melzack R, and Wall PD. 1965. Pain mechanisms: A new theory. Science, 150(699):971–979.

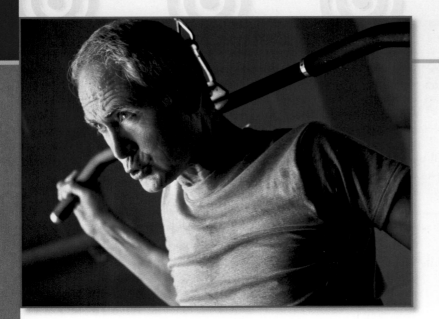

THE HEALING PROCESS

KEY TERMS

- acute
- adhesions
- angiogenesis
- atrophy
- bradykinin
- calor
- chronic
- edema
- exudate
- fibroblasts
- hematoma
- heparin

(continued)

LEARNING OUTCOMES

1. Explain the importance of understanding the healing process.
2. Describe the three phases of the healing process for soft and bone tissue (i.e., the inflammatory phase, the proliferative phase, and the maturation phase).
3. Identify local and systemic factors that can delay the healing process.

KEY TERMS (CONTINUED)

histamine	necrosis	vasodilation
hypertrophy	phagocytosis	zone of primary injury
hypoxia	prostaglandins	zone of secondary injury
inflammation	rubor	
mast cells	vasoconstriction	

The reparative process for injured tissues involves a complex series of interrelated physical and chemical activities. Because the normal healing process takes place in a regular and predictable fashion, knowledge of the various signs and symptoms exhibited at the injury site is essential to determining management and treatment options and monitor healing progress. Ultimately, this information is critical to decisions regarding immediate management, rehabilitation, and return to participation following injury.

This chapter begins with an explanation of the healing process for soft tissue. It is followed by bone and nerve tissue healing.

SOFT TISSUE HEALING

Trauma or physical damage results in the destruction of tissues. **Necrosis** is the death of living cells. It is due to disruption of the oxygen supply (**hypoxia**) to the involved area. The extent or amount of necrosis depends on the cause of the trauma and contributing factors.

The healing of destroyed soft tissues is a three-phase process involving **inflammation**, proliferation, and maturation. Although it is useful to discuss the healing phenomenon in terms these different stages, it should be recognized that there is usually overlap of these processes, both spatially and temporally, within injured tissues.

Inflammatory Phase (0 to 6 days)

The familiar symptoms of inflammation have long been recognized as **rubor** (redness), **calor** (local heat), tumor (swelling), dolor (pain), and in severe cases, loss of function. Although inflammation can be produced by adverse response to chemical, thermal, and infectious agents, the focus of this explanation is on the characteristic course of the inflammatory response following injury.

Depending on the nature of the causative forces, inflammation can be **acute** or **chronic**. An acute inflammatory response is relatively brief and involves the creation of **exudate**, a plasma-like fluid that exudes out of tissues or its capillaries and is composed of protein and granular leukocytes (white blood cells). A chronic inflammatory response, alternatively, is prolonged and is characterized by nongranular leukocytes and the production of scar tissues.

The beginning of the acute inflammatory phase involves the activation of three mechanisms that act to stop blood loss from the wound. First, blood flow is reduced through local **vasoconstriction**, lasting from a few seconds to as long as 10 minutes. The resulting reduction in blood flow volume in the region promotes increased blood viscosity or resistance to the flow, which further reduces blood loss at the injury site. A second response to the loss of blood is the platelet reaction. The platelet reaction causes clotting as individual cells irreversibly combine with each other and with fibrin produced by the coagulation cascade, which is the result of the third response to trauma. When combined, a mechanical plug is formed that occludes the end of a ruptured blood vessel. The platelets also produce an array of chemical mediators that play significant roles in the inflammatory and proliferation phases of healing.

After vasoconstriction, **vasodilation**, or an increase in blood flow, occurs. One process activated during this phase is the attraction of neutrophils and macrophages to rid the injury site of

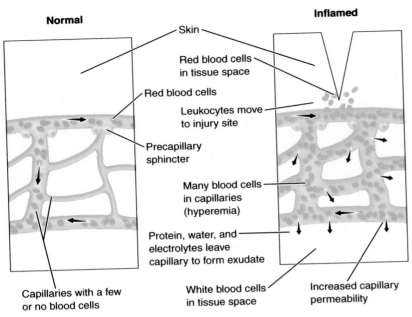

FIGURE 5.1 Acute inflammatory process. Edema forms when histochemical agents open the pores in the vascular walls, allowing plasma to migrate into the interstitial space.

debris and infectious agents through **phagocytosis.** As blood flow to the injured area slows, these cells are redistributed to the periphery, where they begin to adhere to the endothelial lining. **Mast cells** are connective tissue cells that carry **heparin,** which prolongs clotting; **histamine,** which promotes further vasodilation; and **bradykinin,** which promotes vasodilation, increases blood vessel wall permeability, and stimulates nerve endings to cause pain.

The increased blood flow to the region causes swelling or **edema.** Blood from the broken vessels and damaged tissues form a **hematoma** that, combined with necrotic tissue, forms the **zone of primary injury.** Approximately 1 hour post-injury, as the vascular walls become more permeable and increased pressure within the vessels forces a plasma exudate out into the interstitial tissues (between the cells), swelling increases (FIG. 5.1). This increased permeability of the blood vessel walls typically exists for only a few minutes in cases of mild trauma. Normal permeability usually returns in 20 to 30 minutes. More severe trauma can result in a prolonged state of increased permeability and sometimes result in delayed onset of increased permeability; swelling is not apparent until some time has elapsed since the original injury. The tissue exudate provides a critically important part of the body's defense, both by diluting toxins present in the wound and by enabling delivery of the cells that remove damaged tissue and enable reconstruction.

As the body continues to react to the inflammatory process, reparative cells in the exudate arrive at the injury site. Platelets and basophil leukocytes release enzymes that interact with other chemicals in the cell membranes to produce chemical mediators. These mediators include **prostaglandins** and leukotrienes, which attract leukocytes to the damaged area. This chain of chemical activity produces the **zone of secondary injury,** which includes all of the tissues affected by inflammation, edema, and hypoxia. After the debris and waste products from the damaged tissues are ingested through phagocytosis, the leukocytes re-enter the blood stream and the acute inflammatory reaction subsides.

The Proliferative Phase (3 to 21 days)

The proliferative phase involves repair and regeneration of the injured tissue. This phase takes place from approximately 3 days after the injury through the next 3 to 6 weeks, overlapping the later part of the inflammatory phase. The proliferative processes include the development of new blood vessels (**angiogenesis**), the process of fibrous tissue formation, the generation of new epithelial tissue, and wound contraction. This stage begins when the size of the hematoma is sufficiently reduced to allow room for new tissue growth. Although skin and bone can regenerate themselves, other soft tissues replace damaged cells with scar tissues.

Healing through scar formation begins with the accumulation of exuded fluid, which contains a large concentration of protein and damaged cellular tissues. This accumulation forms the foundation for a highly vascularized mass of immature connective tissues that include **fibroblasts,** which are cells capable of generating collagen. The new connective tissue matrix is fueled by nutrients from the blood supply and the newly forming blood vessels, which depend on the mechanical support and protection from the matrix. The matrix rapidly forms cross-links that contribute to stabilization of the wound site. The fibroblasts that have been chemically drawn to the hypoxic sites within the wound region secrete the collagen and promote angiogenesis by helping the growing blood vessels attach to the basement membrane collagen. These cells then fuse and form new vessels.

Other characteristics of the proliferation stage include an increased number of blood vessels, increased water content in the injury zone, and re-epithelialization at the surface caused by epithelial cells migrating from the periphery toward the center of the wound.

Maturation Phase (up to 1+ year)

The final phase of soft tissue wound repair is the maturation, or remodeling, phase. This phase involves the maturation of the newly formed tissue into a scar tissue. The associated characteristics include decreased fibroblast activity, increased organization of the extracellular matrix, decreased tissue water content, reduced vascularity, and a return to normal histochemical activity. In soft tissues, these processes begin about 3 weeks post-injury, overlapping the proliferative phase. Because scar tissue is fibrous, inelastic, and nonvascular, it is less strong and less functional than the original tissues. The development of the scar also typically causes the wound to shrink, resulting in decreased flexibility of the affected tissues. This explains why a person with paraplegia, who has a healed pressure sore from a wheelchair seat in poor condition, can easily redevelop breakdown in the same area, if the pressure stresses reoccur in that same area.[1]

Although the epithelium has typically completely regenerated by 3 to 4 weeks post-injury, the tensile strength of the wound at this time is only approximately 25% of normal.[2] After several more months, strength may still be as much as 30% below preinjury strength.[3] This is partly caused by the orientation of the collagen fibers, which tends to be more vertical during this time than in normal tissue. The collagen turnover rate in a newly healed scar is also high; therefore, failure to provide appropriate support for the wound site can result in a larger scar.

Remodeling continues for a year or more as collagen fibers become oriented to the tissue's normal mechanical stress. The tensile strength of scar tissue may continue to increase for as long as 2 years post-injury. BOX 5.1 summarizes the three stages of the healing process.

BOX 5.1   Phases of Soft Tissue Closed Wound Healing

INFLAMMATION (0 TO 6 DAYS)

- **Vasoconstriction**
  - Initial attempt of the body to stop blood loss.
  - Beginning of coagulation; initiates clotting.
- **Vasodilation**
  - Increased blood flow; swelling; increased capillary permeability.
- **Release of chemicals**
  - Promotes vasodilation.
- **Edema**
  - Large amounts of fluid (plasma and water) and exudate (fluid with cellular debris and high protein content) in the involved area.
- **Clot formation**
  - Fibrin deposits an irregular meshwork of short fibers in the region to contain the area.
- **Phagocytosis**
  - Leukocytes (neutrophils and macrophages) ingest the cellular debris; in doing so, prepares the area for repair.

PROLIFERATION (3 TO 21 DAYS)

- **Angiogenesis**
  - Development of new blood vessels to promote healing.
- **Fibrous tissue formation**
  - Fibroblasts produce a supportive network collagen fiber.
  - Stabilizes the wound site, but the area is significantly weaker that the normal, healthy tissue surrounding the damaged area.

MATURATION (UP TO 1+ YEARS)

- **Development of scar tissue**
  - Initially, fibrous, inelastic, nonvascular scar tissue is formed that is approximately 50% less in strength than its preinjury strength.
  - Scar formation continues modification based of the realignment of collagen fibers, based on the lines of habitual stress; potential for increased strength of scar tissue.
  - Scar tissue formation results in decreased size and flexibility of the involved tissues.
- **Return to normal histochemical activity**
  - Allows reduced vascularity and water content.

Muscles, Tendons, and Ligaments

Muscle fibers are permanent cells that do not reproduce or proliferate in response to either injury or training. However, reserve cells in the basement membrane of each muscle fiber are able to regenerate muscle fiber following injury. Severe muscle injury can result in scarring or the formation of **adhesions** within the muscle, which inhibits the potential for fiber regeneration from the reserve cells. Consequently, following severe injury, muscle may regain only about 50% of its pre-injury strength.[2]

Because tendons and ligaments have few reparative cells, healing of these structures is a slow process that can take more than a year. Regeneration is enhanced by proximity to other soft tissues that can assist with supply of the chemical mediators and building blocks required. For this reason, isolated ligaments, such as the anterior cruciate, have poor chances for healing.[4] If tendons and ligaments undergo abnormally high tensile stress before scar formation is complete, the newly forming tissues can be elongated. If this occurs in ligaments, joint instability may result.

Because tendons, ligaments, and muscles **hypertrophy** and **atrophy** in response to levels of mechanical stress, complete immobilization of the injury leads to atrophy, loss of strength, and decreased rate of healing in these tissues. The amount of atrophy is generally proportional to the time of immobilization. Although immobilization may be necessary to protect the injured tissues during the early stages of recovery, strengthening exercises should be implemented as soon as appropriate during rehabilitation of the injury. Increased risk for re-injury exists as long as the affected tissues are below pre-injury strength.

BONY TISSUE HEALING

Healing of acute bone fractures is a three-phase process, as is soft tissue healing. The acute inflammatory phase lasts approximately 4 days. The formation of a **hematoma** in the medullary canal and surrounding tissues causes damage to the periosteum and surrounding soft tissues. The ensuing inflammatory response involves vasodilation, edema formation, and the histochemical changes associated with soft tissue inflammation.

During repair and regeneration, osteoclasts resorb damaged bone tissues, whereas osteoblasts build new bone. Between the fractured bone ends, a fibrous, vascularized tissue known as a callus is formed (FIG. 5.2). The callus contains weak, immature bone tissues that strengthen with time through bone remodeling. The process of callus formation is known as enchondral bone healing. An alternative process, known as direct bone healing, can occur when the fractured bone ends are immobilized in direct contact with one another. This enables new, interwoven bone tissues to be deposited without the formation of a callus. Unless a fracture is fixed by metal plates, screens, or rods, healing normally takes place through the enchondral process. Because noninvasive treatment is generally preferred, a fixation device is only implanted when it appears unlikely that the fracture will heal acceptably without one.

Maturation and remodeling of bone tissues involves osteoblast activity on the concave side of the fracture, which is loaded in compression, and osteoclast activity on the convex side of the fracture, which is loaded in tension. The process continues until normal shape is restored and bone strength is commensurate with the loads to which the bone is routinely subjected.

Because stress fractures continue to worsen as long as the site is overloaded, it is important to recognize these injuries as early as possible. Elimination or reduction of the repetitive mechanical stress causing the fracture is the primary factor necessary for healing. This allows a gradual restoration of the proper balance of osteoblast and osteoclast activity present in the bone.

NERVE TISSUE HEALING

When a nerve is completely severed, healing does not occur and loss of function is typically permanent. Unless such injuries are surgically repaired, random regrowth of the nerve occurs, resulting in the formation of a neuroma or nerve tumor.

When nerve fibers are ruptured in a tensile injury, but the surrounding myelin sheath remains intact, it is sometimes possible for a nerve to regenerate along the pathway provided by

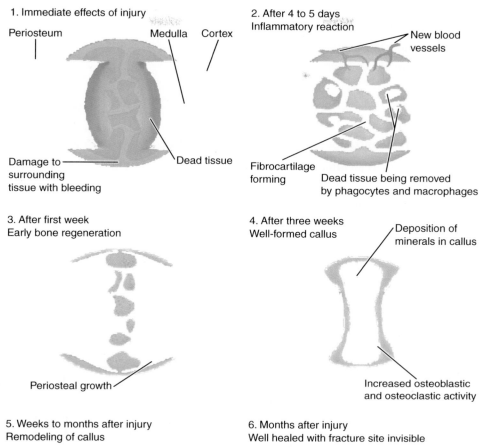

1. Immediate effects of injury

Periosteum   Medulla   Cortex

Damage to
surrounding
tissue with bleeding   Dead tissue

2. After 4 to 5 days
Inflammatory reaction

New blood
vessels

Fibrocartilage
forming   Dead tissue being removed
by phagocytes and macrophages

3. After first week
Early bone regeneration

Periosteal growth

4. After three weeks
Well-formed callus   Deposition of
minerals in callus

Increased osteoblastic
and osteoclastic activity

5. Weeks to months after injury
Remodeling of callus

6. Months after injury
Well healed with fracture site invisible

FIGURE 5.2 Bone healing. The process of endochondral bone healing involves callus formation.

the sheath. However, such regeneration is relatively slow proceeding at a rate of less than 1 mm per day or about 2.5 cm per month.[2]

FACTORS THAT DELAY HEALING

A variety of factors can delay or inhibit the healing of a wound. In general, these factors can be characterized as systemic or local. The ability to manage or influence these factors varies. The coach will likely have minimal influence in controlling or managing most of the factors. However, the coach is positioned to have an impact on some local factors subsequent to their involvement in the immediate management of an **acute injury**. The immediate management of injuries is presented in Chapter 6.

Local factors occur at the site of the wound. Local factors that delay healing include:

- Extent (size) of the injury
- Extent (amount) of hemorrhage and edema
- Muscle spasm
- Inflammation
- Infection
- Poor blood supply
- Prolonged immobilization; excessive motion or repeated adverse stress

Systemic conditions can affect multiple organs, systems, or the entire body. Systemic conditions that can impede wound healing include:

- Poor nutrition—A diet deficient in proteins, vitamins, and minerals is problematic.
- Vascular insufficiencies—These conditions can result in poor circulation and absence of sufficient blood supply to an area.
- Age—Elderly individuals are more susceptible to difficulties.
- Infection—A systemic infection or local infection will delay healing.
- Metabolic disorders—For example, individuals with diabetes mellitus are affected by the regulation of their serum glucose levels.

SUMMARY

1. The healing process takes place in a regular and predictable fashion that includes three phases, namely the inflammatory phase, the proliferative phase, and the maturation phase. An understanding of each phase is essential to determining the appropriate management of an injury and monitor the healing progress.

2. During the inflammatory phase, blood loss is curtailed, clotting takes place, and histochemical reactions promote coagulation, vasodilation, and attraction of specialized cells to rid the wound site of foreign or infectious agents.

3. The proliferative phase includes angiogenesis, bioplasia, re-epithelialization, and wound contraction.

4. The maturation phase involves remodeling of the newly formed tissues.

5. Maturation of bone tissues involves osteoblast activity on the concave side of the fracture, which is loaded in compression, and osteoclast activity on the convex side of the fracture, which is loaded in tension.

6. A variety of local and systemic factors can delay the healing process. Some of these factors can respond to treatment, while others are difficult to control.

APPLICATION QUESTIONS

1. Why is it important for a coach, physical educator, and fitness specialist to understand the healing process?

_____

_____

2. You are a high school physical education teacher. A sophomore student comes to class on Monday using crutches, having sustained a second-degree ankle sprain. The inquisitive student asks you why she needs to be on crutches and when her ankle will be back to "normal." Based on your understanding of the healing process, how would you respond to the student?

_____

_____

3. You are a fitness specialist. A 35-year-old client comes to a training session having sustained a grade II hamstring strain. He is very inquisitive and asks you to explain what is currently taking place and will continue to take place at the injured site. How would you explain the healing process to your client in a manner that is likely to make sense to him?

_____

_____

4. Can the actions of the coach, physical educator, and fitness specialist as the first responder to an acute soft tissue injury influence the primary or secondary injury zone? Why?

_____

_____

REFERENCES

1. Harvey C. 2005. Wound healing. Orthop Nurs, 24(2):143–159.
2. Wong ME, Hollinger JO, and Pinero GJ. 1996. Integrated processes responsible for soft tissue healing. Oral Surg Oral Med Oral Pathol, 82(5):475–492.
3. Orgill D, and Demling RH. 1988. Current concepts and approaches to wound healing. Crit Care Med, 16:899.
4. Hefti F, and Stoll TM. 1995. Healing of ligaments and tendons. Orthopedics, 24(3): 237–245.

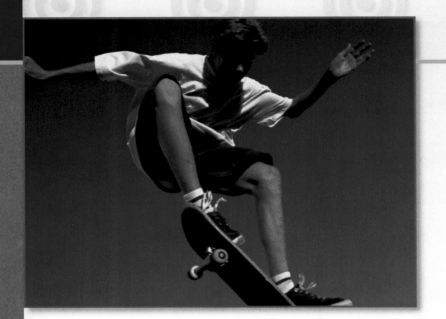

6

INJURY MANAGEMENT

analgesic
contraindications
indication

LEARNING OUTCOMES

1. Identify and explain areas that should be considered in the development and implementation of an emergency/accident plan for use by a coach, physical educator, or fitness specialist.

2. Explain the management of an acute open wound.

3. Identify procedures that should be taken to reduce the risk of transmission of bloodborne pathogens in managing an open wound.

4. Explain the management of an acute soft tissue injury (closed wound), including the use of cold, compression, elevation, protected rest, and movement.

5. Describe the immediate management of injury to a bone.

Accidents and injuries are to be expected. Participants in sport and physical activity need to understand that certain inherent risks are involved with their participation. The coach needs to have that same understanding and, as such, be prepared to provide immediate management for potential injuries/conditions. As the first responder when an injury is sustained, the coach is expected to evaluate the situation, assess the severity of injury, recognize life-threatening conditions, provide immediate care, and initiate procedures, as necessary, to ensure proper referral for ongoing management.

In addressing injury management, two broad areas should be considered. One area is the use of an emergency/action plan to provide direction for the coach in managing a condition. The second area is the on-site treatment appropriate for acute musculoskeletal injuries. Accordingly, this chapter will provide information on the emergency/accident plan, followed by explanation of the acute care of (1) an open wound, (2) a closed soft tissue injury, and (3) injury to bone.

DETERMINATION OF FINDINGS

Following completion of an on-site assessment, the coach must analyze the information obtained and make decisions on the best way to manage the situation. It is especially important to determine whether the situation can be handled on-site or if referral to a physician is warranted. In general, the options available to the coach in managing an acute injury would include:

- Standard acute care (i.e., cold, compression, elevation, protected rest, as appropriate) with no physician referral, but providing the individual with a written instruction sheet identifying signs and symptoms that would necessitate immediate care by a physician
- Standard acute care with physician referral prior to return to activity
- Standard acute care with immediate physician referral (i.e., emergency care facility)
- Summon emergency medical services (EMS)

Regardless of the severity of injury, a written plan should be in place to direct the coach through the implementation of each option.

THE EMERGENCY/ACCIDENT PLAN

Managing acute injuries/conditions is a major responsibility for individuals involved in the instruction, supervision, or administration of programs involving physical activity. In performing this responsibility, the coach must be concerned with providing the appropriate medical care for the participant and it must be within the standards of care of a coach.

An emergency/action plan is a well-developed written process that defines the policies and procedures to be used in the management of an acute injury to a participant. The plan should provide direction to those individuals who will have responsibilities in managing the condition. The plan should not be limited to emergency conditions, but rather it should include injuries of varying severity (e.g., mild; moderate; severe; life-threatening). The emergency/accident plan should be a written document that is comprehensive, yet flexible enough to adapt to any emergency situation at any activity venue. While some items should automatically be included in an emergency/accident plan, no single plan can satisfy the needs of every institution, organization, or facility. As such, every program should design a plan specific to their facility, population served, personnel, and any other factors that could influence injury management.

Note: For the purpose of brevity, the emergency/accident plan will be referred to as the emergency plan.

Developing the Emergency Plan

The development of an emergency plan should be recognized as a significant endeavor that requires input from several sources. It should be developed with input from the personnel at the facility, higher authorities to which the institution reports (e.g., an individual school as part of a school system; a fitness facility as a company-owned entity), medical personnel (e.g., physicians; representatives from local EMS agencies; athletic trainers), and legal personnel (e.g., school lawyer; company lawyer).

In developing the emergency plan, several areas must be addressed, including the population being served, potential injuries/conditions, personnel, availability of medical/first aid equipment, facility access, communication, and documentation.[1]

Population Served

While the immediate on-site treatment for any given musculoskeletal injury may be the same, regardless of the age or gender of the person, the population being served must be considered in developing an emergency plan. By recognizing that a population may have a higher susceptibility to a specific condition, consideration for the potential consequences associated with that condition, as well as the actions to be taken in the immediate management of the condition, can be addressed in advance. For example, elderly participants in an exercise program would be at a greater risk for cardiac-related conditions than third-grade students in a physical education class. In a similar manner, a 12-year-old recreational soccer player presents with a predisposition to musculoskeletal injuries different from those of a 30-year-old recreational soccer player. It is also important to acknowledge the general cognitive awareness of the population being served. For example, the reaction of a third-grade student having sustained an open fracture of the forearm during an activity in a physical education class is likely to be very different from if the same injury were sustained by a tenth-grade student or a 40 year old. In a similar manner, the physical education teacher will have the additional responsibility of supervising and controlling the rest of the third-grade students in the class and, typically, without the initial assistance of another adult.

Potential Injuries/Conditions

Identifying every potential injury or condition that could be sustained by a participant in sport or physical activity and including it in an emergency plan is not a reasonable expectation. However, it is reasonable to anticipate and identify potential emergency conditions that could be associated with some situations. For example, head and neck injuries are more likely to occur in football than in tennis. An elderly population is more vulnerable to a cardiac episode than students in an elementary school. An individual with diabetes must be concerned with maintaining appropriate blood glucose levels during participation in physical activity. As such, establishing written protocols for some injures and conditions can potentially reduce confusion through advanced planning and, in doing so, increase the potential for ensuring appropriate management. Written protocols for specific injuries/conditions should be considered for inclusion in the emergency plan (Box 6.1).

BOX 6.1	**Potential Emergency Conditions that Warrant Written Protocols**

- **On-site management of an unconscious individual**
- **Head and neck injuries**
- **Acute cardiac conditions (e.g., cardiac arrest; commotion cordis)**
- **Acute respiratory distress (e.g., asthma; exercise-induced bronchospasm; exposure to allergen)**
- **Life- or limb-threatening orthopedic injuries (e.g., femoral fracture; hip dislocation; posterior sternoclavicular dislocation)**
- **General medical conditions (e.g., diabetes; sickle cell anemia)**
- **Environmental conditions (e.g., heat illness)**

Personnel

The emergency plan should be developed with an understanding of the qualifications of the personnel that will be part of the emergency plan. The institution/organization would be well advised to require involved personnel to maintain certification in first aid, cardiopulmonary resuscitation (CPR), and automated external defibrillator (AED) training. Institutions should also consider requiring personnel to be trained in the handling of bloodborne pathogens. An emergency plan for an institution that does not require first aid, CPR, and AED training for their staff would necessitate a very different plan from that of an institution requiring such certifications.

Every institution/organization should have an emergency response team. The responsibilities of team members should be clearly defined. In doing so, it is important to recognize that in any given situation, the members of the emergency response team can vary. For example, in a school setting, a nurse may be available during the school day, but not available for after-school activities. In a fitness facility, additional healthcare practitioners (e.g., physician; nurse practitioner) may be available during hours of operation that a cardiac rehabilitation program is conducted rather than the entire time that a facility is open for business.

In establishing the specific responsibilities of personnel, it is necessary to address duties prior to the beginning of a program or event, during the activity, and after the activity. Areas of importance prior to the initiation of a program or event could include

- Identifying the personnel responsible for ensuring that first aid kits are appropriately stocked and restocked after use
- Identifying the personnel responsible for ensuring that emergency equipment are available and operational

During the event, responsibilities that should be defined could include the protocol for the

- Assessment of a condition (e.g., specific protocol for a potential head, neck, or internal injury)
- On-site treatment of a condition (e.g., application of ice and compression for a soft tissue injury; conditions, whereby protective equipment should not be removed: conditions, whereby an injured participant should not be moved; identification of conditions, which warrant activation of the local EMS;
- Implementation of the emergency plan (e.g., if the injury requires contacting the parents, who will make the phone call; if the condition requires obtaining the services of a local EMS agency, who will make the call)
- Proper disposal of items and equipment exposed to blood or other bodily fluids
- Documentation of actions taken in response to an injury/condition

Following the event, the emergency plan should identify the personnel responsible for follow-up communication, as necessary, with (1) the injured participant or their parents and (2) other personnel within the institution/organization. It is also essential that the plan have specific guidelines for documenting the actions taken by personnel in the implementation of the emergency plan. Written documentation should be required for any incident that requires a response by facility personnel, not just for those incidents deemed a "true emergency." If a coach assesses an injury, determines it to be minor, applies ice and compression, and provides instructions for return to play, the coach should be required to document the event.

If external support personnel (e.g., emergency medical technicians (EMTs); athletic trainers; parents) are used in the implementation of the emergency plan, their roles, responsibilities, and protocols should also be defined. For example, if an athletic trainer is hired to provide medical coverage for an event, then there must be a clear delineation of the responsibilities regarding services to be provided by that individual. It should not be assumed that the athletic trainer will provide specific services; rather, the services to be provided must be determined in advance. In a school or recreational setting, parents can be a valuable resource. For example, if a school knows that the coach is responsible for providing medical care for participants during away contests, recruiting parents to serve as members of the emergency medical team during away contests could be extremely beneficial. However, in order to avoid confusion and ensure appropriate implementation of the emergency plan, the decision to use parents should be determined in advance, so they can be informed of their roles and responsibilities.

Availability of Medical/First Aid Equipment and Supplies

In developing the emergency plan, decisions must be made with regard to the specific equipment and supplies that must be available to implement the plan. In making such decisions, it is essential to ensure that the materials are appropriate to the level of expertise or qualifications of the personnel implementing the plan. For example, it may not be appropriate to have an AED available for use in the absence of personnel trained to use the equipment. The same applies to less-sophisticated equipment, such as crutches. If crutches are to be made available for use by an injured participant, the coach must be familiar with the guidelines for the proper fitting of crutches and instructions on the use of crutches. Even the items selected for first aid kits should be predetermined and not left to the discretion of individual personnel. In all instances, personnel should be familiar with the first aid and medical supplies available for their use in advance of making use of them.

Facility Access

In some environments, facility access may not be a major concern. However, in other settings, it should not be overlooked. For example, if an injury occurs during a physical education class being held outdoors, the emergency plan may stipulate that the teacher uses a cell phone to call school personnel for any necessary assistance. If the cell phone is not available, it may become necessary to send a student to the school building to obtain help. In many schools, the outside doors are locked during the school day. If the door closest to the outdoor teaching area is not a door that can be readily accessed, the potential time delay to locate an unlocked door could have serious consequences for the injured individual. Again, the emergency plan is intended to anticipate any potential problems/issues in advance, so access to the facility should be addressed in developing the plan.

The plan should also identify the process for ensuring that emergency vehicles (e.g., EMS) have easy access to the facility and any outdoor venues. In some settings, the exact location of an outdoor venue may not be readily apparent to a responding EMS unit. If the emergency plan has identified a member(s) of the emergency response team to meet the EMS unit at the main entrance and direct them to the appropriate area, it could reduce an otherwise unforeseen delay in reaching the injured participant.

Communication

The availability of a phone is a critical component in the development of an emergency plan. The coach must have access to a working telephone at all times. While the availability of cell phones would seem to negate the importance of this component, it should not be overlooked. A plan must be in place for addressing potential problems with the availability of a cell phone (e.g., the phone loses its charge unexpectedly; phone service is not available in a particular area).

Communication also involves attention to several other areas. These include

- Determining when and who will call 911 (i.e., summon EMS). Again, it becomes important to anticipate potential issues. For example, a school system may already have a plan in place that requires certain personnel be informed before 911 can be called. If so, that policy should be part of the emergency plan. If the decision to call 911 is at the discretion of the coach, there are still items that must be addressed. If the coach is the only adult on-site and is tending to the injured individual, it may become necessary for one of the students on the team to place the call. The role of a student as a member of the emergency response team should be included in the emergency plan.

- Determining when and who will call the parents of a minor to advise them of an injury sustained by their child. Again, if the coach is not available to make the call, it may become necessary for a student to make the call. The plan should not only ensure that a student member of the emergency response team is prepared to make such a phone call, it should also ensure that parents are advised in advance that in some scenarios, a student will be part of the emergency response team.

- The timing of the phone call to the parents should also be determined in advance. For example, if it becomes necessary to activate EMS, it would seem that the parents should be called immediately after the call to 911. An argument could be made that it is not necessary to call the parents until the EMS unit arrives and determines their response. Regardless of the decision, the appropriate timing of a phone call to the parents should be determined in advance and included in the emergency plan.

- Determining when and who will call or inform personnel affiliated with an institution/facility (e.g., athletic director; school principal; fitness facility director) of an incident. An option for ensuring that necessary personnel have been informed is to create a chain of command. This option should allow for an efficient and effective means for disseminating information as necessary.

Documentation

Documentation is essential to verify the implementation of the emergency plan in response to any injury or condition. The actions taken by the coach in assessing and managing the injury should be documented using appropriate forms. These forms should be completed as soon as possible following the incident. Any unnecessary delay in completing the forms could result in failure to accurately recall all the actions that took place.

In addition to documentation of a specific incident, other information pertaining to the emergency plan should be documented. A procedure should be in place for documenting the verification of

- An annual review and rehearsal of the emergency plan, including notations indicating whether the emergency plan was modified and, if so, the changes made
- Personnel training and current certification
- Equipment maintenance and replacement as necessary

Implementing the Emergency Plan

Developing an emergency plan is one part of planning for the management of injuries. In order to ensure the plan is efficient and effective, it must be rehearsed. The emergency response team should practice the emergency plan through regular educational workshops and training exercises. The use of interactive or simulation practice exercises can better prepare individuals to assume their roles in rendering emergency care.

Following any implementation of the emergency plan, personnel other than just those individuals involved in implementing the plan (e.g., administrators) should evaluate the process for the purposes of identifying any areas, which require additional attention. In particular, any obstacles (e.g., breakdown in communication; unforeseen circumstances) that delayed the process should be identified and the appropriate steps taken to rectify the situation in the future implementation of the plan.

SOFT TISSUE WOUND CARE MANAGEMENT

Soft tissue injuries may involve open wounds (e.g., abrasions; blisters; lacerations; puncture wounds) or closed wounds (e.g., contusions; strains; sprains). This section explains immediate care of both broad categories of soft tissue injuries.

Open Wound Injury Care

In general, management of open wounds involves controlling bleeding, evaluating the wound to determine whether emergency treatment is necessary, cleansing the wound, and dressing the wound. In addition, care of open wounds includes following universal precautions to reduce the risk of transmission of bloodborne pathogens.

Bloodborne Pathogens

Bloodborne pathogens, such as Hepatitis B Virus (HBV), Hepatitis C Virus (HCV) and Human Immunodeficiency Virus (HIV) are microorganisms that are present in blood and other body fluids (e.g., semen; vaginal secretions) of infected individuals. The microorganisms can be transmitted when contaminated blood or bodily fluids enter the body of another person.

The risk of exposure to bloodborne pathogens can vary relative to the workplace setting. For example, opportunities for exposure are greater for a registered nurse in an emergency room than an athletic trainer in a high school setting. In an athletic or physical activity setting, transmission of bloodborne pathogens could potentially occur through open wounds subsequent to contact between the damaged skin and infected body fluids, and when contaminated fluids come into contact with the mucous membranes of the eyes, mouth, and nose.

Research suggests that the risk of transmission of bloodborne pathogens in an athletic or physical activity setting is relatively low. Regardless, such guidelines are necessary to minimize health risks and to protect both the coach and participant. In developing the guidelines, several areas should be addressed, including universal precautions, housekeeping, and biohazard waste disposal, accidental exposure, pre-exposure prophylaxis with Hepatitis B vaccine, documentation, and wound management.

Universal precautions should always be practiced in treating any open wound (Box 6.2). Best practice is to treat the blood of any individual as if it is infected with a bloodborne pathogen.

As part of the treatment of an open wound, attention must also be given to managing the treatment setting. In the absence of appropriate housekeeping or environmental control procedures, the risk of infection could still be present. Procedures should include

- Cleaning work surfaces immediately following treatment. An approved biohazard product or a bleach and water solution (mixed at a ratio of 1:10) should be available.
- Cleaning floor spills in accordance with infection control standards. It is important to designate the staff responsible for cleaning various types of spills. For example, if a physical education student sustains an injury that results in blood spots on the gymnasium floor, the physical education teacher should know in advance, if it is their responsibility to clean the floor or if it is their responsibility to inform another staff member (e.g., maintenance personnel) of the spill.
- Making biohazard waste bags and containers available for dispensing of contaminated disposable materials as well as handling of nondisposable contaminated materials (e.g., clothing; towels).
- Establishing protocols for collection of biohazard materials by an appropriate agency.

BOX 6.2 **Universal Precautions**

- **If possible, wash hands before treatment.**
- **If possible, cover any existing personal wounds.**
- **Apply gloves (e.g., latex) before initiating treatment; in some instances, it may be appropriate to give the patient a sterile gauze pad to apply to the wound while the gloves are being applied.**
- **If splattering or splashing of blood is anticipated, wear additional personal protective equipment (e.g., goggles; masks; gowns).**
- **If it becomes necessary to treat another individual, apply a new pair of gloves.**
- **Immediately following treatment, thoroughly wash hands and other skin surfaces with soap and warm water; in the absence of soap and water, disposable towel wipes or sanitizing lotions should be used.**
- **Dispose of all contaminated materials (e.g., gloves; gown; gauze pads) in an appropriate container marked for biohazardous waste.**

Because the potential exists for accidental exposure to blood or other body fluids, a plan must be in place for responding to any such scenario. Areas to be addressed include

- Establishing protocol for obtaining appropriate medical testing and treatment for the individual exposed to the pathogen.
- Developing a reporting system for results of any examinations, medical testing, and follow-up procedures.
- Defining procedures for documentation of the incident (e.g., date of incident; nature of the exposure; amount of blood involved in the exposure; follow-up recommendations).
- Identifying personnel who should be informed about the incident.
- Establishing procedural steps for ensuring confidentiality of the parties involved.

If the nature of a job puts an employee at a reasonable risk of coming into contact with blood or other bodily fluids, employers are required by the Occupational Safety and Health Administration (OSHA) standards to offer Hepatitis B vaccinations to their employees. The Hepatitis B vaccination prophylaxis is considered the best defense against contraction of HBV. The vaccination involves a series of three shots over a 6 month period. The Centers for Disease Control (CDC) reports very small risks of serious side-effects with the vaccination. The most common side-effect is soreness at the injection site. It is believed that the potential risks associated with HBV are far greater than any risk associated with the vaccine.[2] If an employee should decline the vaccination, the decision to decline should be appropriately documented.

The importance of recordkeeping and documentation cannot be overlooked in efforts to prevent the transmission of bloodborne pathogens. The type of records that should be maintained can vary relative to the work setting and practices. In general, records should include

- Verification of completion of OSHA training
- HBV vaccination or decline of the vaccination
- Medical records for individuals exposed to blood or other body fluids; information required as part of a medical report (e.g., exam results; medical testing)

Policies and procedures for ensuring the documentation and maintenance of appropriate information must be regulated. In particular, a process must exist for maintaining confidentiality of medical reports.

Open Wound Management

The first step in managing an open wound is to control the bleeding. In order to initiate the healing process, the blood must clot. Clotting will not take place when blood is flowing. The best method for controlling bleeding is the application of direct pressure. Using gauze pads to apply the pressure to the wound will promote the clotting process. While applying direct pressure, elevating the wound to a position above the heart will slow the flow of blood and make it easier to control the bleeding. If bleeding cannot be controlled using direct pressure and elevation, indirect pressure should be applied. Specifically, pressure should be applied to sites where the blood vessel is relatively superficial and at a spot between the wound and the heart. Common sites for indirect pressure include

- The upper arm for the brachial artery.
- The groin region for the femoral artery.
- The posterior knee for the popliteal artery.

The next step in managing an open wound is to clean the wound. Mild soap and water should be used to clean the wound and the area around it (i.e., at least twice the size of the wound). The area should be cleaned and rinsed thoroughly, ensuring removal of any debris or soap. Saline water can also be used to cleanse the wound. In fact, saline is often preferred over water as it is less irritating than water.

BOX 6.3	**Open Wound Conditions That Warrant Immediate Referral**

- **Life-threatening wounds (EMS should be activated).**
- **Uncontrolled bleeding.**
- **Inability to cleanse all the debris from the wound.**
- **A wound that potentially requires stitches.**
- **A penetrating wound (a tetanus shot may be necessary to avoid serious infection).**

In the process of cleaning the wound, the coach must evaluate the wound to determine whether immediate or emergency care is required. Conditions that warrant immediate medical attention at an emergency room or urgent care center can be found in BOX 6.3.

When the wound is clean and the bleeding has stopped, the next step is to dress the wound with a sterile bandage. The bandage could be a simple gauze pad or an occlusive type pad. In addition, an antiseptic ointment can be used to reduce bacterial growth. If the wound is a laceration, incision, or avulsion, butterfly strips can be used to join the edges of the wound. If the wound is deep enough that subcutaneous fat is visible or wide enough that it cannot be easily closed, it may require stitches. In addition, location of the wound can be a factor in determining the need for stitches. Specifically, if the wound site is an area that readily stretches or moves, a medical professional should evaluate the condition.

If the coach suspects that a wound requires stitches, arrangements should be made to have the individual seek medical attention at an emergency room or urgent care center. If necessary, stitches should be applied within 6 hours to avoid contamination of the wound. If a physician's evaluation suggests contamination, a wound cannot be stitched, as doing so would compromise the healing process.

If the evaluation suggests that the wound does not require immediate medical attention, the individual may be permitted to return to activity after the wound has been dressed and bandaged securely. If the wound resulted in blood on the individual's clothing, the clothing should be changed prior to return to activity if it appears wet or has soaked through the fabric. If the blood presents as small droplets of dried blood, it is not necessary to change the clothing.

The individual should be instructed to change the dressing daily. As part of that process, potential signs of infection should be assessed, including localized heat, swelling, redness, pus, and pain. Body temperature should also be taken as an elevated temperature could be indicative of infection. If signs of infection are present, the individual should seek medical attention.

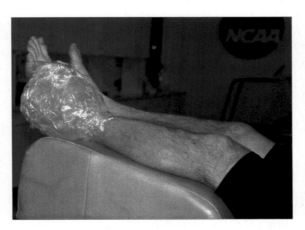

FIGURE 6.1 Standard acute protocol. Ice, compression, and elevation can reduce acute inflammation in response to a closed soft tissue injury.

Closed Soft Tissue Injury Care

Closed wound care focuses on immediately reducing inflammation, pain and secondary **hypoxia**. The process for providing immediate management for an acute closed soft tissue injury includes several components, commonly referred to as the PRICE principle (i.e., protected rest, ice, compression, and elevation) (FIG. 6.1). The focus of the information that follows is the immediate (e.g., on-the-field; onsite) management of a closed soft tissue injury.

Application of Cold

The extent of a soft tissue injury can be significantly affected by altering the temperature of the injured tissues. Within minutes of an injury, the application of cold can lead to vasoconstriction at the cellular level and decreased tissue metabolism (i.e., decreases the need for oxygen), which reduces secondary hypoxia. Capillary permeability and pain are decreased, and the release of inflammatory mediators and prostaglandin synthesis are inhibited. As the temperature of

BOX 6.4   Application of Cold

INDICATIONS

- Acute or chronic pain
- Acute or chronic muscle spasm/guarding
- Acute inflammation or injury
- Postsurgical pain and edema
- Neuralgia
- Superficial first-degree burns
- Used with exercises to
  - Facilitate mobilization
  - Relieve pain
  - Decrease muscle spasticity

CONTRAINDICATIONS

- Decreased cold sensitivity and/or hypersensitivity
- Cold allergy/cold-induced urticaria
- Circulatory or sensory impairment
- Raynaud's phenomenon
- Advanced diabetes
- Hypertension
- Uncovered open wounds
- Cardiac or respiratory disorders
- Nerve palsy
- Arthritis

peripheral nerves decreases, a corresponding decrease is seen in pain perception. Because nerve impulses are inhibited and muscle spindle activity is decreased, muscles in spasm are relaxed, breaking the pain–spasm cycle and leading to an **analgesic**, or pain-free, effect. As such, cold is the modality of choice during the acute phase of injury. **Indications** and **contraindications** associated with the use of cold can be found in Box 6.4.

While there are a variety of options for applying cold (e.g., cold packs; ice massage; cold whirlpool; vapocoolant sprays), coaches should consider using an ice bag (e.g., crushed or cubed) or an instant cold pack. For practical reasons, these methods are relatively convenient options. From a physiological perspective, it is not appropriate to use ice massage or whirlpool in the immediate management of an injury. The massaging effect produced by these techniques is not a desirable effect, until bleeding has subsided.

Plastic bags filled with crushed ice or small cubes can be safely applied to the skin without danger of frostbite. Ice bags can be molded to the body's contours, held in place by a cold compression wrap, and elevated above the heart to minimize swelling and pooling of fluids in the interstitial tissue spaces.

Instant (chemical) cold packs are convenient to carry in a first aid kit, disposable after a single use, and can conform to a body part. Each bag contains two chemicals separated by a plastic barrier. When the barrier is ruptured, the chemicals mix, producing cold. Disadvantages of this type of application are the short duration of the cold application, the expense in using the pack only once, and the potential for the pack tearing or leaking. The chemical substance that produces the cold has an alkaline pH, which can cause burns, if the liquid substance comes in contact with the skin. As such, the packs should never be squeezed or used about the face, and if possible, should be placed inside another plastic bag.

The cold pack should be applied to the injured area as soon as possible following the injury. The length of application time can range from 15 to 30 minutes. The time for a larger muscle mass, such as the quadriceps, would be 30 minutes and for a smaller site, such as a finger, 15 minutes should be sufficient. Cold applications should be repeated every 1 to 2 hours while the patient is awake and continue for at least 72 hours postinjury. During the application, the patient can expect to experience progressive sensations, namely cold, burning, aching, and analgesia (Box 6.5).

BOX 6.5   Stages of Cold Sensation

- Initial cold sensation (0 to 3 minutes)
- Burning and aching sensation (2 to 7 minutes)
- Numbing sensation (anesthesia) (5 to 12 minutes)

Application of Compression

The application of a compression following an acute injury can aid in the reduction of swelling to the injured site. Compression decreases hemorrhage, reduces the space available for fluid seepage, and encourages fluid absorption. In doing so, it promotes rather than delays healing. An exception for the use of compression in managing a soft tissue injury is any injury in which the additional compression would compound the trauma. For example, the addition of compression to an acute compartment syndrome in the lower leg is contraindicated.

The most common method of compression application requires an elastic wrap or bandage. The wrap should be applied in a distal-to-proximal direction to avoid forcing extracellular fluid into the distal aspect of an extremity. The wrap should be applied with sufficient tension to ensure compression without impairing blood supply. As a general rule, the patient should feel the firmness of the wrap, but should not experience a throbbing sensation. Another way to ensure that a wrap is not overly tight is to assess the distal pulse of the involved limb. If a wrap is too tight, it should be removed and re-applied, not simply removed.

In the immediate management of injury, the use of a cold, wet compression wrap is advantageous. Using an elastic wrap to secure the cold agent to the body part produces a significant reduction in subcutaneous tissue temperatures as compared with simply placing the cold agent on the skin.[3] One layer of the wrap should be applied to the injured site prior to placing an ice bag over the area. The remainder of the wrap should be used to secure the ice bag in place. When the treatment time for the cold pack is complete, a dry compression wrap should be applied. The compression wrap should be worn throughout the day and night.

Elevation of the Injured Site

Elevation of an injured body part at least 6 to 10 inches above the heart can reduce bleeding in the area, encourage venous return, and prevent pooling of blood in the extremities. Elevation should be performed as often as possible during the 72 hours postinjury. If the injury is to the lower extremity, in preparation for sleeping, raising the end of mattress (using a hard object, e.g., a suitcase) will permit elevation throughout the night. While the use of several pillows under the lower extremity is a viable option, there could be a tendency for the pillows to move and compromise the elevation.

Protected Rest

Following injury, the area should be rested to avoid further damage to the involved tissues. If continued unrestricted activity is permitted, it could result in increased bleeding, increased pain, and delayed healing. If the injury is to a lower extremity and the individual is unable to walk pain-free without a limp, the individual should be placed on crutches and an appropriate protective device applied to limit unnecessary movement of the injured joint. If the injury is to an upper extremity and the individual is unable to move the limb without pain, then the individual should be fitted with an appropriate splint or brace.

The length of the time for the protected rest will vary relative to the severity of the injury. Mild injuries may only require 24-hour rest, while a major injury could require at least 72 hours of rest. Protected rest does not imply cessation of activity, but simply means "relative rest," decreasing activity to a level below that required in participation in sport or physical activity, but tolerated by the recently injured tissue or joint.

While the protected rest is an important component of injury management, it is equally as important to appreciate the effects of both immobilization and remobilization on injured tissues. In certain instances, immobilization can prolong the repair and regeneration of damaged tissues, while early controlled mobilization can optimize the healing process. For example, immobilization can lead to a loss of muscle strength within 24 hours. This is manifested with decreases in the muscle fiber size, total muscle weight, mitochondria (energy source of the cell) size and number, muscle tension produced, and resting levels of glycogen and adenosine triphosphate, which reduces muscle endurance. In comparison, muscle regeneration begins within 3 to 5 days after mobilization. In a similar manner, ligaments adapt to normal stress by remodeling in response to the mechanical demands placed on them. Stress leads to a stiffer, stronger ligament, whereas immobilization leads to a weaker, more compliant structure.

This causes a decrease in the tensile strength, thus reducing the ability of ligaments to provide joint stability.

In general, soft tissues respond to the physical demands placed on them, causing the formation of collagen to remodel or realign along the lines of stress, thus promoting healthy joint biomechanics (Wolff's law). Continuous passive motion can prevent joint adhesions and stiffness, and decrease joint **hemarthrosis** (blood in the joint) and pain. Early motion, and loading and unloading of joints, through partial weight-bearing exercises maintain joint lubrication to nourish articular cartilage, menisci, and ligaments. This leads to an optimal environment for proper collagen fibril formation.

The Role of Movement in the Healing Process of Soft Tissue

It is not within the standards of care of a coach to prescribe therapeutic exercises. However, a general understanding of the role of movement in the healing of soft tissue injury enables the coach to educate and advocate for injured individuals. In particular, it would be advantageous for the coach to understand the importance of movement during the inflammatory phase of healing.

During the inflammatory phase of healing, movement can be initiated when bleeding has stopped. Bleeding can persist for up to 36 hours. The type of movement should be gentle and controlled motions that progress to routine activities of daily living. For example, if the injury is an ankle sprain, the movements could include wiggling the toes, performing plantar flexion and dorsiflexion within pain-free limits, and using the foot and ankle to make the letters of the alphabet. The next step in the progression would be to initiate walking within the parameters of being pain-free and maintaining a normal gait (i.e., without a limp). The advantages of movement in the inflammatory phase include

- Encouraging venous return
- Encouraging fluid resorption
- Encouraging phagocytosis
- Preventing contracture and loss of range of motion

BONE INJURY MANAGEMENT

A fracture can range in severity from a minor injury to a life-threatening emergency. As such, the immediate management of a fracture must take into consideration the nature and severity of the fracture. In all instances, medical attention is required.

If a suspected fracture to an extremity is associated with minor trauma, the initial focus of the immediate management should include splinting the extremity in the position in which it is found and immobilizing the joint above and below the fracture site. There should be no attempt to realign the bone or move the individual until the suspected fracture is stable. Immobilization is necessary to prevent any further damage to the bone and surrounding tissues (e.g., blood vessels; nerves; muscle) and it should aid in reducing pain. Consideration should be given to purchasing commercial-type splints as part of an institution's first aid supplies. It is important that the splints purchased are suited for use by the coach as compared to those splints (e.g., air splints) that should only be used by trained medical personnel (e.g., EMTs; athletic trainers). In the absence of commercial splints, splints can be made from materials that will provide rigidity, such as magazines, strips of wood, and cardboard. In a similar manner to the treatment of closed wound injuries, cold packs can be applied to reduce swelling, and the area elevated, as the physiological effects of both will minimize the secondary injury zone and optimize the healing process. Individuals with a suspected fracture should be advised to seek treatment at an urgent care center or emergency room. Fractures, even those minor in nature, should be treated as soon as possible to avoid complications and optimize the conditions for proper healing.

If a suspected fracture is associated with a major trauma or injury, it should be treated as a medical emergency. Such a condition warrants activation of the emergency medical plan, including summoning of 911. In assessing the individual, the presence of any "red flags" would indicate the need for emergency medical assistance (Box 6.6).

BOX 6.6	Suspected Fracture "Red Flags" that Indicate Need to Summon EMS

- **An open, or compound, fracture**
- **Suspected multiple fractures**
- **Suspected fracture of the femur, hip, pelvis, vertebra (e.g. cervical; lumbar), or skull**
- **A limb or joint presents with significant deformation**
- **The toes or fingers of the involved extremity are pale, blue, cold, or numb (suggesting circulatory compromise)**
- **Signs and symptoms of shock**

In situations considered a medical emergency, it is best to avoid moving or transporting the individual. Because movement could aggravate the condition, the individual should remain in the position found and the paramedics should handle transport. While waiting for medical assistance to arrive, the following actions should be considered in managing the condition:

- Controlling any bleeding (e.g., application of gentle pressure)
- Immobilizing the injured area in the position in which it was found
- Applying cold to the area
- If shock is suspected, then providing treatment for shock

SUMMARY

1. An emergency/accident plan should be developed for the purpose of providing direction to the coach and other individuals who will have responsibilities in managing an injury/condition. The plan should not be limited to emergency conditions, but rather it should include injuries of varying severity (e.g., mild; moderate; severe; life-threatening).

2. In developing the emergency plan, the institution/facility should design a plan specific to their facility, population served, personnel, and any other factors (e.g., availability of medical/first aid equipment; communication; facility access; documentation) that could influence injury management.

3. Every facility/institution should have an emergency response team. The emergency response team should practice the emergency plan through regular educational workshops and training exercises.

4. Because the potential does exist for exposure to blood or other infectious fluids among coaches and participants, guidelines must be in place to ensure compliance with the OSHA universal precautions and infection control standards to minimize health risks, including the transmission of HBV and HIV.

5. The management of an open wound includes application of pressure to control bleeding, cleansing the wound, evaluating the wound to determine, if referral is necessary, and dressing the wound.

6. The standard acute care for the management of a closed soft tissue injury includes the application of ice, compression, elevation, and protected rest. In addition, for some injuries, the performance of gentle and controlled motions during the inflammatory phase of healing can optimize healing conditions.

7. If a fracture is suspected, there should be no attempt to realign the bones or move the injured individual, until the site is stabilized.

8. While any suspected fracture requires medical attention, a suspected fracture associated with a major trauma or injury should be treated as a medical emergency.

APPLICATION QUESTIONS

1. You are a high school cross-country coach. A runner falls and sustains an abrasion to the knee. Explain your management of this condition. Is it necessary to document your actions?

2. You are a physical education teacher. During a soccer unit on an outdoor field, a sixth-grade student sustains an ankle injury. Your assessment suggests that the student has a mild inversion ankle sprain. Should there be a plan in place to provide you with guidelines for managing the injury? Explain your response. If there is no plan, what strategies could you use to ensure appropriate care of the student and minimize the potential for litigation?

3. You are the manager of a fitness facility that provides programs for adults aged 21 years and older. What items would you include in a first aid kit for your facility? Explain the rationale for each of your choices.

4. A ninth-grade student in your physical education class sustains a suspected forearm fracture. What signs and symptoms would indicate the need for summoning EMS?

5. You are a high school volleyball coach. During away contests, you are the only staff member from the school that goes with the team? How could you use parents to provide assistance in the area of injury management? What steps should be taken to avoid any confusion concerning the role of parents in providing assistance?

6. During a training session, one of your clients accidently falls and sustains an injury to the forearm. Your assessment suggests a mild contusion. Explain your on-site management of this condition (i.e., standard acute care).

REFERENCES

1. Anderson JC, Courson RW, Kleinert DM, and McLoda TA. 2002. National Athletic Trainers' Association Position Statement: Emergency planning in athletics. J Ath Train, 37(1):99–104.
2. Centers for disease control. (n. d.) Retrieved from http://www.cdc.gov/hepatitis/HBV/Vacc Adults.htm.
3. Danielson R, Jaeger J, Rippetoe J, et al. 1997. Differences in skin surface temperature and pressure during the application of various cold and compression devices. J Ath Train, 32(2): S34.

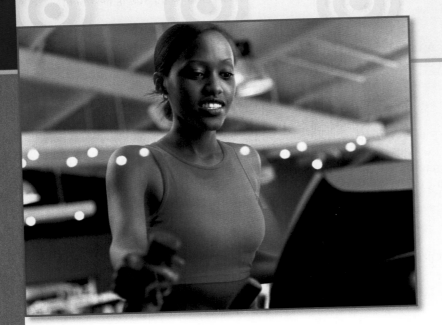

INJURY ASSESSMENT

KEY TERMS

acute
chronic
disposition
HOPS
referred pain
primary survey
sign
somatic pain
symptom
triage
visceral pain
diplopia

LEARNING OUTCOMES

1. Describe the use of the HOPS (i.e., history of the injury, observation and inspection, palpation, and special tests) format in the assessment of an injury.

2. Describe the use of the HOPS format by the coach in the on-site assessment of an acute injury or condition.

3. Apply the HOPS format in completing an on-site assessment of a nonorthopedic condition.

4. Apply the HOPS format in completing an on-site assessment of a musculoskeletal injury.

A coach, physical educator, or fitness specialist is often the first respondent in an injury situation, and as such, must be able to perform an injury assessment. The assessment is necessary to determine the appropriate management of the condition. The coach must be prepared to respond to a range of injuries, from a seemingly minor orthopedic condition to a potentially life-threatening emergency. In completing an assessment, the coach must ensure that their actions are consistent with their standard of care.

This chapter will address the role of the coach in performing both a primary and a secondary injury assessment. A systematic approach to assessment that includes history, observation, palpation, and testing components will be presented. The assessment approach will be adapted for use by the coach, physical educator, or fitness specialist.

THE INJURY EVALUATION PROCESS

When evaluating any injury or condition, diagnostic signs and symptoms are obtained and interpreted to determine the type and extent of injury. A diagnostic **sign** is an objective, measurable physical finding regarding an individual's condition. A sign is what the evaluator hears, feels, sees, or smells when assessing the patient. A **symptom** is information provided by the injured individual regarding their perception of the problem. Examples of these subjective feelings include blurred vision, ringing in the ears, fatigue, dizziness, nausea, headache, pain, weakness, and the inability to move a body part. Obtaining information about signs and symptoms can determine if the individual has an **acute injury** resulting from a specific event leading to a sudden onset of symptoms, or a **chronic injury** characterized by a slow, insidious onset of symptoms that culminates in a painful inflammatory condition.

As part of the injury evaluation process, healthcare professionals (e.g., physicians; emergency medical technicians; athletic trainers) use standardized clinical practices to make decisions relative to the nature and severity of an injury or illness. The injury evaluation process typically includes several key components, namely taking a history of the current condition, visually inspecting the area for noticeable abnormalities, physically palpating the region for abnormalities, and completing functional, stress, or special tests.

While the background of the coach does not permit evaluation at the level of care of a healthcare professional, the coach should still be prepared to perform an on-site evaluation of acute injuries sufficient to determine the nature and severity of the condition and, subsequently, the immediate management of the condition. An injury assessment should follow a consistent, sequential order to ensure that as much information as possible is obtained. Such an assessment can be completed by the coach adapting an assessment format known as **HOPS** (i.e., history, observation, palpation, and special testing). The HOPS format uses both subjective information (i.e., history of the injury) and objective information (i.e., observation and inspection, palpation, and special testing) to recognize and identify problems contributing to the condition. This format is easy to use and follows a basic consistent format.

The HOPS Format—An Overview

For reference purposes, a general overview of the HOPS format as a tool for assessing an acute condition will be provided. This will be followed by adapting the format for use by a coach in the on-site evaluation of an acute injury.

History

Identifying the history of the injury can be the most important step in injury assessment. A complete history includes information on the primary complaint; cause or mechanism of injury; characteristics of the symptoms; and related medical history that may have a bearing on the specific condition. This information can provide potential reasons for the symptoms and identify injured structures prior to initiating the physical examination.

Although information provided by the individual is subjective, examiners attempt to gather and record information as quantitatively as possible. This is accomplished by using numbers to establish the intensity of the described symptoms. For example, the individual can rate the severity of pain using a scale from 1 to 10. The patient can also be asked to quantify the length of time the pain lasts. In using such measures, the progress of the injury can be determined. If the individual reports that pain begins immediately after activity and lasts for 3 to 4 hours, a baseline of information has been established. As the individual undergoes treatment for the injury, a comparison with baseline information can determine if the condition is getting better, worse, or remained the same.

Although the intent of taking a history is to narrow the possibilities of conditions causing the injury, the history is to be taken with an open mind. If too few factors are considered, premature conclusions may be reached, resulting in failure to adequately address the nature and severity of injury. It is essential to document in writing the information obtained during the history.

Primary Complaint

The primary complaint focuses on the injured individual's perception of the current injury. As such, the individual is asked questions that permit responses that describe the current nature, location, and onset of the condition. The questions posed are simple and open-ended, such as "what is the problem?" and "what hurts?" While listening to the response to questions, additional information about the condition can be obtained by noting the words and gestures used to describe the condition as they may provide clues to the quality and intensity of the symptoms.

Mechanism of Injury

The mechanism of injury is the physical cause or circumstance under which the injury occurred. For example, a mechanism could be a hit in the head by a thrown ball that results in an acceleration force involving the brain. Another possible mechanism of injury could be tension that results from stress placed on the lateral ankle due to landing on another person's foot while attempting to rebound a basketball shot. An understanding of the mechanism of injury aids in identifying possible injured structures and, subsequently, guides the ongoing assessment and directs the objective component of the evaluation. In the case of an acute injury, questions used to determine the mechanism of injury include "what happened?" "what were you doing?" and "are you able to demonstrate how the injury happened?"

Characteristics of the Symptoms

The primary complaint is explored in detail to discover the evolution of symptoms, including the location, onset, severity, frequency, duration, and limitations caused by the pain or disability. The individual's pain perception can indicate which structures may be injured. There are two categories of pain: somatic and visceral.

Somatic pain arises from the skin, ligaments, muscles, bones, and joints, and is the most common type of pain encountered in musculoskeletal injuries. It is classified into two major types: deep and superficial. Deep somatic pain is described as diffuse or nagging, as if intense pressure is being exerted on the structures, and may be complicated by stabbing pain. Deep somatic pain is longer lasting and usually indicates significant tissue damage to bone, internal joint structures, or muscles. Superficial somatic pain results from injury to the epidermis or dermis, and is usually a sharp, prickly type of pain that tends to be brief.

Visceral pain results from disease or injury to an organ in the thoracic or abdominal cavity, such as compression, tension, or distention of the viscera. Similar to deep somatic pain, it is perceived as deeply located, nagging, and pressing, and it is often accompanied by nausea and vomiting. **Referred pain** is a type of visceral pain that travels along the same nerve pathways as somatic pain. It is perceived by the brain as somatic in origin. In other words, the injury is in one region but the brain considers it in another. For example, referred pain occurs when an individual has a heart attack and feels pain in the chest, left arm, and sometimes the neck.

In the case of an acute injury, questions used to obtain information about pain could include "where is the pain?" "is there one spot in particular that is painful?" "is the pain limited to an area or does it radiate into the extremities?" "how bad is the pain on a scale from 1 to 10?" and "how would you describe the pain (e.g., dull, sharp, aching)?"

If pain is localized, it suggests limited bony or soft tissue structures may be involved. Diffuse pain around the entire joint may indicate inflammation of the joint capsule or injury to several structures. If pain radiates into other areas of the limb or body, it may be traveling up or down the length of a nerve or it could be indicative of an internal injury (e.g., heart attack; ruptured spleen).

In assessing the primary complaint and characteristics of the symptoms of an acute injury, it is also important to determine if the individual experienced other unusual sensations at the time of injury. Responses to the questions "did you hear anything?" and "did you feel anything?" can provide valuable input regarding the type of injury and the structures involved. For example, the unusual sound of hearing a "pop" is characteristic of a rupture to a ligament or tendon, while report of a snapping or cracking sound may suggest a fracture. An unusual feeling can be presented in various ways. For example, having sustained a tear to the anterior cruciate ligament, an individual may report a feeling of the knee giving way or following a rupture of the Achilles tendon, an individual may report a feeling of being shot or kicked in the lower leg.

Related Medical History

In many scenarios involving acute conditions, obtaining information regarding other problems or conditions that may affect the current condition is also advantageous. For example, awareness of a previous history of exercise-induced bronchospasm (EIB) or determining no previous history of EIB may offer insight into the individual's response to the condition and, ultimately, influence the ongoing assessment and immediate management. While knowledge of a history of ankle sprains may not change the continued assessment of the injury or its immediate management, it may offer explanation relative to the individual's ability to provide efficient and insightful responses to questions.

Observation

Observation and inspection begins the objective evaluation in an injury assessment. It is initiated the moment the injured person is seen and continues throughout the assessment. The initial observation focuses on the individual's state of consciousness and body language, which may indicate pain, disability, fracture, dislocation, or other conditions. Valuable information is also obtained by noting the individual's general posture, willingness and ability to move, ease in motion, and general overall attitude.

In acute injury, the localized injury site is inspected for any deformity, swelling, or discoloration (e.g., redness, pallor, bruising, or ecchymosis). More detailed observation as deemed appropriate given to the potential injury includes a visual analysis of symmetry, general motor function, posture, and gait to ascertain information that could aid in identifying the structures involved and the seriousness of the condition. The injured area should be compared to the opposite side if possible. A bilateral comparison helps to establish normal conditions for the individual.

Palpation

Palpation involves the healthcare provider physically touching and feeling the body of the injured individual. Palpation begins with gentle, circular pressure followed by gradual, deeper pressure. It is initiated on structures away from the injury site and progresses toward the injured area. Palpating the most painful area avoids any carryover of pain into noninjured areas.

Palpation of anatomical structures can detect eight physical findings, namely temperature, swelling, point tenderness, crepitus, deformity, muscle spasm, cutaneous sensation, and pulse. Each of these findings provides information that helps to determine the nature and severity of the injury. For example, skin temperature can be noted when the fingers first touch the skin. Increased temperature at the injury site could indicate inflammation or infection, whereas decreased temperature could indicate a reduction in circulation. In a similar manner, feeling an area with the fingers can determine the presence of localized or diffuse swelling as well as general or precise point tenderness. Localized swelling and precise point tenderness could be indicative of a fracture.

Testing

Once fractures and/or dislocations have been ruled out, soft tissue structures, such as muscles, ligaments, the joint capsules, and bursae, are assessed using a variety of tests. Testing includes functional tests (i.e., active, passive, and resisted range of motion), stress tests, special tests, neurologic testing, and sport or activity-specific functional testing.

Functional Tests

Functional tests identify the patient's ability to move a body part through the range of motion (ROM) actively, passively, and against resistance. Active range of motion (AROM) is joint motion performed voluntarily by the individual through muscular contraction. Unless contraindicated, AROM is performed before passive range of motion (PROM). AROM indicates the individual's willingness and ability to move the injured body part. Active movement determines possible damage to contractile tissue (i.e., muscle, muscle-tendon junction, tendon, and tendon-periosteal union), and measures muscle strength and movement coordination. The individual's willingness to perform a movement, the fluidity of movement, and extent of movement (joint ROM) is assessed. Limitation in motion may result from pain, swelling, muscle spasm, muscle tightness, joint contractures, nerve damage, or mechanical blocks, such as a loose body. If the individual has pain or other symptoms with movement, it can be difficult to determine if the joint, muscle, or both are injured.

If the individual is unable to perform active movements at the injured joint due to pain or spasm, passive movement can be performed. In passive movement, the injured limb or body part is moved through the ROM with no assistance from the injured individual. PROM distinguishes injury to contractile tissues from noncontractile or inert tissues (i.e., bone, ligament, bursae, joint capsule, fascia, dura mater, and nerve roots). If no pain is present during passive motion but is present during active motion, injury to contractile tissue is involved. If noncontractile tissue is injured, passive movement is painful and limitation of movement may be present.

Resisted manual muscle testing can assess muscle strength and detect injury to the nervous system. Resistance testing is performed by applying an overload pressure in a stationary or static position, sometimes referred to as a break test, or throughout the full ROM. Muscle weakness and pain indicates a muscular strain. Muscle weakness in the absence of pain may indicate nerve damage.

Stress Tests

Each body segment has a series of tests to assess joint function and integrity of joint structures, primarily noncontractile tissues (e.g., ligaments, intra-articular structures, and joint capsule). Stress tests occur in a single plane and are graded according to severity. Specifically, sprains of ligamentous tissue are generally rated on a three-degree scale after a specific stress is applied to a ligament to test its laxity. Laxity describes the amount of "give" within a joint's supportive tissue. Instability is a joint's inability to function under the stresses encountered during functional activities.

Special Tests

Special tests have been developed for specific body parts or areas as a means for detecting injury or related pathology. In general, special tests occur across planes and are not graded. For example, Speed's test is used as a technique for assessing pathology related to bicipital tendonitis; Thompson's test is used to assess potential rupture of the Achilles tendon.

Neurologic Testing

A segmental nerve is the portion of a nerve that originates in the spinal cord and is referred to as a nerve root. Most nerve roots share two components: (1) a somatic portion, which innervates a series of skeletal muscles and provides sensory input from the skin, fascia, muscles, and joints; and (2) a visceral component, which is part of the autonomic nervous system. The autonomic system supplies the blood vessels, dura mater, periosteum, ligaments, and intervertebral discs, among many other structures.

The motor component of a segmental nerve is tested using a myotome, a group of muscles primarily innervated by a single nerve root. The sensory component is tested using a dermatome, an area of skin supplied by a single nerve root. An injury to a segmental nerve root often affects more than one peripheral nerve and does not demonstrate the same motor loss or sensory deficit as an injury to a single peripheral nerve. Dermatomes, myotomes, and reflexes are used to assess the integrity of the central nervous system (CNS). Peripheral nerves are assessed using manual muscle testing and noting cutaneous sensory changes in peripheral nerve patterns.

Neurologic testing is only necessary in orthopedic injuries when an individual complains of numbness, tingling, or a burning sensation, or suffers from unexplained muscular weakness.

Activity-Specific Functional Testing

Before permitting an individual to return to sport and physical activity after an injury, the individual's condition must be fully evaluated so risk of reinjury is minimal. Activity-specific tests involve the performance of active movements typical of the movements executed by the individual during sport or activity participation. These movements should assess strength, agility, flexibility, joint stability, endurance, coordination, balance, and activity-specific skill performance. For example, in a lower leg injury, testing should begin by assessing walking, jogging, and then running forward and backward. If these skills are performed pain-free and without a limp, the individual might then be asked to run in a figure eight or zigzag pattern. Each test must be performed pain-free and without a limp.

Injury Assessment and the Coach

The coach should be prepared to assess a range of acute conditions as the first respondent. It is not within the duty of care of a coach to assess and manage post-acute, chronic, or stress-related injuries. Rather, it is the responsibility of the coach to refer those injuries to healthcare professionals.

While the medical background of a coach limits their ability to accurately and definitively assess a condition, adapting the HOPS method provides a means by which the coach can follow an established step-by-step plan of action. By following a deliberate and planned approach to assessment, the coach is more likely to be more effective and efficient. Lack of organization can readily transfer to confusion and loss of valuable time.

When faced with assessing an on-site injury, the coach must remain calm at all times. It is also important that the injured individual remains calm. The individual is less likely to remain calm and cooperative, if the coach is panicked and disorganized.

Primary Survey

Assessment of acute on-site injuries, regardless of their perceived severity, should always include a primary survey. The purpose of the primary survey is to identify and initiate management of any life-threatening conditions. The **primary survey** determines the level of responsiveness and assesses airway, breathing, and circulation (ABCs). The primary survey begins as the coach approaches the individual by observing their body language (e.g., movement; absence of movement) and observing any talking (e.g., absence of any talking or sounds; screams or statements attributed to pain). Level of responsiveness is sometimes referred to as the "shake and shout" action. If the individual is not responsive when the coach arrives, the coach should try to arouse the individual by gently shaking or pinching (without moving the head or neck) and by shouting (APPLICATION STRATEGY 7.1). The arousal actions

APPLICATION STRATEGY 7.1

Assessment of an Unconscious Individual

If the individual appears to be unconscious:

- Do not move the individual if there is any possibility of a spinal injury!
- Call their name loudly and gently touch the arm.
- If this does not elicit a response, pinch the soft tissue in the armpit and note any withdrawal from the painful stimuli.
- If there is no response, immediately initiate the primary survey.
- If the individual is not breathing and there is no pulse, activate the emergency plan, including summoning of emergency medical services (EMS), and initiate cardiopulmonary resuscitation (CPR).
- If the individual is breathing and has a pulse, activate the emergency plan, including summoning of EMS and monitoring the condition of the individual through continued assessment of their vital signs.

BOX 7.1	"Red Flags" Indicating a Serious Emergency Where Activation of Emergency Medical Plan Should Be Initiated

- Airway obstruction
- Respiratory failure
- Severe shock
- Severe chest or abdominal pains
- Excessive bleeding

- Suspected spinal injury
- Head injury with loss of consciousness
- Severe heat illness
- Fractures involving several ribs, the femur, or pelvis

---

will determine whether the person is alert, restless, lethargic, or nonresponsive. Assessment of the ABCs involves

- A—Airway: The first step in the process is to assess and ensure an open airway. The assessment involves listening for any abnormal sounds or noises as well the total absence of any sounds (i.e., complete silence). Maintaining an open airway is typically accomplished by placing the individual's head in a position of hyperextension by tilting the head and lifting the chin. This technique should only be performed if a neck injury has been ruled out. If a neck injury is suspected, a modified jaw thrust can be used to establish an open airway.
- B—Breathing: Breathing is assessed by using the "look, listen, and feel" technique. The examiner looks at the chest to determine any movement, while listening for any sounds and feeling for any air coming from the nose/and or mouth.
- C—Circulation: Assessment of circulation involves determining the presence of a pulse. The carotid and radial pulses are typically used.

If at any time during the assessment, conditions exist that are an immediate threat to life or "red flags" are noted (Box 7.1), the assessment process should be terminated and the emergency medical plan activated. If more than one individual is injured, triage must be performed. **Triage is the rapid assessment of all injured individuals followed by return to the most seriously injured.**

It is not within the scope of this textbook to address cardiopulmonary resuscitation (CPR) or advanced first aid. Rather, the coach should enroll in an appropriate class sponsored by the American Red Cross, National Safety Council, or American Heart Association to receive CPR and advanced first aid training.

Secondary Survey

Once it has been determined that a life-threatening condition does not exist, a secondary survey is performed to identify the type and extent of any injury, and the immediate **disposition** of the condition (APPLICATION STRATEGIES 7.2 and 7.3). Decisions must be made regarding the on-site management of the injury (e.g., controlling bleeding or immobilizing a possible fracture or dislocation), the safest transportation from the field (e.g., manual conveyance, stretcher, or spine board), and the need for rapid referral of the individual for further medical care.

Vital Signs

When warranted, the vital signs should be assessed to establish a baseline of information. Vital signs indicate the status of the cardiovascular and CNS. These signs include the pulse, respiratory rate and quality, temperature, and blood pressure. Although not specifically cited as vital signs, assessment of skin color, pupillary response to light, and eye movement can also provide valuable information regarding the status. Abnormal vital signs can indicate a serious injury or illness (BOX 7.2). As such, the coach should be familiar with the normal parameters for vital signs in order to recognize any abnormalities.

Pulse. Normal adult resting pulse rates range from 60 to 100 beats a minute; children from 120 to 140 beats per minute. Aerobically conditioned individuals may have a pulse rate as low as 40 beats per minute. Factors such as age, aerobic physical condition, degree of physical

APPLICATION STRATEGY 7.2

On-Site Assessment of a Potential Nonorthopedic Condition—Conscious Individual

HISTORY
- Chief complaint
  - What's wrong?
  - What happened?
  - What were you doing?
- Pain
  - Are you experiencing any pain? If so, where? (Consider potential referred pain.)
  - Do you have a headache?
- Sounds/feelings
  - Did you hear anything?
  - Did you feel any unusual sensations (e.g., tearing, tingling, numbing, cracking)?
  - Are you nauseous?
  - Are you dizzy?
- Previous history
  - Has this ever happened to you before? If so, what happened? Were you treated for it?

ASSESS VITAL SIGNS
- Pulse
  - Site: carotid artery
  - Rate: 30 seconds × 2
  - Volume (e.g. weak; strong/bounding)
  - Capillary refill test

- Respiration
  - Look for the rise and fall of the chest Listen for the sounds of breathing Feel for air from exhalation on your facial cheek
  - Rate: 30 seconds × 2
  - Character (e.g., rapid; shallow; deep; gasping; labored)
- Skin temperature
  - Site: forehead; appendages
  - Character (e.g., dry; moist; clammy; hot; cool)
- Skin color
  - Site: face; mucous membranes (mouth, tongue, and inner eyelids), lips, and nail beds.
  - Character (e.g., red; white/pale/ashen; blue/cyanotic)
- Pupils
  - Appearance: constricted/dilated; equal in size
  - Response to light
  - Ability to focus (i.e., no double vision)

OBSERVATION
- General presentation (e.g., body language, willingness and ability to move)

exertion, medications or chemical substances being taken, blood loss, and stress can influence the pulse rate and volume.

Pulse is usually taken at the carotid artery because a pulse at that site is not normally obstructed by clothing or equipment. Pulse rate is assessed by counting the carotid pulse rate for a 30-second period and then doubling it. It is also important to assess the pulse volume, which reflects the sensation of the contraction (e.g., strong/weak).

If difficulty is encountered in taking the pulse, capillary refill can be assessed as a means for measuring the effective functioning of the vascular system in the extremities. The capillary refill test is performed by applying pressure to the nail beds of the fingers or toes until it turns white (this action should only take a couple of seconds). The pressure is then removed. If the blood flow to the area is good, the normal pink color of the nail bed should return within 2 seconds of removing the pressure.

Respiration. Respiration rate refers to the number of breaths a person takes per minute. Normal respiration is 10 to 25 breaths per minute in an adult and from 20 to 25 breaths per minute in a child. Breathing rate is assessed by counting the number of respirations in 30 seconds and then doubling it. The character of the respiration (e.g., rapid; shallow; deep; gasping; labored) should also be noted.

Temperature. Normal body temperature is 98.6°F(37°C), but it can fluctuate considerably. In the early morning hours, it may fall to as low as 96.4°F (35.8°C); in the late afternoon or evening, it may rise to as high as 99.1°F (37.3°C).

APPLICATION STRATEGY 7.3

On-Site Assessment of a Potential Musculoskeletal Injury

HISTORY
- Chief complaint
  - What's wrong?
- Mechanism of injury
  - What happened?
  - What were you doing?
  - Are you able to demonstrate how it happened?
- Pain
  - Location
    - Where is the pain?
    - Can you point with one finger to indicate where it hurts the most?
    - Do you have pain anywhere else in your body?
  - Type
    - Can you describe the pain (i.e., sharp, shooting, dull, achy, diffuse)?
  - Intensity
    - What is the level of pain on a scale from 1 to 10?
- Sounds
  - Did you hear anything?
- Feelings
  - Did you feel any unusual sensations (e.g., tearing, tingling, numbing, cracking)?

- Previous history
  - Have you ever injured this body part?
  - If so, what happened? What was the injury? Were you treated for it?
- Is there anything else you would like to tell me about your condition?

OBSERVATION
- General presentation (e.g., guarding; moving easily; posture)
- Injury site appearance—deformity, swelling, discoloration, scars, and general skin condition

PALPATION
(Only palpate as a way to confirm a potential sign noted during inspection AND only if you are familiar with the anatomy such that the palpation would provide useful information.)

TESTING
- Range of Motion
  - Active
  - Resisted (manual muscle testing)
- Activity/sport-specific functional testing

The body temperature is typically measured by a thermometer placed under the tongue, in the ear or armpit, or in the case of unconsciousness, the rectum. However, these options are not normally viable as part of an on-site assessment. In fact, as part of an on-site assessment, placing an object in the individual's mouth is contraindicated and, as such, the action should not be performed. Because the skin plays a key role in regulating the body temperature, it can be used to aid in assessing the body temperature. Skin temperature is assessed by placing the back of the hand against the individual's forehead or by palpating appendages bilaterally. While the skin temperature does not provide the precision of a thermometer, it still offers potentially valuable information. For example, the presence of cool, clammy skin is a sign of heat exhaustion, while hot, dry skin is a sign of heat stroke.

Skin Color. Skin color can indicate abnormal blood flow and low blood oxygen concentration in a particular body part or area. Three colors are commonly used to describe light-skinned individuals: red, white or ashen, and blue. The colors and their potential indications can also be seen in Box 7.2. In dark-skinned individuals, skin pigments mask cyanosis. However, a bluish cast can be seen in mucous membranes (e.g., mouth; tongue; and inner eyelids), the lips, and nail beds. Fever in these individuals can be seen by a red flush at the tips of the ears.

Pupils. The pupils are extremely responsive to situations affecting the CNS. Rapid constriction of pupils when the eyes are exposed to intense light is called the pupillary light reflex. The pupillary response to light can be assessed by holding a hand over one eye and then moving the hand away quickly, or shining the light from a penlight into one eye and observing the pupil's reaction. A normal response would be constriction with the light shining in the eye, and dilation

BOX 7.2	**Abnormal Vital Signs and Possible Causes**

PULSE

Rapid: Weak shock, internal hemorrhage, hypoglycemia, heat exhaustion, or hyperventilation

Rapid: Bounding heat stroke, fright, fever, hypertension, apprehension, hyperglycemia, or normal exertion

Slow: bounding skull fracture, stroke, drug use (barbiturates and narcotics), certain cardiac problems or some poisons

No pulse: Blocked artery, low blood pressure, or cardiac arrest

RESPIRATION

Shallow: Shock, heat exhaustion, insulin shock, chest injury, or cardiac problems

Irregular: Airway obstruction, chest injury, diabetic coma, asthma, or cardiac problems

Rapid, deep: Diabetic coma, hyperventilation, some lung diseases

Slowed: Stroke, head injury, chest injury, or use of certain drugs

Wheezing: Asthma, EIB

Apnea: Hypoxia (lack of oxygen), congestive heart failure, head injuries

No breathing: Cardiac arrest, poisoning, drug abuse, drowning, head injury, or intrathoracic injuries with death imminent, if action is not taken to correct conditions

SKIN TEMPERATURE

Dry, cool: Exposure to cold or cervical, thoracic, or lumbar spine injuries

Cool, clammy: Shock, internal hemorrhage, trauma, anxiety, or heat exhaustion

Hot, dry: Disease, infection, high fever, heat stroke, or overexposure to environmental heat

Hot, moist: High fever

Isolated hot spot: Localized infection

Cold appendage: Circulatory problem

Goose pimples: Chills, communicable diseases, exposure to cold, pain, or fear

SKIN COLOR

Red: Embarrassment, fever, hypertension, heat stroke, carbon monoxide poisoning, diabetic coma, alcohol abuse, infectious disease, inflammation, or allergy

White or ashen: Emotional stress (fright, anger, etc.), anemia, shock, heart attack, hypotension, heat exhaustion, insulin shock, or insufficient circulation

Blue or cyanotic: Heart failure, some severe respiratory disorders, and some poisoning. In darkskinned individuals, a bluish cast can be seen in the mucous membranes (mouth, tongue, and inner eyelids), lips, and nail beds.

PUPILS

Constricted: Use of opiate-based drug or ingestion of poison

Dilated: Shock, hemorrhage, heat stroke, use of a stimulant drug, coma, cardiac arrest, or death

Unequal: Head injury or stroke

BLOOD PRESSURE

Systolic < 100 mm Hg: Hypotension caused by shock, hemorrhage, heart attack, internal injury, or poor nutrition

Systolic > 140 mm Hg: Hypertension caused by certain medications, oral contraceptives, anabolic steroids, amphetamines, chronic alcohol use, and obesity

as the light is removed. The pupillary reaction is classified as brisk (normal), sluggish, nonreactive, or fixed. The eyes may appear normal, constricted, unequal, or dilated.

Eye movement is tested by asking the individual to focus on a single object. An individual experiencing **diplopia** sees two images instead of one. This condition is attributed to failure of the external eye muscles to work in a coordinated manner. The tracking ability of the eyes can be assessed by asking the individual to follow the examiner's fingers as they are moved through the six cardinal fields of vision. The individual's depth perception can be assessed by placing a finger several inches in front of the individual and asking the person to reach out and touch the finger. The examiner should move the finger to several different locations.

Blood Pressure. Blood pressure is the pressure or tension of the blood within the systemic arteries, generally considered to be the aorta. Measurements of blood pressure include both a systolic and diastolic reading. The systolic pressure is the pressure in the arteries when the heart is beating. It is approximately 120 mm Hg for a healthy adult and 125 to 140 for healthy children aged 10 to 18. Diastolic blood pressure is the residual pressure present in the aorta between heart beats and averages 70 to 80 mm Hg in healthy adults and 80 to 90 in healthy children aged 10 to 18.

Blood pressure reflects the effectiveness of the circulatory system. Changes in blood pressure are very significant. High blood pressure, or hypertension, is a systolic pressure of 140 mm Hg or higher or a diastolic pressure of 90 mm Hg or higher. High blood pressure or low blood pressure that presents suddenly can be indicative of a serious underlying condition.

While assessment of blood pressure can provide valuable information, it is the one sign that the coach is not likely to be able to obtain. Measurement of blood pressure as part of an on-site assessment should only be performed by a qualified healthcare practitioner.

On-Site History

During the history component of the assessment, the coach should be positioned close to the individual. Before asking any questions, the coach should make sure the individual is attentive (i.e., calm; focused). During the history, the coach should listen and observe for any clues that may indicate the nature and severity of the injury.

On-site history is not as detailed as the history in a comprehensive evaluation. As such, there will not be as many questions. The questions should be open-ended to allow the individual to provide as much clues as possible. Questions that should be asked include:

- What is wrong? What hurts? (establish the primary complaint)
- How did it happen? What were you doing (identify mechanism of injury—establish the position of the injured body part at the point of impact and the direction of force)
- Where is your pain? Is there one spot where it hurts the most? Can you describe the pain? Can you rate the pain on a scale of 1 to 10?
- Do you have pain in any other areas? (identifying potential for more than one injury and/or referred pain)
- Do you hear anything at the time of the injury?
- Did you feel anything? (e.g., tearing sensation; snapping sensation; unusual movement of a joint)
- Are you experiencing any unusual sensations in your arms or legs?
- Has this ever happened to you before? (identify any pre-existing conditions that may have exacerbated the current injury or complicate the injury assessment)

On-Site Observation

As previously stated, the coach should begin the observation component while en route to the injured individual. Initially, the focus should be on observing the individual's state of consciousness, body language, willingness and ability to move, general body posture, and overall attitude. In doing so, signs indicating pain and disability could become evident and aid in directing the ongoing assessment. For example, an individual holding an injured body part and expressing pain indicates consciousness as well as an intact CNS and cardiovascular system. In comparison, if an individual is not moving or is having a seizure, possible systemic, psychological, or neurologic dysfunction should be suspected.

Once the coach reaches the individual, the next step is to inspect the site of the actual injury for any deformity, swelling, or discoloration (e.g., redness, pallor, or ecchymosis). The injured area should be compared to the opposite side if possible. A bilateral comparison helps to establish normal conditions for the individual. If the history and initial observation suggest that it is safe for the individual to move the injured area, observation of motor function is appropriate.

On-Site Palpation

The palpation component of the assessment will be limited, in part, by the coach's background in anatomy and their ability to identify anatomical structures. In addition, palpation is a skill that becomes more effective with experience.

In the absence of understanding or being knowledgeable about the structures being palpated, the value of a coach performing palpation is questionable. The coach should consider the potential physical findings that can be detected with palpation (i.e., temperature, swelling, point tenderness, crepitus, deformity, muscle spasm, cutaneous sensation, and pulse) and determine if palpation is appropriate or necessary. For example, in assessing a potential lateral sprain of the ankle, unless the coach is familiar with the key anatomical structures of the ankle, there is arguably no need to palpate the region. In fact, it could be argued that improper palpation might unnecessarily increase the pain. In that same scenario, if an observation suggests swelling, there is not necessarily a need for the coach to confirm the swelling through palpation. In a similar manner, determining the presence of precise point tenderness is of minimal value, if the coach cannot identify the structure (e.g., soft tissue; bone) being palpated. In comparison, if a coach suspects that an individual is experiencing some form of heat illness, palpation to determine skin temperature provides extremely important information. Ultimately, the coach needs to decide whether or not any palpation performed can contribute to determining the nature and severity of the injury. Palpation in the absence of understanding and using the findings as part of an assessment is not necessarily advantageous.

Finally, it is important to understand that informed consent must be granted prior to making physical contact with the injured individual. If the patient is under 18 years of age, permission must be granted by the parent or guardian. In some cultures and religions, the act of physically touching an exposed body part may present certain moral and ethical issues. Likewise, some individuals may feel uncomfortable being touched by a coach of the opposite gender. If a same-gender coach is not available, the evaluation should be observed by a third party (e.g., another coach, parent, or guardian).

On-Site Physical Examination Tests

When not contraindicated, the coach should identify the individual's willingness to move the injured body part. Movement is contraindicated in the presence of a possible head or spinal injury, fracture, dislocation, or muscle/tendon rupture.

If the findings from the history, observation, and palpation components of the assessment suggest that there is no harm associated with movement, the coach should initiate the testing component with ROM testing.

- **Active range of motion:** As previously noted, AROM is performed voluntarily by the individual. As such, the coach is not providing any assistance in the effort to move an injured body part. Rather, the individual is asked to move the injured body part through the available ROM. The coach should note the quantity and quality of movement in the absence of pain.

- **Passive range of motion:** The value of the coach performing PROM is questionable. While a trained clinician can obtain valuable information in performing PROM, a lack of understanding of the proper technique for completing the movement could result in additional harm. As such, if an injured individual is unable to perform full and pain-free AROM, the coach should consider the examination complete.

- **Resisted range of motion:** In comparison, if the individual is able to perform full and pain-free AROM, the coach may want to consider assessment of resisted range of motion as a means for detecting muscle strength. In performing a break test, the individual is instructed to contract the involved muscle(s), while the coach applies gentle, but firm resistance to the movement. In doing so, the coach should place one hand just proximal to the involved joint to stabilize the area and the hand providing resistance should be placed distally on the bone comprising the joint. The pressure should be held for at least 5 seconds and repeated at least three times to determine any weakness or pain. The decision to perform resisted range of motion should be carefully considered. It may be more appropriate to perform resisted range of motion only when all other findings suggest the absence of any serious injury.

- **Weight bearing:** If the individual successfully completes active and resisted motion, walking may be permitted. However, if the individual is unable to perform these tests, or if signs and symptoms of moderate to severe injury are apparent, the individual should not be permitted to bear weight.

BOX 7.3	Reasons for Avoiding The Removal of a Helmet

- **Removal of the face mask allows full airway access. The face mask should be removed immediately when the decision is made to transport, regardless of the current respiratory status.**
- **Most injuries can be visualized with the helmet in place.**
- **Neurologic tests can be performed with the helmet in place. The eyes may be examined, the nose and ears checked for fluid or blood, and the level of consciousness determined.**
- **The individual can be immobilized on a spine board with the helmet in place.**
- **When both a helmet and shoulder pads are worn, removing the helmet without removing the shoulder pads results in cervical hyperextension.**
- **Many helmets are radiographic translucent. Therefore, a definitive diagnosis can be made prior to removal.**

The continued physical examination testing component of the assessment will be significantly different for the coach in comparison to a qualified healthcare practitioner. Simply stated, the coach should not attempt to perform any stress or special tests. The only additional testing that a coach should consider is activity-specific functional testing. If the findings from the assessment to this point suggest the absence of injury, activity-specific functional testing can be used to confirm or refute those findings. In doing so, the coach is better situated to make a decision concerning immediate management, including whether or not return to activity should be permitted.

Equipment Considerations

A potential concern during an on-site assessment of an injured individual is that of equipments. In some cases, the equipment being worn by the individual could interfere with some aspects of the assessment. However, the solution is not the automatic removal of the equipment. For example, if there is a potential cervical spine injury, removal of a helmet may worsen the condition or lead to additional injury. Therefore, removal of any helmet should be avoided, unless individual circumstances dictate otherwise (see Box 7.3).[1] Policies and procedures for determining the conditions under which equipments should be removed and guidelines for any such removal should be defined within the emergency medical plan. It is important to recognize that policies and procedures can vary based on the qualifications of the individual performing the assessment. As such, there can be scenarios in which qualified healthcare professionals may opt to remove equipments, but a coach would be ill-advised to do the same.

DISPOSITION

Information gathered during the assessment must be analyzed and decisions made based on the best interests of the injured individual. It is especially important to determine whether the situation can be handled on-site or referral to a physician is warranted. As a general rule, the individual should always be referred to the nearest trauma center or emergency clinic if any life-threatening situation is present, if the injury results in loss of normal function, or if no improvement is seen in injury status after a reasonable amount of time. Examples of these injuries are provided in Box 7.1. Other conditions that are not necessarily life-threatening, but serious enough to warrant referral to a physician for immediate care, include

- Eye injuries
- Dental injuries in which a tooth has been knocked loose or knocked out
- Minor or simple fractures

- Lacerations that might require suturing
- Injuries in which a functional deficit is noticeable
- Loss of normal sensation
- Noticeable muscular weakness in the extremities
- Any injury if you are uncertain about its severity or nature

The immediate management of specific injuries and conditions is provided in the chapters that address the various areas of the body.

SUMMARY

1. In an injury assessment, signs and symptoms are obtained and interpreted to determine the extent and type of injury.

2. The HOPS format includes history, observation and inspection, palpation, and special tests.

3. The information gathered during the history taking should include the primary complaint, mechanism of injury, characteristics of the symptoms, and related medical history.

4. The observation component should include assessment of the general presentation of the individual (e.g., body language; willingness and ability to move; overall attitude) and the localized injury site for abnormalities.

5. The palpation of anatomical structures can detect eight physical findings, namely temperature, swelling, point tenderness, crepitus, deformity, muscle spasm, cutaneous sensation, and pulse.

6. Testing includes functional tests (i.e., active, passive, and resisted range of motion), stress tests, special tests, neurologic testing, and sport or activity-specific functional testing.

7. The coach should only complete components of an assessment that are within their standard of care. As such, in using the HOPS format, it must be appropriately adapted.

8. The coach should be prepared to assess acute conditions. The coach should not engage in the assessment of post-acute, chronic, or stress-related injuries. In those scenarios, the coach should refer the individual to a healthcare professional.

9. In an emergency injury assessment, the presence of a head or spinal cord injury should be assumed. As such, the individual should not be moved.

10. Assessment of all injuries, no matter how minor, should include a primary injury assessment to determine level of responsiveness and assess the ABCs. A secondary assessment determines the presence of moderate to severe injuries.

11. As a general rule, an individual should always be referred to the nearest trauma center or emergency clinic if any life-threatening situation is present or if the injury results in loss of normal functioning.

APPLICATION QUESTIONS

For each of the following questions, the coach, physical educator, or fitness specialist is the individual responsible for assessing and managing the situation. No healthcare professionals (e.g., athletic trainer; emergency medical technician) are available on-site to assist with the assessment.

1. During practice, a high school soccer player collapses on the field. When the coach reaches the individual, the player appears to be unconscious. How should the coach proceed? If the individual remains unconscious, how should the coach manage the condition?

2. During a physical education class, a fifth-grade student falls, landing on an outstretched arm. As the teacher approaches the student, he observes her to be visibly upset and holding her forearm in a guarded manner. When the teacher reaches the student, he observes an obvious deformity in the forearm. What questions should be asked by the instructor as part of the history component of the assessment? Following the history and observation components of the assessment, the signs and symptoms strongly suggest a forearm fracture. Should the instructor perform the palpation and testing components of the assessment? Why or why not?

3. Following 20 minutes of running on a treadmill, a 35-year-old female informs one of the fitness specialists on staff that she is experiencing discomfort in the lower leg. The fitness specialist initiates the history component of an assessment. During the history, the female reveals that the pain began about 2 weeks earlier. How should the fitness specialist proceed? Why?

4. During a physical education class, two third-grade students on scooter boards accidently collide. Both students appear to be injured. How should the teacher proceed?

5. During a practice, a 12 year old on a recreational basketball team falls after rebounding the ball. Initially, she reports mild pain to the lateral aspect of her ankle. Following the completion of the history and observation components of the exam, the participant appears to be fine. She is not experiencing any pain or any other abnormalities. How should the coach proceed in completing the testing component of the assessment?

REFERENCE

1. Klossner D (ed.) NCAA Sports Medicine Handbook: 2009–10. Indianapolis: National Collegiate Athletic Association, 2009.

CHAPTER

8

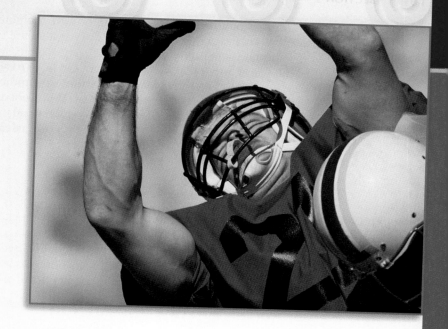

EMERGENCY CONDITIONS

KEY TERMS

anaphylaxis

angina

arrhythmia

atherosclerosis

cyanosis

hypertrophic cardiomyopathy

myocardial infarction

syncope

LEARNING OUTCOMES

1. Differentiate between a partial and total airway obstruction. Describe the management for each condition.

2. Describe the situations that can lead to sudden death from cardiac arrest. Identify the signs and symptoms of heart attack or cardiac arrest. Describe the management for suspected cardiac condition.

3. Identify the actions of the coach in the assessment and management of an unconscious individual.

4. Describe shock, including its signs and symptoms. Explain the management of shock.

5. Describe anaphylaxis, including its signs and symptoms. Explain the management of anaphylaxis.

6. Explain the effects of hemorrhage. Describe the management for external and internal hemorrhage.

Injuries or conditions that impair, or have the potential to impair, vital functions of the central nervous system and cardiorespiratory system are considered emergency conditions. Many serious injuries are clearly evident and recognizable, such as lack of breathing or absence of a pulse. However, other serious injuries may not be as easy to determine.

This chapter provides information on conditions that may pose a threat to the life of an athlete or physically active individual. While not a comprehensive list of emergency conditions, the conditions presented are more common and, as such, a coach should be familiar with each of them. Information pertaining to the onsite assessment of emergency conditions is provided in Chapter 7.

OBSTRUCTED AIRWAY

The airway can become partially or totally blocked by a solid foreign object (e.g., mouthguard, bridgework, chewing gum, chaw of tobacco, or mud), fluids (e.g., blood clots from head injuries or vomitus), swelling in the throat caused by allergic reactions, or, more commonly, the back of the tongue (e.g., due to unconsciousness). An obstructed airway prevents adequate oxygen from being exchanged in the lungs and can lead to **cyanosis** and death.

Partial Airway Obstruction

When a person has a partial airway obstruction, there is still some air exchange in the lungs.

Signs and Symptoms

The individual is able to cough. The individual typically grasps the throat in the universal distress signal for choking.

Management

If the individual is able to cough forcefully, there should be no action taken by the coach other than to encourage the individual to continue coughing in an attempt to dislodge the obstruction. An ineffective cough or a high-pitched noise during breathing indicates poor air exchange and should be treated as a total airway obstruction.

Total Airway Obstruction

In a total airway obstruction, no air is passing through the vocal cords.

Signs and Symptoms

The individual is unable to speak, breathe, or cough. In a conscious person, the universal distress signal is usually apparent.

Management

The Heimlich maneuver is used to dislodge the foreign object so breathing may resume. However, if the individual becomes unconscious, the coach must react quickly to clear the airway and stimulate the breathing process. The emergency plan should be activated, including summoning of emergency medical services (EMS). While waiting for EMS to arrive, the coach should continue to perform rescue breathing and if breathing begins again, then monitor the individual's airway, breathing, and circulation.

CARDIOPULMONARY EMERGENCIES

Cardiac arrest can result from strenuous physical activity in a dehydrated state, direct trauma, electrical shock, excessive alcohol or other chemical substance abuse, suffocation, drowning, or heart anomalies. Sudden cardiac death (SCD) has been termed the "silent killer." It is defined as an unexpected death, owing to sudden cardiac arrest within 6 hours of an otherwise normal clinical healthy state.[1]

The prevalence of SCD during physical activity is uncertain. It is estimated that 1 in 180,000 high school–aged athletes experiences sudden death. Males have an estimated death rate five times that of females, with the highest rates seen in basketball and football players.[1] Explanation for the low occurrence in female athletes is inconclusive. However, some researchers postulate that the decreased incidence can be attributed to[2-4]:

- Fewer females participate in sports.
- Fewer females participate in highly intense sports that require full-body protective equipment (e.g., football, ice hockey).
- Gender differences exist regarding cardiac adaptation to training demands.
- Females have smaller hearts.

SCD is often precipitated by physical activity and may be caused by an array of cardiovascular conditions; the most common is **hypertrophic cardiomyopathy** (HCM). The age of the individual appears to dictate the underlying physiologic pathology for the occurrence of SCD. Congenital cardiac abnormalities are responsible for the vast majority of SCDs in individuals younger than 30 years, whereas an atherosclerotic coronary artery disease is the leading cause of SCDs for individuals older than 35 years, accounting for up to 80% of such events.[5] Other reported cardiac-related causes include mitral valve prolapse, myocarditis, acquired valvular heart disease, coronary artery disease, and Marfan syndrome.

HCM, characterized by an abnormal thickening of the left ventricle wall, develops before the age of 20 years and typically goes undetected during routine physical examination. Symptoms of cardiac dysfunction, which do not appear until early adulthood if at all, result in impaired ventricle filling. As a result, periods of **arrhythmia** (irregular heartbeats) or blood flow obstruction can occur that may produce **syncope** (fainting and lightheadedness) during physical exertion.

Atherosclerosis involves an excessive buildup of cholesterol within the coronary arteries, which narrows the diameter of the arteries and impedes blood flow. In turn, the amount of oxygen supplied to the heart is reduced. Because of the diminished oxygen, **angina** or chest pain during physical exertion is a common symptom. If excessive cholesterol buildup blocks a coronary artery, the person is at risk for a **myocardial infarction** (heart attack). If the blockage exists in a major coronary artery, death often occurs.

Signs and Symptoms

The signs and symptoms that indicate a possible heart attack or cardiac arrest can be found in Box 8.1.

Management

The emergency plan should be activated, including summoning of EMS. While waiting for EMS to arrive, the coach should monitor the individual's airway, breathing, and circulation. As necessary, the coach should perform rescue breathing and CPR.

BOX 8.1   Warning Signs for Heart Attack and Cardiac Arrest

- Chest discomfort (e.g., uncomfortable pressure; squeezing; pain)
- Pain originating behind the sternum and radiating into either or both arms (usually the left)
- Pain radiating into the neck, jaw, teeth, or upper back
- Shortness of breath
- Nausea
- Lightheadedness

UNCONSCIOUS INDIVIDUAL

While unconsciousness can be attributed to a variety of causes (e.g., medication overdose; diabetic coma; seizure), head injuries are the leading cause of loss of consciousness in sport activity and are discussed in more detail in Chapter 9. Being fully alert and conscious implies that the individual is aware of the surroundings and can respond to questions.

Signs and Symptoms

Unconsciousness identifies an individual who lacks conscious awareness and is unable to respond to superficial sensory stimuli, such as pinching in the armpit. Coma, the most depressed state of consciousness, occurs when the individual cannot be aroused even by stimuli as powerful as pin pricks.

Management

The coach must proceed on the basis that an unconscious individual has a life-threatening condition that requires an immediate primary survey and, as appropriate, continue with an assessment of vital signs (refer to Chapter 7). This condition requires the activation of the emergency plan, including summoning of EMS. APPLICATION STRATEGY 8.1 provides additional information pertaining to the assessment management of an unconscious individual.

SHOCK

Shock occurs if the heart is unable to exert adequate pressure to circulate enough oxygenated blood to the vital organs. This condition may result from a damaged heart that fails to pump properly, low blood volume from blood loss or dehydration, or dilation of blood vessels that leads to blood pooling in larger vessels away from vital areas. The result is a lack of oxygen and nutrition at the cellular level. The heart pumps faster, but because of reduced volume, the pulse rate is weakened and the blood pressure drops (i.e., hypotension). A rapid, weak pulse is the most prominent sign of

---

APPLICATION STRATEGY 8.1

Assessment and Management of an Unconscious Individual

- Do not move the individual, if there is any possibility of a spinal injury!
- If the individual appears to be unconscious:
  - Call their name loudly and gently touch the arm.
  - If this does not elicit a response, pinch the soft tissue in the armpit and note any withdrawal from the painful stimuli.
  - If there is no response, immediately initiate the primary survey.
  - If the individual is breathing and has a pulse, activate the emergency plan, including summoning of EMS, and monitor the condition of the individual through continued assessment of their vital signs. Regardless of whether the individual is supine (i.e., face up) or prone (i.e. face down), the individual should not be moved.
  - If the individual is not breathing and there is no pulse, activate the emergency plan, including summoning of EMS, and initiate CPR. In this scenario, if the individual is prone, the coach will have to move the individual into a supine position in order to initiate CPR. A logroll technique should be used to move the person into a supine position.
  - If a helmet is worn, it should not be removed until a full assessment is completed to determine the presence or absence of a cervical neck injury. The removal of a helmet without removal of the shoulder pads leads to hyperextension of the cervical spine. If CPR is necessary, the jersey and shoulder pad laces can be cut and spread to access the sternum for hand placement.
- Any necessary life support should be maintained and monitored until emergency personnel arrive.

BOX 8.2   Types and Causes of Shock

- **Hypovolemic**—From excessive blood or fluid loss leading to inadequate circulation and oxygen supply to all body organs. Possible causes include hemorrhage, dehydration, multiple trauma, and severe burns.
- **Respiratory**—From insufficient oxygen in the blood as a result of inadequate breathing. Possible causes are spinal injury to the respiratory nerves, airway obstruction, or chest trauma, such as from a pneumothorax, hemothorax, or punctured lung.
- **Neurogenic**—Occurs when peripheral blood vessels dilate and an insufficient blood volume cannot supply oxygen to the vital organs. This may occur in a spinal or head injury when nerves that control the vascular system are impaired, thereby altering the integrity of blood vessels.
- **Psychogenic**—Refers to a temporary dilation of blood vessels, resulting in the draining of blood from the head with pooling of blood in the abdomen. A common example is an individual fainting from the sight of blood.
- **Cardiogenic**—Occurs when the heart muscle is no longer able to sustain enough pressure to pump blood through the system. Possible causes are injury to the heart or previous heart attack.
- **Metabolic**—Results from a severe loss of body fluids because of an untreated illness that alters the biochemical equilibrium. Possible causes are insulin shock, diabetic coma, vomiting, or diarrhea.
- **Septic**—Derives from severe, usually bacterial, infection whereby toxins attack the walls of small blood vessels, causing them to dilate and, therefore, decreasing blood pressure.
- **Anaphylactic**—Refers to a severe allergic reaction of the body to a foreign protein that is ingested, inhaled, or injected (e.g., foods, drugs, or insect stings).

---

shock. As an individual's condition deteriorates, breathing becomes rapid and shallow, and sweating is profuse. Vital body fluids pass through weakened capillaries, thereby causing further circulatory distress. If not corrected, circulatory collapse can lead to unconsciousness and even death.

Shock is associated with injuries involving severe pain, bleeding, the spinal cord, fractures, or intra-abdominal or intrathoracic regions, but shock also may occur, to some degree, with minor injuries. The severity of shock depends on the age, physical condition, pain tolerance, fatigue, dehydration, presence of any disease, extreme cold or heat exposure, or handling of an injured area. Types of shock include anaphylactic, cardiogenic, hypovolemic, metabolic, neurogenic, respiratory, psychogenic, and septic (BOX 8.2).

Signs and Symptoms

The signs and symptoms of shock can develop over time (BOX 8.3). Initially, the individual may have a feeling of uneasiness or restlessness, increased respirations, and increased weakened

---

BOX 8.3   Signs and Symptoms of Shock

- Restlessness, anxiety, fear, or disorientation
- Cold, clammy, moist skin
- Profuse sweating
- Extreme thirst
- Eyes are dull, sunken, and with the pupils dilated
- Skin that is chalk-like but that later may appear to be cyanotic
- Nausea and/or vomiting
- Shallow, irregular breathing; breathing also may be labored, rapid, or gasping
- Dizziness
- Rapid and weak pulse

APPLICATION STRATEGY 8.2

Management of Shock

- Activate emergency action plan, including summoning EMS. Secure and maintain an open airway. Control any major bleeding. Monitor vital signs.
- Body position
  - If a head or neck injury or a leg fracture is not suspected, elevate the feet and legs 8 to 12 inches.
  - If there are breathing difficulties, the individual might be more comfortable with the head and shoulders raised in a semireclining position.
  - If a head injury is suspected, elevate the head and shoulders to reduce pressure on the brain. The feet also may be slightly elevated.

- In a suspected neck injury, keep the individual lying flat.
- An individual who vomits or is unconscious should be placed on their side to avoid blocking the airway with any fluids. This allows the fluids to drain from the mouth.
- Maintain normal body temperature. This action may require removing any wet clothing, if possible, and covering the individual with a blanket.
- Keep the individual quiet and still. Avoid rough or excessive handling of the individual.
- Do not give the individual anything by mouth.
- Monitor vital signs every 2 to 5 minutes until EMS arrives.

heart rate. The skin turns pale and clammy, which usually is accompanied by profuse sweating. The lips, nail beds, and membranes of the mouth appear to be cyanotic. Thirst, weakness, nausea, and vomiting may then become apparent. During later stages, a rapid, weak pulse and labored, weakened respirations may lead to decreased blood pressure and possible unconsciousness.

Management

The emergency action plan should be activated, including summoning EMS. While waiting for EMS to arrive, the coach should maintain the airway, control any bleeding, and maintain normal body temperature. If a head or neck injury is not suspected, the feet and legs should be elevated 8 to 12 inches. APPLICATION STRATEGY 8.2 summarizes the immediate care of shock.

ANAPHYLAXIS

For most individuals, allergies cause simple rashes, itching, watery eyes, and some short-term discomfort. However, for some individuals, a more powerful reaction to allergens, either eaten or injected, can lead to a life-threatening condition called **anaphylaxis**. Anaphylaxis is a severe allergic reaction that affects the entire body. Commonly known substances that cause anaphylaxis in hypersensitive individuals include

- Medications (e.g., penicillin and related drugs, aspirin, sulfa drugs)
- Food and food additives (e.g., shellfish, nuts, berries, eggs, monosodium glutamate [MSG], nitrates, nitrites)
- Insect stings (e.g., honeybee, yellow jacket, wasp, hornet, fire ant)
- Inhaled substances (e.g., plant pollens, dust, chemical powders)
- Radiographic dyes

The individual may have a history of such reactions, wear a medical identification tag, and have a self-administered epinephrine device (EpiPen®).

BOX 8.4	Signs and Symptoms of Anaphylactic Shock

- Initially, a general feeling of warmth accompanied by intense itching, especially on the soles of the feet and palms of the hands
- Skin reactions (e.g., localized rash or swelling)
- Choking, wheezing, and shortness of breath
- Rapid and weak pulse
- Dizziness, light headedness, or fainting
- Tightness and swelling in the throat and chest
- Blueness around the lips and mouth
- Swelling of the mucous membranes (tongue, mouth, nose), which can lead to respiratory distress and unconsciousness
- Nausea, vomiting, or diarrhea
- Anxiety
- Confusion

Signs and Symptoms

The signs and symptoms can develop within seconds or minutes of exposure to the allergen (Box 8.4). In rare cases, they may be delayed 30 minutes or longer.

Management

Immediate treatment involves activating the emergency plan, including summoning EMS. While waiting for EMS to arrive, the coach should monitor the individual's airway, breathing, and circulation and perform rescue breathing and CPR, as necessary. If the individual has medication, such as a self-administered epinephrine device (EpiPen®), it should be administered immediately.

HEMORRHAGE

Severe hemorrhage causes a decrease in blood volume and blood pressure. In an attempt to compensate for this factor, the heart's pumping action must increase. Because there is less blood in the system, the strength of the pumping action is weakened, resulting in a characteristic rapid, weak pulse.

Signs and Symptoms

Arterial bleeding from an oxygen-rich vessel is characterized by a spurting, bright red color. Major arteries, when completely severed, often constrict and seal themselves for a short period. However, if the artery is only punctured or partially severed, bleeding can be severe. Venous bleeding from an oxygen-depleted vessel is a dark, bluish-red, almost maroon color. The continuous steady loss of blood can be heavy. Most superficial veins collapse if they are cut, but bleeding from deep veins can be as profuse and difficult to control as arterial bleeding. Capillary bleeding is usually very slow and often described as oozing. The blood is red, but has a duller shade than arterial blood. This type of bleeding clots easily.

Management

External bleeding is best controlled with direct pressure and elevation. Using universal safety precautions (refer to Chapter 6), pressure is applied directly over the wound with a sterile gauze pad, compressing the region against the underlying bone. Elevation uses gravity to reduce blood pressure, and in doing so, aids blood clotting. In more severe bleeding, indirect pressure points can also help control hemorrhage, but they should not be used, if a fracture is suspected, because of possible movement of the fractured bone ends.

Internal bleeding can result from blunt trauma or certain fractures (such as those of the pelvis, rib, or skull). Because internal hemorrhage is not visible, it can be overlooked, which can lead to shock. The history of injury (i.e., a fall, a deceleration injury, or severe blunt trauma), coupled with signs and symptoms of shock (Box 8.3), can be indicative of internal bleeding. The emergency plan should be activated, including either immediate referral to a physician or emergent care facility or summoning of EMS.

SUMMARY

1. In assessing an airway obstruction, it is important to differentiate between a partial and a total obstruction. If the individual is able to cough (partial obstruction), the coach should encourage coughing. If the individual is unable to speak or cough, it should be treated as a total obstruction. The coach must act to clear the airway and activate EMS.

2. Cardiac anomalies are the most direct cause of sudden death in athletes. Hypertrophic cardiomyopathy is the most common cause of death in athletes younger than 30 years. In athletes older than 30 years, an atherosclerotic coronary artery disease is the more likely cause of sudden death.

3. Unconsciousness can be due to various reasons. In assessing and managing an unconscious individual, the coach must proceed on the basis that the individual has a life-threatening condition. This condition requires summoning of EMS.

4. Shock, regardless of the type, is a medical emergency. It can occur with injuries involving severe pain, bleeding, the spinal cord, fractures, or intra-abdominal or intrathoracic regions, but shock also may occur, to some degree, with minor injuries. The signs of shock include a rapid, weak pulse; labored, weakened respirations; and decreased blood pressure.

5. Anaphylaxis is a severe allergic reaction that can be life-threatening. Signs and symptoms can develop within seconds of exposure to the allergen. Some individuals who know that they are hypersensitive to a substance carry medication (e.g., epinephrine) to manage the condition.

6. External hemorrhage is best controlled with direct pressure and elevation. The danger with internal hemorrhage can be overlooked as it is not visible.

APPLICATION QUESTIONS

1. While walking on a treadmill, a male adult grabs his chest and stops the exercise. The individual is conscious but has severe chest pain. How should the fitness specialist manage this situation? Why?

2. A physical education teacher is holding their second-grade class on one of the school fields that is approximately 500 yards from the school building. One of the students gets stung by a bee on the left forearm. The teacher tells the student to sit on the bleachers and watch the remainder of the class. Five minutes later, the student tells the teacher that he is experiencing intense itching on the soles of the feet and the palms of the hands. In addition, the student reports feeling dizzy and having nausea. How should the physical education teacher manage this situation? Why?

3. A high school varsity basketball coach is holding an evening practice (6:00 PM to 7:30 PM). Except for the janitorial staff, the coach is the only adult in the building. During a water break halfway through a relatively strenuous practice, one of the players comes running into the gym stating that another player has just collapsed in the locker room. When the coach reaches the individual, he finds him unconscious and has a difficult time assessing his pulse. How should the coach manage this situation? Why?

4. A personal trainer is working with a client at the fitness center, which is part of the apartment complex where the client lives. While moving from one piece of equipment to the next, the client accidentally trips and hits her head on a piece of equipment. The individual is unconscious. There is no one else in the fitness center. The only available phone is the personal trainer's cell phone, but it is not getting reception. How should the personal trainer manage this situation? Why?

5. A third-grade physical education class is using floor scooters as part of a lesson. Two students have a head-on collision. One student is bleeding profusely from the head; the other is not bleeding, but is lying on the floor rubbing her head. How should the physical education teacher manage this situation? Why?

6. While in the dugout, a high school varsity baseball player grabs his throat with both hands. He appears to be choking. The athlete is coughing. How should the coach manage this situation? Why?

REFERENCES

1. Van Camp SP, et al. 1995. Non-traumatic sports death in high school and college athletes. Med Sci Sports Exerc, 27(5):641–647.
2. Maron BJ, et al. 1996. Sudden death in young competitive athletes: clinical, demographic, and pathological profiles. JAMA, 276(3):199–204.
3. Kronisch RL. 1996. Sudden cardiac death in sports. Athl Ther Today, 1(4):39–41.
4. Thompson PD. 1996. The cardiovascular complications of vigorous physical activity. Arch Intern Med, 156(20):2297–2302.
5. Hosey RG, and Armsey TD. 2003. Sudden cardiac death. Clin Sports Med, 22(1):51–66.

Specific Conditions

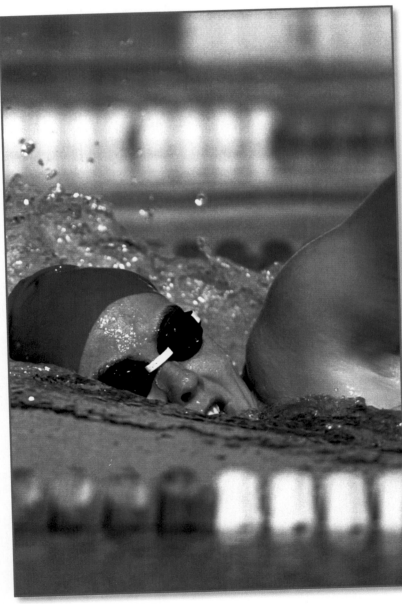

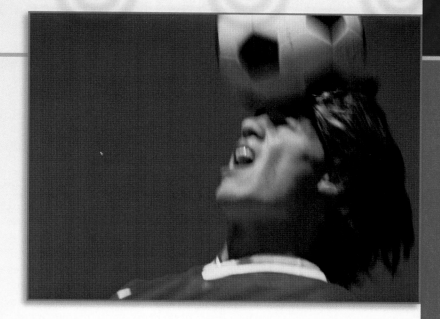

CRANIAL AND FACIAL CONDITIONS

KEY TERMS

anterograde amnesia
Battle's sign
blowout fracture
cauliflower ear
concussion
conjunctivitis
contrecoup-type injury
coup-type injury
detached retina

(continued)

LEARNING OUTCOMES

1. Identify the important bony and soft tissue structures of the head and facial region.

2. Explain the importance of wearing protective equipment to prevent injury to the head and facial region.

3. Describe the forces responsible for cranial injuries.

4. Identify the signs and symptoms associated with specific head and cerebral injuries and explain how to manage these conditions.

5. Describe the role of the coach in the assessment and management of a concussion.

6. Identify common facial injuries. Describe the signs and symptoms as well as the management for these conditions.

KEY TERMS (CONTINUED)

diffuse injuries	intruded	photophobia
diplopia	malocclusion	postconcussion syndrome
dural sinuses	meninges	raccoon eyes
epistaxis	meningitis	retrograde amnesia
extruded	nystagmus	tinnitus
focal injuries	otitis externa	
hyphema	periorbital ecchymosis	

The head and facial areas are sites for injuries ranging from mild to potentially catastrophic in nature. Given the potential for catastrophic injuries related to head-trauma, it is essential for the coach, physical educator, and fitness specialist to have a clear understanding of cranial injuries, their prevention, and management. While facial injuries may not produce catastrophic results, eye, nose, and dental injuries can result in functional as well as cosmetic problems.

This chapter begins with information on cranial and facial anatomy. It is followed by cranial injuries, their management, and protocol for a basic assessment of a **concussion**. Finally, common injuries to the facial area and their management are presented.

HEAD ANATOMY

This review of anatomy focuses on the bones of the skull, the brain and its coverings, the 12 cranial nerves that emerge from the brain stem, and the arterial blood vessels that nourish the skull. A basic understanding of this anatomy can help the coach understand the reasons for particular signs and symptoms occurring with damage to specific anatomic structures of the region.

Bones of the Skull

The skull is primarily composed of flat bones that interlock at immovable joints called sutures (FIG. 9.1). The bones that form the portion of the skull known as the cranium protect the brain. The facial bones provide the structure of the face and form the sinuses, orbits of the eyes, nasal cavity, and mouth. The large opening at the base of the skull that sits atop the spinal column is called the foramen magnum.

The Scalp

The scalp is the outermost anatomical structure of the cranium. The scalp is composed of three layers: the skin, subcutaneous connective tissue, and pericranium. The protective function of these tissues is enhanced by the hair and looseness of the scalp, which enables some dissipation of force when the head sustains a glancing blow. The scalp and face have an extensive blood supply; as a result, superficial lacerations tend to bleed profusely.

The Brain

The four major regions of the brain are the cerebral hemispheres, diencephalon, brainstem, and cerebellum. The entire brain and spinal cord are enclosed in three layers of protective tissue collectively known as the **meninges** (FIG. 9.2). The outermost membrane is the dura mater, a thick, fibrous tissue containing **dural sinuses** that act as veins to transport blood from the brain to the jugular veins of the neck. The arachnoid mater is a thin membrane internal to the dura mater, separated from the dura mater by the subdural space. Beneath the arachnoid mater is the subarachnoid space, which is filled with cerebrospinal fluid (CSF). This space contains the largest of the blood vessels supplying the brain. The arachnoid mater is connected to the inner pia mater by weblike strands of connective tissue. The dura mater and arachnoid mater are rather loose membranes, but the pia mater is in direct contact with the cerebral cortex. The pia mater contains several small blood vessels.

FACIAL ANATOMY

The Bones of the Face

In addition to protecting the brain, the facial skeleton provides the bony framework and protection for the eyes, nose, mouth, and ears. The primary bones of the face are the mandible, maxilla, frontal bone, nasal bones, and zygoma.

The mandible, often referred to as the jaw bone, forms the lower jaw. It holds the lower teeth in place and because it is a mobile bone, it enables the chewing process. The mandible articulates with the upper temporal bone to form the temporomandibular joint (TMJ), or what is commonly called the lower jaw. The maxilla, sometimes referred to as the mustache bone, forms the upper jaw. In addition to holding the upper teeth, the maxilla forms the roof of the mouth, the floor of the eye orbit, and the lateral wall and roof of the nasal cavity. The frontal bone consists of two segments. The vertical component of the frontal bone comprises the area known as the forehead; the horizontal component forms the sinus cavities and the orbital cavities. The nasal bones are paired bones that form the roof of the nasal cavity. These bones vary in size and shape and, as such, produce a variety of appearances of the nose. The zygoma, typically referred to as the cheek bone, forms the lateral portion of the eye orbit.

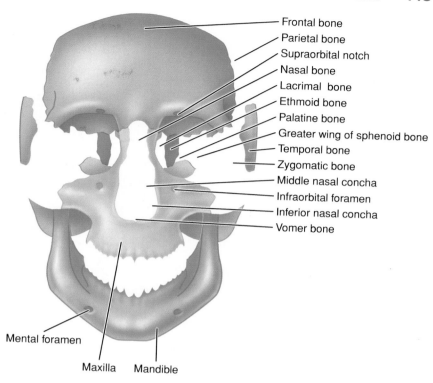

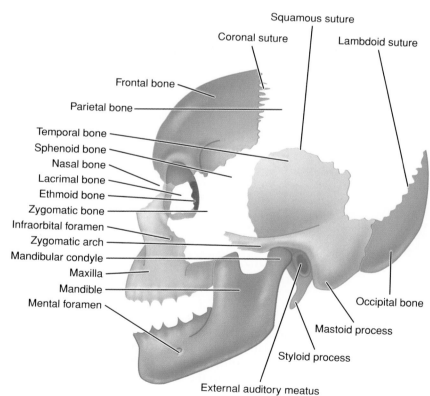

FIGURE 9.1 Bones of the skull. **A**. Frontal view. **B**. Lateral view.

The Eyes

The eye is a hollow sphere, approximately 2.5 cm (1 in.) in diameter in adults (FIG. 9.3). The anterior eye surface receives protection from the eyelids, eyelashes, and the attached conjunctiva. The conjunctiva lines the eyelids and the external surface of the eye, and secretes mucus to

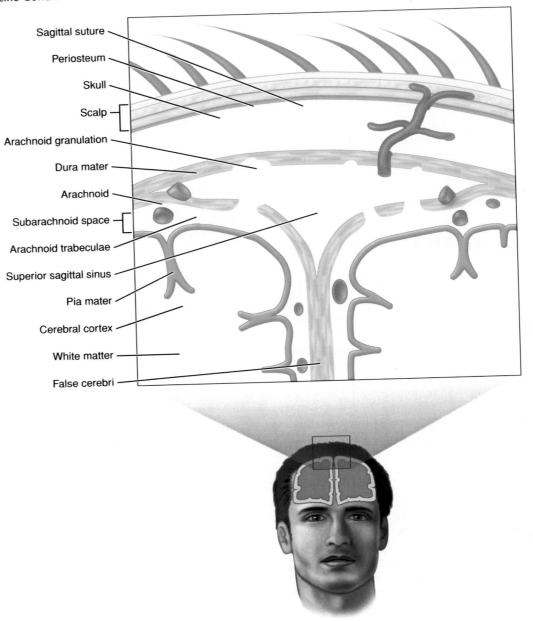

FIGURE 9.2 Meninges. Three layers of protective tissue, known as the meninges, enclose the brain and spinal cord.

lubricate the external eye. The lacrimal glands, located above the lateral ends of the eyes, continually release tears across the eye surface through several small ducts. The lacrimal ducts, located at the medial corners of the eyes, serve as drains for the moisture. These ducts funnel the moisture into the lacrimal sac and eventually into the nasal cavity.

The eye is surrounded by three protective tissue layers, called tunics. The outer tunic is a thick white connective tissue called the sclera and forms the "white of the eye." The cornea, found in the central anterior part of the sclera, is clear to permit passage of light into the eye. The choroid, the middle covering, is a highly vascularized tissue, which usually appears blue or brown on the anterior eye and contains the pupil. The inner protective layer is the retina, which contains light-sensitive photoreceptor cells that stimulate nerve endings to provide sight.

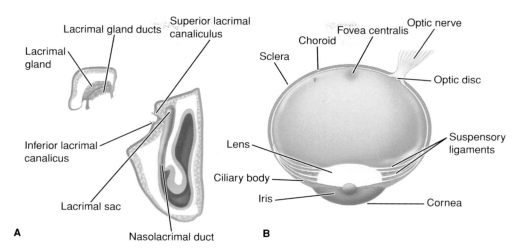

FIGURE 9.3 Eye. **A.** The lacrimal structures of the eye. **B.** Internal structures of the eye globe.

The Nose

The nose is composed of bone and hyaline cartilage. The roof is formed by the cribriform plate of the ethmoid bone. The nasal bones form the bridge of the nose. The nasal cavity is separated into right and left halves by the nasal septum, which is made of cartilage.

The Ear

The ear is divided into three major areas: the outer ear (auricle and external auditory canal), middle ear (tympanic membrane), and inner ear (labyrinth) (FIG. 9.4). Assisting the middle and inner ear in the process of hearing and equalizing pressure between the two areas is the eustachian tube, a canal that links the nose and middle ear.

The Teeth

The 20 primary teeth seen in children are replaced between the ages of 6 and 14 with 32 permanent teeth. The visible part of the tooth is the crown. It lies almost entirely above the exposed

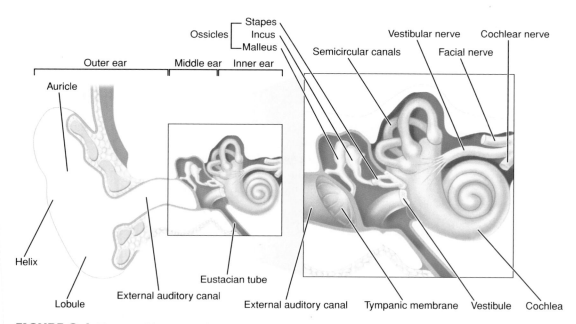

FIGURE 9.4 The ear. The ear is divided into three major areas: the outer ear (auricle and external auditory canal), the middle ear (tympanic membrane), and the inner ear (labyrinth).

TABLE 9.1	**The Cranial Nerves**			
NUMBER	NAME	SENSORY	MOTOR	FUNCTION
I	Olfactory	X (smell)		Sense of smell
II	Optic	X (vision)		Vision
III	Oculomotor		X	Control of some of the extrinsic eye muscles
IV	Trochlear		X	Control of the remaining extrinsic eye muscles
V	Trigeminal	X (general sensation)	X	Sensation of the facial region and movement of the jaw muscles
VI	Abducens		X	Control of lateral eye movement
VII	Facial	X (taste)	X	Control of facial movement, taste, and secretion of tears and saliva
VIII	Vestibulocochlear	X (hearing and balance)		Hearing and equilibrium (acoustic)
IX	Glossopharyngeal	X (taste)	X	Taste, control of the tongue and pharynx, secretion of saliva
X	Vagus	X (taste)	X	Taste, sensation to the pharynx, larynx, trachea, and bronchioles
XI	Accessory		X	Control of movements of the pharynx, larynx, head, and shoulders
XII	Hypoglossal		X	Control of tongue movements

gum line. The nonvisible root serves to anchor the tooth into the bone (i.e., mandible or maxilla). The major components of the teeth include the dentin, enamel, cementum, and pulp. Enamel covers the crown and, in doing so, provides resistance to mechanical and chemical damage. Cementum is relatively soft bony tissue that covers the root of the tooth. It assists in holding the tooth in its socket. Dentin is a hard, but porous, substance that provides strength. It is covered by enamel at the crown of the tooth and cemetum on the root. The center of the tooth is known as the pulp. The pulp contains blood vessels and nerves and serves to nourish the dentin.

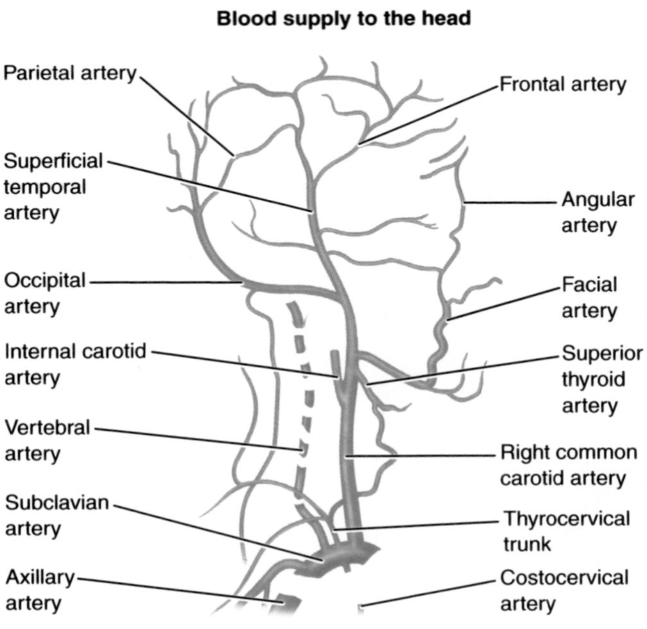

NERVES OF THE HEAD AND FACE

Twelve pairs of cranial nerves emerge from the brain, some with motor functions, some with sensory function, and some with both. Knowledge of their function is important in assessing a cranial injury. The cranial nerves are numbered and named according to their functions (TABLE 9.1).

BLOOD VESSELS OF THE HEAD AND FACE

The major vessels supplying the head and face are the common carotid and vertebral arteries (FIG. 9.5). The common carotid artery ascends through the neck on either side to divide into the external and internal carotid artery just below the level of the jaw. The external carotid arteries and

Blood supply to the head

Parietal artery
Superficial temporal artery
Occipital artery
Internal carotid artery
Vertebral artery
Subclavian artery
Axillary artery

Frontal artery
Angular artery
Facial artery
Superior thyroid artery
Right common carotid artery
Thyrocervical trunk
Costocervical artery

FIGURE 9.5 Blood supply to the head. The common carotid and vertebral arteries are the major vessels supplying blood to the brain.

their branches supply most regions of the head external to the brain. The middle meningeal artery supplies the skull and dura mater; if this artery is damaged, serious epidural bleeding can result. The internal carotid arteries send branches to the eyes and portions of the brain. The left and right vertebral arteries and their branches supply blood to the posterior region of the brain.

PROTECTIVE EQUIPMENT FOR THE HEAD AND FACE

The most important injury preventive measure for the head and facial area is the use of protective equipment. Many sports, such as baseball/softball, competitive bicycling, fencing, field hockey, football, ice hockey, lacrosse, and wrestling, require some type of head or facial protective equipment for participation. Protective equipment, when used properly, can protect the head and facial area from accidental or routine injuries. It is important to recognize that protective equipment cannot prevent all injuries.

Protective equipment may include a helmet, face guard, mouth guard, eye wear, ear wear, and throat protector. Helmets protect the cranial portion of the skull by absorbing and dispersing impact forces, thereby reducing cerebral trauma. Face guards protect and shield the facial region. Mouth guards have been shown to reduce dental and oral soft tissue injuries, as well as cerebral concussions, jaw fractures, and TMJ injuries. Eye wear, ear wear, and throat protectors reduce injuries to their respective regions.

In order to be effective, a variety of considerations must be followed in the use of protective equipments. These considerations should include

- Ensuring that equipment is properly fitted, clean, and in good condition.
- Ensuring that equipment is used in the manner for which it was designed. (e.g., instruct football players that the head is not to be used as a battering ram)
- Following manufacturer's guidelines and recommendations for using the equipment (e.g., recommended time for replacing or refurbishing a helmet; guidelines for fitting a helmet; guidelines for fitting a mouth guard)
- Maintaining accurate records pertaining to the equipment purchase date, use, and reconditioning history

It is critical to use equipment that meets the recommended standards as determined by the appropriate agency [e.g., football, baseball, and softball helmets must be approved by the National Operating Committee on Standards for Athletic Equipment (NOCSAE); and ice hockey helmets should be approved by the American Society for Testing and Materials (ASTM) and the Hockey Equipment Certification Council (HECC)]. The responsible agency ensures that a helmet meets the minimum impact standards and can tolerate forces applied to several different areas.

HEAD INJURIES

Scalp Injury

As the outermost anatomical structure of the cranium, the scalp is the first area of contact in trauma. The scalp is highly vascular and bleeds freely, making it a frequent site for abrasions, lacerations, contusions, or hematomas between the layers of tissue. The primary concerns with any scalp laceration are to control bleeding, prevent contamination, and assess for a possible skull fracture.

Management

In keeping with universal precautions, latex gloves should be worn in the assessment and management of any open wound. Mild direct pressure should be applied to the area with sterile gauze until bleeding has stopped and the wound is visible. The wound should be inspected for any foreign bodies or signs of a skull fracture. If a skull fracture is ruled out, the wound should be cleansed with a saline solution, covered with a sterile dressing, and the individual referred to a physician for possible suturing.

If a closed wound is sustained, a hematoma, or "goose egg," may develop. In this situation, a collection of blood develops between the layers of the scalp and skull. These injuries should be managed with crushed ice and gentle pressure to control hemorrhage and edema. The individual should be referred to a physician (1) if there are any signs of cerebral trauma or (2) if the hematoma does not improve in 24 hours.

Skull Fracture

A fracture or intracranial injury of the skull depends on the material properties of the skull, thickness of the skull in the specific area of impact, magnitude and direction of the sustained force, and size of the impact area. When the head is struck by another object, such as a baseball, two phenomena occur—deformation and acceleration. The bone deforms and bends inward, placing the inner border of the skull under tensile strain, whereas the outer border is placed in compression. If the force of impact is sufficient and the skull is thin in the region of impact, a skull fracture can occur where tensile loading occurs. In contrast, if the skull is thick and dense enough at the area of impact, it may sustain inward bending without fracture. Fracture may then occur some distance from the impact zone where the skull is thinner (FIG. 9.6).

Whenever a severe blow to the head occurs, a skull fracture should always be suspected. Skull fractures can be linear (in a line), comminuted (in multiple pieces), depressed (fragments are driven internally toward the brain), or basilar (involving the base of the skull) (FIG. 9.7). If there is a break in the skin adjacent to the fracture site and a tear to the underlying dura mater, the risk of bacterial infection into the intracranial cavity is high and can result in septic **meningitis**.

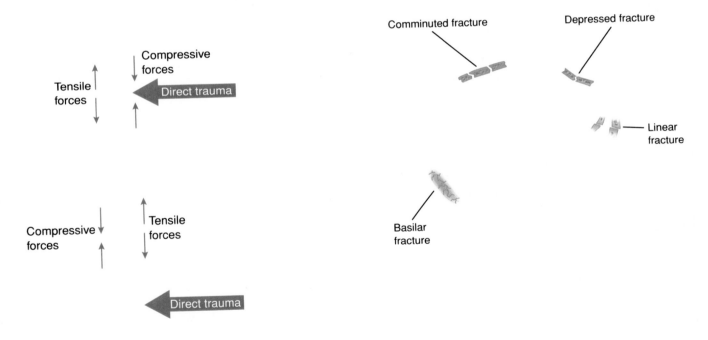

FIGURE 9.6 Mechanical failure in bone. When a blow impacts the skull, the bone deforms and bends inward, placing tensile stress on the inner border of the skull. **A.** If an impact is of sufficient magnitude and the skull is thin in the region of the impact, a skull fracture occurs at the impact site. **B.** If the skull is thick and dense enough at the area of impact, it may sustain bending without fracture; however, the fracture may occur some distance from the impact zone, in a region where the skull is thinner.

FIGURE 9.7 Skull fractures. Fractures of the skull are categorized as linear, comminuted, depressed, or basilar.

Signs and Symptoms

Complaints of a severe headache and nausea, as well as changes in pupils (i.e., unequal size; not reactive to light) are symptoms associated with a skull fracture regardless of the fracture site. Depending on the fracture site, different signs and symptoms may appear including:

- Discoloration around the eyes (**raccoon eyes**)
- Blood or CSF may leak from the nose
- Blindness or loss of smell (due to bony fragments may damage the optic or olfactory cranial nerves)
- **Battle's sign,** a discoloration that can appear within minutes behind the ear (due to a basilar fracture above and behind the ear)
- Blood or CSF may leak from the ear canal
- A hearing loss
- Facial paralysis; slurred speech

Management

A skull fracture can be a life-threatening condition. If any of the signs and symptoms become apparent, activation of the emergency plan, including summoning emergency medical services (EMS), is warranted. While waiting for EMS to arrive, the coach should

- Avoid moving the individual (unless absolutely necessary); if the individual must be moved, the head and neck must be stabilized. The head should not be allowed to flex, extend, bend, or rotate.
- Check airway, breathing, and circulation. If necessary, perform rescue breathing and CPR.
- Cover any open wounds with a sterile dressing without applying pressure to the area; the area should not be probed and any foreign materials or objects should not be removed.
- Monitor the individual until EMS arrives. Regardless of any complaints by the individual, the coach should not administer any medication.

CEREBRAL INJURIES

A force that is not sufficient to lead to a skull fracture can still produce an intracranial injury. The impact can cause a shock wave to pass through the skull to the brain, causing acceleration. This acceleration can lead to shear, tensile, and compression strains within the brain substance. Shear is the most serious type of strain. If the brain is traumatized at the point of impact, it is called a **coup-type injury.** The brain can be injured further as the full force of the brain's weight accelerates and hits the opposite side of the skull, leading to **contrecoup-type injury,** or an injury away from the actual impact site. In this type of injury, the head is typically moving and strikes a stationary object or a more slowly moving object. In an acceleration-deceleration injury, such as whiplash, the head is hurled forward, traumatizing the brain by the accelerated skull. The brain is then smashed against the halted skull, which leads to further rebounding within the confines of the skull (FIG. 9.8).

Several terms are used to describe acute head trauma. The most common is traumatic brain injury (TBI). TBIs are classified into two categories, namely focal and diffuse.

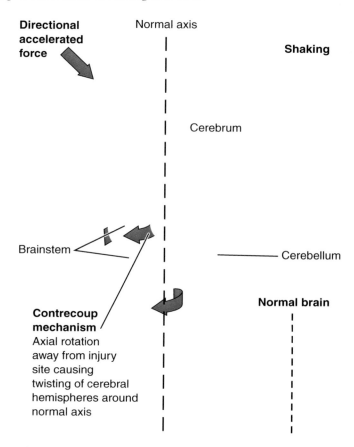

FIGURE 9.8 Cranial mechanisms. Trauma can produce a coup- or contrecoup-type injury.

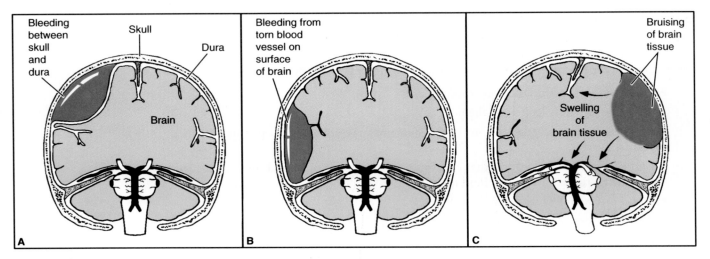

FIGURE 9.9 Focal cerebral injuries. **A.** Focal injuries can involve an epidural hematoma in which bleeding occurs outside the dura mater. **B.** A subdural hematoma in which bleeding occurs deep to the dura mater. **C.** A cerebral contusion in which the microhemorrhaging does not form a space-occupying lesion.

Focal injuries involve localized damage, whereas **diffuse injuries** involve widespread disruption and damage to the function or structure of the brain. Although diffuse injuries account for only 25% of fatalities caused by head trauma, they are the most prevalent cause of long-term neurologic deficits in individuals.

Focal Cerebral Injuries

Focal cerebral injuries usually result in a localized collection of blood or hematoma (FIG. 9.9). Because the skull has no room for additional accumulation of blood or fluid, any additional foreign matter within the cranial cavity increases pressure on the brain, leading to significant alterations in neurologic function. Depending on the location of the accumulated blood relative to the dura mater, these hematomas are classified as epidural (outside the dura mater) or subdural (deep to the dura mater). A cerebral contusion is also classified as a focal injury; however, there is no mass-occupying lesion associated with this condition.

Epidural Hematoma

An epidural hematoma is very rare in sport or recreational physical activity. Typically, the condition is caused by a direct blow to the side of the head and is almost always associated with a skull fracture. If the middle meningeal artery or its branches are severed, the subsequent arterial bleeding leads to a "high-pressure" epidural hematoma (FIG. 9.10A).

Signs and Symptoms

The individual may experience an initial loss of consciousness at the time of the injury, followed by a lucid interval in which the individual feels relatively normal and asymptomatic. However, within 10 to 20 minutes, a gradual decline in mental status occurs as the hematoma outside the brain reaches a critical size and compresses the underlying brain. Other signs and symptoms may include increased headache, drowsiness, nausea, vomiting, decreased level of consciousness; an ipsilateral dilated pupil on the side of the hematoma; and subsequently contralateral weakness and decerebrate posturing. This condition may require immediate surgery to decompress the hematoma and control arterial bleeding.

Subdural Hematoma

A subdural hematoma is approximately three times more frequent than an epidural hematoma, and is the leading cause of catastrophic death in football players.[1] Hemorrhaging occurs when the bridging veins between the brain and the dura mater are torn (FIG. 9.10B). It is caused by acceleration forces of the head, rather than the impact of the force. Subdural hematomas may

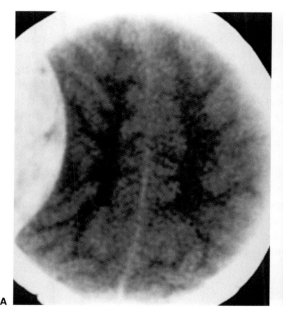
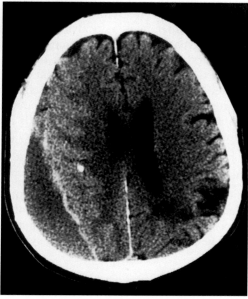

FIGURE 9.10 Cerebral hematomas. **A.** This epidural hematoma resulted from a fracture that extended into the orbital roof and sinus area, leading to rapid hemorrhage in the right frontal lobe of the brain. **B.** The subdural hematoma on the right side of the brain is fairly evident. A chronic subdural hematoma can be seen on the left side of the brain.

be classified as either acute, which presents 48 to 72 hours after injury, or chronic, which occurs in a later time frame with more variable clinical manifestations, simple or complicated. In a simple subdural hematoma, blood collects in the subdural space but no underlying cerebral injury occurs. Complex subdural hematomas are characterized by contusions of the brain's surface and associated cerebral swelling that increase intracerebral pressure. The mortality rate for simple subdural hematomas is approximately 20%, whereas complicated subdural hematomas have a 50% mortality rate.[2]

Signs and Symptoms

In a complicated subdural hematoma, the individual is typically knocked out and remains unconscious. In a simple subdural hematoma, the individual is less likely to be rendered unconscious. These individuals seldom demonstrate deterioration in level of consciousness, and fewer than 15% have a lucid interval. Signs and symptoms of increasing intracranial pressure include

- Pupillary dilation and retinal changes on the affected side
- Irregular eye tracking or eye movement
- Severe headache
- Nausea and/or vomiting
- Confusion and/or drastic changes in emotional control
- Progressive or sudden impairment of consciousness
- Rising blood pressure
- Falling pulse rate
- Irregular respirations
- Increased body temperature

Signs and symptoms may not become apparent for hours, days, or even weeks after injury. Early diagnosis of a subdural hematoma is essential for a successful recovery. A loss of consciousness implies a poor prognosis with an overall mortality rate of 35 to 50%.[3]

Cerebral Contusion

A cerebral contusion is a focal injury, but a mass-occupying lesion is not present. Instead, microhemorrhaging, cerebral infarction, necrosis, and edema of the brain occur.

Cerebral contusions occur most often from an acceleration-deceleration mechanism from the inward deformation of the skull at the impact site. For example, an acceleration force is generated when another individual or an object (e.g., ball; hockey puck) hits an individual's head, resulting in injury at the point of impact (i.e., coup injury). In comparison, deceleration forces are generated when an individual's head strikes the ground, producing injury opposite the point of impact (i.e., contrecoup injury). The injury may be limited to small, localized areas or it can involve large, extensive areas.

Signs and Symptoms

Clinical signs and symptoms vary greatly, depending on the location, number, and extent of the hemorrhagic lesions. Most individuals experience a loss of consciousness. The individual may subsequently become alert or may become comatose. The individual may have a normal neurologic examination, but symptoms such as headaches, dizziness, or nausea may be present.

Management of Focal Cerebral Injuries

Epidural hematomas, subdural hematomas, and cerebral contusions are emergency conditions, As such, activation of the emergency plan, including summoning EMS, is warranted. While waiting for EMS to arrive, the coach should

- Check airway, breathing, and circulation. If necessary, perform rescue breathing and CPR.
- Monitor the individual. Regardless of any complaints by the individual, the coach should not administer any medication.

Diffuse Cerebral Conditions

Diffuse cerebral injuries involve trauma to widespread areas of the brain rather than one specific site. The range of these injuries can vary from mild to severe, involving impairment of neural function, structural damage, or both. Common diffuse cerebral injuries include concussion, posttraumatic headaches, **postconcussion syndrome**, and second-impact syndrome.

Concussions

A **concussion** is a TBI that can occur from a mild to severe blow to the head. The data concerning the number of concussions sustained on a yearly basis in the United States is staggering:

- A suggested 3,000,000 concussions occurred in 2008 as a result of participation in youth sport.[4]
- 1 in 10 high school athletes participating in contact sports will sustain a concussion.[5]
- 50% of college athletes have a history of concussion.[5]

It is important to note that on any number of occasions, a concussion can be sustained during participation in sport and physical activity and may go undiagnosed and, as such, untreated.

The rising number of concussions attributed to participation in sport and physical activity has drawn the attention of the medical community. In November 2001, the First International Symposium on Concussion in Sport was held in Vienna to provide recommendations to improve the safety and health of athletes who suffer concussive injuries. Several issues were discussed, including protective equipment, epidemiology, basic and clinical science, grading systems, cognitive assessment, and management. A second international symposium was held in 2004 in Prague.[6] Subsequently, sport-related concussions have been defined as a complex pathophysiological process affecting the brain and induced by traumatic biomechanical forces.[7] Most recently, experts from varied fields, including professional associations (e.g., NATA), the medical/healthcare community, and sport-related bodies (e.g., NCAA; NFL), have increased their attention to concussion-related issues, including prevention, assessment, management, and

BOX 9.1   Typical Signs and Symptoms of a Concussion

- Vacant stare (e.g., befuddled facial expression; glassy eyed)
- Visual problems (e.g., seeing stars or flashing lights, double vision)
- Headache or pressure in the head
- Delayed verbal and motor responses (e.g., slow to answer questions or follow instructions)
- Confusion and inability to focus attention (e.g., easily distracted; unable to follow through with normal activities)
- Disorientation (e.g., walking in the wrong direction; unaware of time, date, and place)
- Slurred or incoherent speech (e.g., making disjointed or incomprehensible statements)

- Gross observable incoordination with balance of dizziness (e.g., stumbling, inability to walk tandem/straight line)
- Emotions out of proportion to circumstances (e.g., distraught, crying for no apparent reason, laughing)
- Memory deficits (e.g., exhibited by the individual repeatedly asking the same question that has already been answered, or inability to memorize and recall three of three words or three of three objects in 5 minutes)
- Any period of loss of consciousness (e.g., unresponsiveness to arousal)

long-term effects. However, the efforts of the professional associations are not sufficient. It is essential that individuals involved in administering physical activity and sports programs increase their awareness and understanding of concussion. A coach is often the first person to respond to an individual with a potential concussion. As such, their actions or inactions can have a significant impact on the immediate and subsequent outcome of the situation.

What is a Concussion?

A concussion is a disturbance in brain function caused by a direct blow to the head or an indirect force that produces a violent jarring of the brain. The injury may cause an immediate and transient impairment of neural function, such as alteration of consciousness and disturbance of vision and equilibrium. Under normal conditions, the brain balances a series of electrochemical events in billions of brain cells. When the brain is shaken or jarred, brain function can be disrupted temporarily without causing injury or damage to brain tissue. For example, mild trauma can result in interruption of cerebral function. Signs and symptoms range from mild to moderate and are transient and reversible. This can be attributed to the minimal damage to soft tissue structures. As the impact magnitude increases with an acceleration injury, both cerebral function and structural damage may occur, resulting in more serious signs and symptoms. These include varying degrees of loss of consciousness (LOC), headache, confusion, memory loss, nausea, **tinnitus**, pupillary changes, dizziness, and loss of coordination (BOX 9.1).

Classifications of Concussions

There are numerous and different classification schemes that attempt to define the various degrees of brain dysfunction in cerebral concussions. None of the scales has been universally accepted and followed, which has led to much confusion over determining the severity of a TBI. It is critical to understand that no two concussions will be identical nor will the signs and symptoms be the same. Each injury will vary depending on the magnitude of force to the head, the level of metabolic dysfunction, the tissue damage and duration of time needed to recover, the number of previous concussions, and the time between injuries.

There are currently three main approaches to grading sports-related concussions. One approach is to grade the TBI at the time of injury based on the existing signs and symptoms within 15 minutes of injury. The American Academy of Neurology (AAN) Concussion Grading Scale (TABLE 9.2) is widely used in this approach.[8] Although confusion and amnesia remain the most frequently cited symptoms, not all injuries behave as expected in the initial evaluation, making the return-to-play (RTP) decision more challenging.

TABLE 9.2	Grading Scales for Athletic Head Injury		
	GRADE I/MILD	GRADE II/MODERATE	GRADE III/SEVERE
AAN	Transient confusion; no LOC; symptoms and mental status resolve <15 minutes.	Transient confusion; no LOC; symptoms and mental status resolve >15 minutes.	Any LOC
Cantu	No LOC; PTA <30 minutes; PCSS <24 hours.	LOC <1 minute **or** PTA ≥30 minutes. <24 hours or PCSS ≥24 hours <7 days	LOC ≥1 minute **or** PTA ≥24 hours **or** PCSS ≥7 days

AAN = American Academy of Neurology; LOC = loss of consciousness; PTA = posttraumatic amnesia (anterograde/retrograde); PCSS = postconcussion signs and symptoms other than amnesia.

Another popular approach is the Cantu Evidence-Based Grading Scale, which grades the injury only after all concussion signs and symptoms have resolved.[9] Less emphasis is placed on LOC as a predictor of potential impairment and additional weight is placed on overall symptom duration.

The third approach in grading a concussion is not to use any grading scale, but rather attend to the individual's recovery based on their symptoms, neuropsychological tests, and postural-stability tests. This allows the supervising healthcare provider to determine when the patient is symptomatic or asymptomatic. Once asymptomatic, the individual can begin a progressive regimen of activity that increases demands over several days. This progression will differ in individuals who are withheld from activity for only a few days versus individuals withheld for several weeks. This multitiered approach was summarized and supported by consensus at the 2001 Vienna Conference on Concussion in Sport and reaffirmed at the 2004 Conference. Their recommendation was to abandon the continued use of grading scales in favor of combined measures of recovery in order to determine injury severity (and/or prognosis) and to guide individual RTP decisions.[6,7]

Given the controversy that surrounds establishing a universal grading criterion for concussion, the concept of simple concussion and complex concussion will be presented in lieu of a graded scale.

Simple Concussion

Although the most common concussion, it is the most difficult to recognize. The individual may simply report "I had my bell rung." Use of this phrase or the term "ding" should not be used to determine the severity of injury, as they carry a connotation that may underestimate the severity of injury. The individual is not rendered unconscious, and the only neurologic deficit is a brief period of posttraumatic confusion (e.g., inattentiveness, poor concentration, an inability to process information or sequence tasks), or posttraumatic amnesia (PTA). Usually the concussion symptoms or mental status abnormalities on examination resolve within a 30 minute period.[9] If significant disorientation, confusion, memory disturbance, dizziness, headache, or other neurologic abnormality persists after 30 minutes of observation, a more serious concussion is present.[10] In a simple concussion, the injury progressively resolves without complications over 7 to 10 days.

Complex Concussion

In a complex concussion, the individual suffers persistent symptoms (including persistent symptoms that recur with exertion), specific sequelae (e.g., prolonged LOC [>1 minute]), or prolonged cognitive impairment following the injury. This classification also includes those individuals who suffer multiple concussions over time or where repeated concussions occur with progressively less impact force.[7] Less frequently, no loss of consciousness occurs; however, the individual experiences a protracted period of PTA lasting more than 30 minutes, but less than 24 hours. This PTA may involve loss of memory of events immediately preceding the injury (**retrograde amnesia**) or the loss of memory of events following the injury (**anterograde amnesia**). This memory loss may diminish somewhat, but the individual will always have some degree of permanent, although short, memory loss about the injury. Other signs that may be present include moderate dizziness and unsteady gait, blurred vision, tinnitus, and headache.

Posttraumatic Headaches

Posttraumatic vascular headaches can be confused with a simple concussion or postconcussive headache. A vascular headache is a result of vasospasm and does not usually occur with impact but, rather, develops shortly afterward.

Signs and Symptoms

Common symptoms include a localized area of blindness that may follow the appearance of brilliantly colored shimmering lights. In addition, migraines are characterized by recurrent attacks of severe headache with sudden onset, with or without visual or gastrointestinal problems.

Management

This individual should be immediately referred to a physician for evaluation and care.

Postconcussion Syndrome

Postconcussion syndrome may develop after any concussion. Cognitive impairments may extend from the time of injury to 48 hours after trauma and last for several weeks to months.

Signs and Symptoms

The syndrome is characterized by persistent headaches, blurred vision, vertigo, memory loss, irritability, decreased attention span, and inability to concentrate on even the simplest task.

Management

No definitive treatment exists other than symptomatic measures to control the headaches. The individual should not be permitted to return to activity until all symptoms have resolved. A physician should determine the individual's readiness to return to activity and supervise their gradual return.

Second Impact Syndrome

Second impact syndrome occurs when an individual who has sustained an initial head injury, usually a concussion, sustains a second head injury before the symptoms associated with the previous one have totally resolved. This second trauma may be relatively minor and does not have to be the result of direct contact. As such, any individual who reports headache, lightheadedness, visual disturbances, or other neurologic symptoms should not be allowed to participate in any physical activity in which head trauma may occur until asymptomatic.

Signs and Symptoms

Following the trauma, the individual may appear to be stunned but often completes the current action or play and, in some cases, can walk unassisted. However, there is an associated increase in intracranial pressure which results in compromise of the brainstem. Subsequently, the individual collapses and presents with rapidly dilating pupils, progressing to loss of eye movement, coma, and respiratory failure. The usual interval from second impact to brainstem failure is short—usually 2 to 5 minutes.

Management

Immediate activation of the emergency plan, including summoning EMS, is warranted. While waiting for EMS to arrive, the coach should administer basic life support as necessary.

The Coach and Concussion

Simply stated, a concussion can occur in any sport or physical activity. While contact and collision sports place an individual at a greater risk for concussion, an individual who trips while running on a hard surface could fall, hit their head, and subsequently sustain a concussion.

All too often, qualified medical personnel are not on site for sporting events (e.g., practices and game), physical education classes, recreational physical activities, or fitness training activities. As such, the coach, the physical educator, or the fitness specialist is often the first respondent in an injury situation. It is essential that coaches not be naïve about the possibility of a participant sustaining a head injury, but rather that they understand and respect their responsibility to the individuals with whom they are working. Coaches, physical educators, and fitness specialists must have a clear understanding of their roles and responsibilities in the prevention, assessment, and management of concussions. The assessment, management, and prevention information that follows is intended for use by coaches, physical educators, and fitness specialists. The information reflects the level of care that is appropriate for the coach (as compared to a trained medical specialist).

Assessment

The primary responsibility of the coach is to recognize potential signs and symptoms of a concussion. It is not the responsibility of the coach to determine the level of a concussion, but rather to note the presence of any signs and/or symptoms that could be indicative of a concussion. Any time an individual sustains a blow to the head as a result of either direct or indirect trauma, the coach should assume the potential for head injury and be prompted to perform an assessment. The initial assessment should take place immediately following the trauma (e.g., it should not wait until the end of a drill or the class period) and should be repeated at regular intervals (i.e., 5 to 10 minutes) until the symptoms have resolved or the individual is released to the care of someone else (e.g., athletic trainer; physician; parent; school nurse).

A concussion can't be seen, per se. However, there are specific signs that can be observed by a coach and symptoms reported by the individual that should be noted in assessing a possible concussion. The coach should initially take vital signs to establish a baseline of information that can be rechecked periodically to determine if status is improving or deteriorating. The vital signs should include pulse, respiration, blood pressure, pupil abnormalities (i.e., size; accommodation to light; presence of **nystagmus**—inability to track smoothly), and skin temperature.

Throughout the assessment the coach should be attentive to observing potential signs of concussion. These include

- Any period of loss of consciousness (It is important to note whether it occurred immediately on direct impact or whether the person progressed to unconsciousness. In addition, the length of time of unconsciousness should be recorded.)
- The presence of a vacant stare (e.g., befuddled facial expression; glassy eyed)
- Disorientation (e.g., walking in the wrong direction)
- Gross observable incoordination with balance or dizziness (e.g., stumbling; inability to walk tandem/straight line)
- Slurred or incoherent speech (e.g., making disjointed or incomprehensible statements)
- Emotions out of proportion to circumstances (e.g., distraught; crying for no apparent reason; laughing)

The coach should determine the presence of any symptoms being experienced by the individual. This can be accomplished by having the individual simply describe their symptoms. However, if certain symptoms aren't volunteered by the individual, the coach should ask about their presence. In particular, the coach should make note of the following symptoms which could be indicative of a concussion:

- Headache
- Nausea/or vomiting
- Dizziness
- Feeling of confusion

- Feeling of sluggishness
- Sensitivity to light or noise
- Blurred vision
- Balance problems
- Inability to concentrate
- Inability to recall things

The next part of the assessment process should include mental status testing. The coach must understand that some signs can be manifested immediately after the trauma, while others could be delayed in presentation. The following can be used to gather a history of the injury and test the mental status of the individual:

- Determine level of orientation: Ask the individual about the time, place, person, and situation (e.g., the circumstances surrounding the mechanism of injury).
- Assess ability to concentrate: Recite three digits and ask the individual to recite them backward. Move to four digits, and then to five digits (e.g., 3–1-7, 4–6-8–2, and 5–3-0–7-4). Ask the individual to list the months of the year in reverse order.
- Assess memory: Name three words or identify three objects, and ask the individual to recall these words or objects. Every 5 minutes, ask the individual to recall those same words again. Additionally, ask the individual to recall recent newsworthy events or provide details of the current activity (e.g., plays, moves, and strategies). The individual should also be asked to recall events prior to the incident and following the incident.

In continuing the assessment, the coach can assess the coordination and balance proprieties of the individual. While a variety of tests can accomplish this task, the following are relatively easy to perform:

- Finger-to-nose test: This test can assess balance, depth perception, and ability to focus on an object. While the individual's eyes are open and their arms are out to the side, the examiner should instruct the individual to touch the index finger of one hand to the nose and then alternate with the other hand to the nose (Fig. 9.11). The examiner should observe for any swaying or inability to touch the nose. Then, standing a few feet from the person, the examiner should hold a finger in front of the injured individual. The individual should alternate between the right and left hand to reach out and touch the examiner's finger. The examiner can change the position of the finger after two or three touches. The speed of touch between the nose and finger is then progressively increased.
- Gait: Observing the individual walking in a straight line, the examiner should note any sway-ing or unsteadiness of gait. Heel-to-toe walking (tandem walking) may also be performed.
- Romberg test: The individual is asked to stand with the feet together, arms at the side, and eyes closed while maintaining balance (Fig. 9.12). While stand-ing lateral or posterior to the individual—to support the patient, if needed—the examiner observes for any body sway, indicating a positive test. Variations include the individual raising their arms to 90°, standing on the toes, touching the nose with the hand while the eyes are closed (finger-to-nose test), standing in a tandem position on a foam surface, and tilting the head backward while lifting one foot off the ground. Recently, the standard Romberg test has been criticized for its lack of sensibility and objectivity, because a considerable amount of stress is required to produce a positive test.

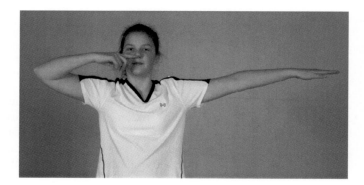

FIGURE 9.11 Finger-to-nose test. The individual should be standing with their eyes open and arms out to the side. The examiner instructs the individual to touch their index finger to the nose and then alternate with the other hand to the nose. Inability to perform this test indicates physical disorientation and lack of coordination and should preclude reentry to activity.

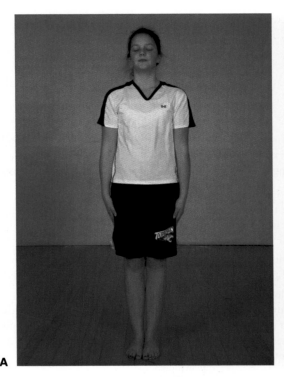
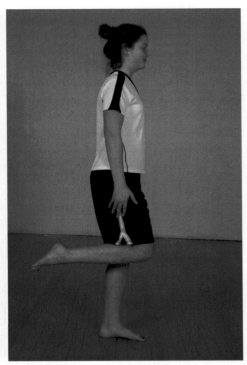

A   B

FIGURE 9.12 Romberg test. The individual should be standing with their eyes closed and arms at the side. The examiner instructs the individual to maintain a standing position. Any sway indicates lack of balance and sensation and should preclude reentry to activity.

As a final component of the assessment, the use of external provocative tests may or may not be warranted. If the assessment has already determined a possible intracranial injury, the individual should not be subjected to these tests. These tests require the individual to perform exertional activities, such as running or push-ups. Any appearance of associated symptoms (e.g., headaches, dizziness, nausea, unsteadiness, **photophobia**, blurred or double vision, loss of emotional control, or mental status changes) associated with exertion is abnormal. If a possible intracranial injury has not yet been determined, the following tests can be performed:

- 40-yard sprint
- Five jumping jacks
- Five sit-ups
- Five push-ups
- Five knee bends

Management

Subsequent to the assessment, the coach must make a determination as to the appropriate course of action. The possibility exists for several scenarios in response to findings. If at any point during or following the assessment, sign and symptoms of a serious head injury become apparent, the coach should activate the emergency action plan, including summoning EMS. While waiting for EMS to arrive, the coach should

- Check airway, breathing, and circulation. If necessary, perform rescue breathing and CPR.
- Monitor the individual. Regardless of any complaints by the individual, the coach should not administer any medication.

In some cases, it may be determined that signs and symptoms do not warrant summoning of EMS, but immediate referral to a physician or an emergency medical facility is necessary. In these scenarios, the emergency action plan should be appropriately followed regarding contact of parents/guardians (if necessary) and method of transport to the medical facility (i.e., who will be responsible for driving the individual to the medical facility).

In some instances, it may be determined that while potential signs of a concussion are present, the injury appears to be mild and there are insufficient indicators to suggest the need for immediate referral to a physician (e.g., mild headache in the absence of other symptoms; individual initially appears stunned and dazed, but otherwise is asymptomatic). In these scenarios, for the period of time that individual continues to be under the care of the coach, a system must is in place that will allow for the continued observation and monitoring of the individual. The individual should not be left alone under any circumstances. A reassessment should be completed every 5 to 10 minutes. If their condition starts to deteriorate, the original decision for handling the situation must be reexamined.

Prior to sending home an individual who may have experienced signs and symptoms of concussion, the coach should provide an instruction sheet to the individual. The sheet should provide a list of signs and symptoms which would necessitate that the individual seek immediate medical attention (Box 9.2). In addition, the sheet could provide information on use of medication, rest, eating and performance of activities of daily living (ADLs). This instruction sheet should be approved by a qualified healthcare provider prior to distribution. If the individual is of age, it's advisable for the individual to give a copy of the document to a friend or roommate who could follow up on their condition. If the individual is a minor, the sheet should be given to their parent/guardian. In the case of a minor, the parent/guardian should always be informed of any trauma (direct or indirect) to the head.

BOX 9.2	Information Sheet on Follow-up Care for a Head Injury

_____ (Name)_____ sustained a head injury during __ (event)_____. It does not appear to be serious at this time. However, in many cases, signs and symptoms from a head injury do not become apparent until hours after the initial trauma. As such, we want to alert you to appropriate guidelines to follow for the next 24 hours. For the rest of the day _____(Name)_____ should

- **Rest quietly for at least 24 hours.**
- **Consume a liquid diet for the next 8 to 24 hours. Avoid spicy foods.**
- **Apply ice to the head and neck as needed for comfort.**
- **Use acetaminophen (e.g., Tylenol) for headaches. Do not use aspirin or other medication without a physician's approval.**
- **Not consume alcohol or drive a vehicle.**

Have someone awaken the individual every 2 hours during the next 24 hours. If any of the following signs or symptoms are observed, medical help should be sought immediately:

- **Persistent or increasing headache, particularly if it becomes localized or persists after 48 hours**
- **Persistent or increasing nausea and/or vomiting**

- **Mental confusion, disorientation, irritability, or forgetfulness that gets progressively worse**
- **Loss of appetite**
- **Drowsiness, lethargy, sleepiness, or difficulty in awakening**
- **Any visual difficulties, dizziness, or ringing in the ears**
- **Unequal pupil size; slow or no pupil reaction to light**
- **Bleeding and/or clear fluid from the nose or ears**
- **Progressive or sudden impairment of consciousness**
- **Alterations in breathing pattern or irregular heartbeat**
- **Difficulty speaking or slurring of speech**
- **Convulsions or tremors**

____(Name)_____ should not participate in physical activity without medical clearance by a doctor.

Emergency Phone Numbers:

Ambulance 911
Hospital _____

Remember: If any of the symptoms or signs listed in the preceding becomes apparent, medical treatment should be sought immediately.

Return to Play

If an individual experiences any signs or symptoms of a concussion, the person should be removed from activity. The person should not be permitted to return to activity that day. In fact, the individual should not be permitted to return to activity until having been seen and released by an appropriate healthcare professional. The medical release should be in written form and include parameters for returning to play and discontinuing play.

Ultimately, the decision for RTP is based on a variety of factors. In fact, a concussion is often best diagnosed and managed by a team of healthcare providers bringing their expertise to the situation (e.g., family or general practitioner; neurologist; pediatrician, athletic trainer). RTP is a decision that must be made on a case-by-case basis.

In general, RTP is progressive in nature. Following an established period of being symptom-free at rest, the individual is required to complete a series of exertional tests. If the individual becomes symptomatic, the testing should be stopped and RTP is not to be permitted. If the individual remains symptom-free during and after the testing, gradual return to sport-specific activities that are void of any contact may be initiated. In this phase, the activities must be deliberately selected and performance monitored at all times.

FACIAL INJURIES

Eye Injuries

The eyes are exposed daily to potential trauma and injury. Trauma can range in severity from mild to severe with complications. The coach should be able to recognize "red flags" that indicate a potentially serious injury that warrants immediate referral to an appropriate healthcare provider (Box 9.3).

The incidence of eye injuries can be reduced by wearing protective eyewear. Protective eyewear and/or face masks should be worn during participation in any sport or physical activity with a high risk of injury to the eye. For example, racquetball, whether played at a professional or recreational level, involves players confined to a limited space with swinging racquets and balls traveling at high speeds. The potential for eye injury in such an environment is extremely high in the absence of proper protection.

There are three types of protective eye wear: goggles, face shields, and spectacles. Goggles have two designs. One is the eyecup design seen in swimming, which completely covers the eye socket. These goggles are made of hard, impact-resistant plastic that is water-tight. The other style can be worn over spectacles, such as a ski goggle. These goggles are usually well ventilated to allow air currents to minimize fogging. Face shields are secondary protective devices that can

---

BOX 9.3	**Eye "Red Flags" Requiring Further Examination by a Physician**

- **Visual disturbances or loss of vision**
- **Unequal pupils or bilateral, dilated pupils**
- **Irregular eye movement or failure to accommodate to light**
- **Severe ecchymosis and swelling (raccoon eyes)**
- **Suspected corneal abrasion or corneal laceration**
- **Blood in the anterior chamber**
- **Embedded foreign body**
- **Individual complaining of floaters, light flashes, or a "curtain falling over the eye"**
- **Itching, burning, watery eye that appears pink**
- **Displaced contact lens that cannot be removed easily**

be attached to specific helmets. Individuals who wear contact lenses often prefer the shield, because there is less chance that a finger or hand can hit the eye. The shield can be tinted to reduce glare from the sun; however, the plastic can become scratched and may fog up in cold weather. Spectacles (eye glasses) contain the lenses, frames, and side shields commonly seen in industrial eye protective wear. The lenses and frames should meet industry standards—these standards are available through an optician.

Any individual with monocular vision or vision in only one eye should consult an ophthalmologist before participating in any sport or physical activity because of the reduced visual fields and depth perception. If a decision is made to participate, the individual should follow the instructions of the ophthalmologist concerning appropriate protection.

Hemorrhage into the Anterior Chamber

Hemorrhage into the anterior chamber (**hyphema**) usually results from blunt trauma from a small ball (squash or racquetball), hockey puck, stick (field hockey or ice hockey), or swinging racquet (squash or racquetball). The small size of the object can fit within the confines of the eye orbit, thereby inflicting direct damage to the eye.

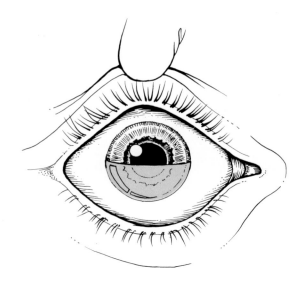

FIGURE 9.13 Hyphema. Blood in the anterior chamber of the eye signals a serious eye injury.

Signs and Symptoms

Initially, a red tinge in the anterior chamber may be present, but within a few hours, blood begins to settle into the anterior chamber (FIG. 9.13). Other possible symptoms include pain in the injured eye and visual disturbances (e.g., blurred vision).

Management

A hyphema can be a medical emergency. The individual should be referred to an ophthalmologist for an immediate appointment. If an ophthalmologist is not available for an immediate appointment, the individual should be referred to an emergency medical facility.

Detached Retina

The retina, a layer of tissue which lines the inside of the eye, sends messages to the brain via the optic nerve. If a retina detaches, it has been displaced from its normal position. A **detached retina** can occur at any age, but it is more common in people over the age of 40. It can be due to trauma or several eye diseases/disorders (e.g., degenerative myopia).

Signs and Symptoms

The classic symptoms of retinal detachment are seeing "floaters" (i.e., specks that float in the visual field) and/or light flashes. The individual frequently describes the condition with phrases like, "A curtain fell over my eye," or "I keep seeing flashes of light going on and off."

Management

The individual should be referred to an ophthalmologist for an immediate appointment. If an ophthalmologist is not available for an immediate appointment, the individual should be referred to an emergency medical facility.

Periorbital Ecchymosis (Black Eye)

A "black eye" is a relatively common injury that results from a blow to the eye. The accumulation of blood and other fluids in the interstitial spaces around the eye produce the characteristic discoloration or "black eye." Most black eyes are minor injuries. However, it is essential that a complete ocular examination be performed to rule out an underlying fracture or injury to the globe.

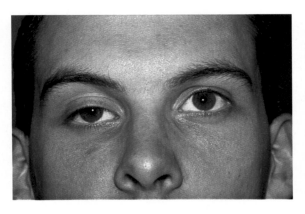

FIGURE 9.14 Orbital "blowout" fracture. An orbital fracture can entrap the inferior rectus muscle, leading to an inability to elevate the eye.

Signs and Symptoms

Hemorrhage and swelling ranging from mild to severe accompanied by pain are characteristic of this condition. In some instances, there may be reports of blurred vision.

Management

Treatment involves controlling the swelling and hemorrhage by applying ice to the area. The use of chemical ice bags is discouraged as leakage of the bags contents would result in potentially serious injury. This condition requires referral to an ophthalmologist for further examination to rule out an underlying fracture or injury to the globe.

Orbital "Blowout" Fracture

Direct trauma to the eye from an object, usually larger than the eye orbit, can lead to a **blowout fracture**. Upon impact, forces drive the orbital contents posteriorly against the orbital walls. The force typically results in the area of least resistance, namely the orbital floor. In some cases, an increase in intraorbital pressure associated with the trauma is sufficient to produce a fracture.

Signs and Symptoms

This injury can present with a range of signs and symptoms. The individual could present with seemingly minor symptoms, such as mild swelling and ecchymosis. In other cases, the signs and symptoms could include **diplopia** (double vision), absent eye movement, numbness (hypoesthesia) of the cheek and gum of the involved side, and a recessed, downward displaced globe. The lack of eye movement becomes evident when the individual is asked to look up and only one eye is able to move (Fig. 9.14).

Management

The immediate management of this injury involves limiting the swelling by applying ice to the area without applying pressure over the suspected fracture site. The individual should immediately be referred to an emergency medical facility. A complete ocular examination is necessary to determine any damage to the globe or the ocular nerve.

Conjunctivitis (Pinkeye)

Conjunctivitis is an inflammation of the conjunctiva, the membrane between the inner lining of the eyelid and anterior eyeball. There are several possible causes of conjunctivitis, including viral infection, bacterial infection, allergy, and environmental irritants. Conjunctivitis caused by a virus is a highly contagious condition.

Signs and Symptoms

Itching, burning, and watering of the eye causes the conjunctiva to become inflamed and red. It gives a "pinkeye" appearance. Another classic symptom is that eyelids appear stuck together upon waking up after sleeping.

Management

As soon as signs and symptoms are evident, precaution should be taken to avoid contact with the other eye and other people to prevent the spread of the infection. This condition requires immediate referral to a physician to ensure accurate assessment and appropriate treatment.

Subconjunctival Hemorrhage

The conjunctiva have several small capillaries that are barely visible. These blood vessels have the potential to become irritated and rupture. A specific cause of the condition is not typically readily apparent. Potential causes include the strain associated with coughing, sneezing, or vomiting. In most cases, the individual does not realize that the condition is present until looking in a mirror or having another person observe a red area on the sclera (i.e., white of the eye).

Signs and Symptoms

The classic sign of this injury is the appearance of a bright red area over the sclera. Otherwise, the condition is asymptomatic. In spite of its pronounced appearance, the condition is relatively harmless.

Management

This condition requires no treatment and resolves spontaneously in 1 to 3 weeks. However, if there is blurred vision, pain, limited eye movement, blood in the anterior chamber, or other abnormalities, immediate referral to an ophthalmologist is warranted.

Foreign Bodies

Foreign bodies can enter the eye for a variety of reasons. For example, an eyelash call move into the eye or debris can blow into the eye. Depending of the actual substance, damage to the structures of the eye may or may not occur.

Signs and Symptoms

Signs and symptoms will vary depending on the actual substance. Typical symptoms include burning, irritation, tearing, and redness. Occasionally, a foreign body scratches the cornea, resulting in a sudden onset of pain, tearing, and photophobia. Blinking and movement of the eye only aggravate the condition. Examination may not reveal a foreign object, but the individual continues to complain that something is in the eye.

Management

In minor situations, rinsing the eye is normally sufficient for removing the foreign body. While saline is preferable, water can be used to flush the eye. If rinsing the eye is not successful, using a gauze pad or the tip of a cotton swab is the next option for removing the object. In cases involving a large piece of debris or debris that is sharp in nature, it is not typically advisable to remove the body. Rather, the individual should be taken immediately to an emergency medical care facility. If a corneal abrasion is suspected, the individual should be referred to an ophthalmologist or an appropriate medical facility.

Nasal Injuries

The nose can be vulnerable to injury during sports and physical activity that involve contact and do not require facial protection. Box 9.4 identifies the signs and symptoms of nasal conditions that warrant further examination by a physician.

Fractures

Fractures to the nasal bone are the most common facial fracture in sport. Blunt trauma is the leading mechanism of injury with lateral forces producing the greatest amount of visible deformity.

Signs and Symptoms

Bleeding is usually profuse, and the nose may appear flattened and lose its symmetry, particularly if a lateral force caused the fracture. Swelling is rapid. The nasal airway can be obstructed

---

BOX 9.4	**Nasal "Red Flags" Requiring Further Examination by a Physician**

- **Bleeding or CSF from the nose**
- **Loss of smell**
- **Nasal deformity or fracture**
- **Nosebleeds that do not stop within 5 minutes**
- **Foreign objects that cannot be removed easily**

with bony fragments, or the fracture can extend into the cranial region and cause a loss of CSF. There may be crepitus over the nasal bridge and ecchymosis under the eyes. Severity can range from a slightly depressed greenstick fracture (seen in adolescents) to total displacement or disruption in the bony and cartilaginous parts of the nose.

Management

Treatment involves controlling the swelling and hemorrhage by applying ice and, if tolerable, mild pressure to the area. This condition requires immediate referral to a physician to ensure accurate assessment and appropriate treatment.

Epistaxis (Nosebleed)

A nosebleed, or **epistaxis**, occurs when superficial blood vessels on the anterior septum are lacerated. Common causes of epistaxis include direct trauma, nasal infection, and dry nasal membranes due to prolonged inhalation of dry air. Because the nose is rich in blood vessels, bleeding can range from mild to profuse often dependent on the cause.

Management

In most cases, bleeding stops suddenly by applying mild pressure at the nasal bone. Ice may be applied to stop more persistent bleeding. The head should be tilted slightly forward to reduce the risk of blood traveling down the oropharynx. A nasal plug (rolled gauze) may be used to assist in clotting. However, if used, the plug should protrude from the nostrils at least 1/2 inch to facilitate removal. If bleeding continues for more than 10 minutes despite manual pressure and ice, the individual should be referred to a physician. The individual should be instructed to avoid blowing their nose following a nosebleed, as the forces could restart the bleeding.

Facial Injuries

Injuries to the cheek, nose, lips, and jaw are common in sports and physical activities with moving projectiles (e.g., racquets, bats, or balls), in contact sports (e.g., football, rugby, or ice hockey), or in sports involving collisions with objects (e.g., diving, skiing, hockey, or swimming). In some cases, facial injuries can be prevented by wearing properly fitted face masks and mouth guards; however, in many cases, face masks are not appropriate for the activity. Box 9.5 identifies signs and symptoms of facial conditions that necessitate further examination by a physician.

Fractures

Fractures to the upper or lower jaw caused by direct trauma occur more often in collision activities. The lower jaw, or mandible, is particularly susceptible to fracture at the jaw's frontal angle because of its limited padding and sharp contour.

Signs and Symptoms

Mandibular or jaw fractures seldom occur as an isolated single fracture, but rather occur as a double fracture or fracture-dislocation (FIG. 9.15). **Malocclusion** is the classic sign. Because the

---

BOX 9.5	Facial "Red Flags" Requiring Further Examination by a Physician

- **Obvious deformity or crepitus**
- **Appearance of a long face**
- **Increased pain on palpation**
- **Irregular eye movement or failure to accommodate to light**
- **Malocclusion of the teeth**

articulation of words is impossible, changes in speech are apparent. Oral bleeding may occur even though a mouthguard is properly fitted and worn.

If the upper jaw, or maxilla, is fractured, the maxilla may be mobile, giving the appearance of a longer face. Nasal bleeding is also commonly seen. With direct impact forces, a fracture to the zygomatic arch (cheek bone) may result in the cheek appearing flat or depressed. Swelling and ecchymosis around the eye may occlude vision and hide damage to the eye orbit. Occasionally, the eye on the side of the fracture may appear sunken in, or the eye opposite the fracture may appear to be raised. Double vision is common, and numbness may be present on the affected cheek.

Management

If a fracture is suspected, the individual should be referred to an emergency medical facility. Prior to transport, the immediate treatment involves controlling the swelling and hemorrhage by applying ice and, if tolerable, mild pressure to the area.

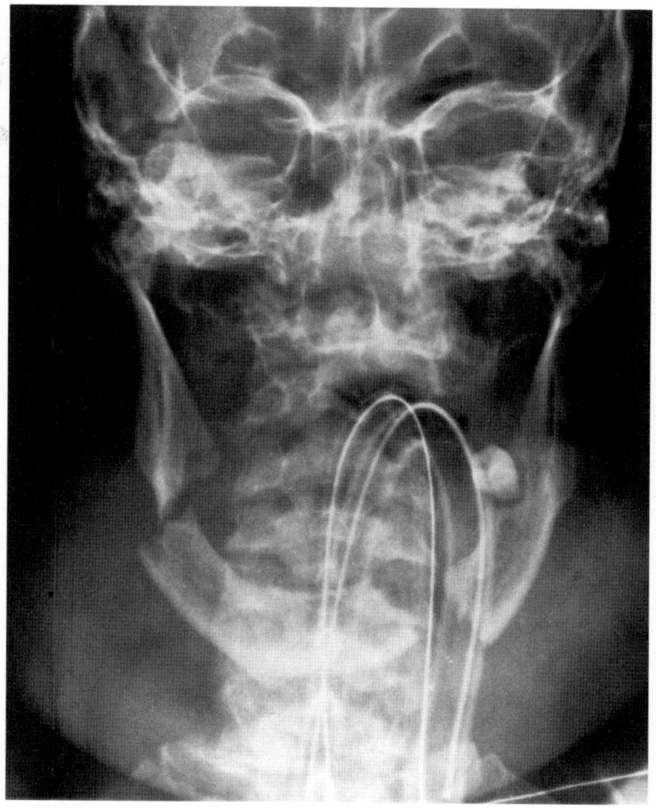

Oral and Dental Injuries

Any force great enough to cause a tooth fracture or loose teeth can also cause a jaw fracture or even a concussion. Therefore, an assessment of the individual's overall condition should be conducted to ensure that one is only dealing with an isolated tooth injury. BOX 9.6 identifies signs and symptoms of oral and dental conditions that necessitate further examination by a physician.

FIGURE 9.15 Mandibular fracture. The most common site for a mandibular fracture is near the angle of the jaw, which leads to malocclusion of the teeth.

For sport participants, nearly all dental injuries are preventable through regular use of mouth protectors. Although certain sports (e.g., football, boxing, field hockey, and lacrosse) require mouthguards, few coaches or league officials require the devices in other contact and collision sports (e.g., basketball).

Properly fitted across the upper teeth, a mouthguard can absorb energy, disperse impact, cushion contact between the upper and lower teeth, and keep the upper lip away from the incisal edges of the teeth. This action significantly reduces dental and oral soft tissue injuries, and to a lesser extent jaw fractures, cerebral concussions, and TMJ injuries. The practice of cutting down mouthguards to cover only the front four teeth invalidates the manufacturer's warranty, cannot prevent many dental injuries, and can lead to airway obstruction if the mouthguard becomes dislodged.

BOX 9.6 Oral and Dental "Red Flags" Requiring Further Examination by a Physician

- Lacerations involving the lip, outer border of the lip, or tongue
- Loose teeth either laterally displaced, intruded, or extruded
- Chipped, cracked, fractured, or dislodged teeth
- Any individual complaining of persistent toothache or sensitivity to heat and cold
- Inability to close the jaw
- Malocclusion of the teeth

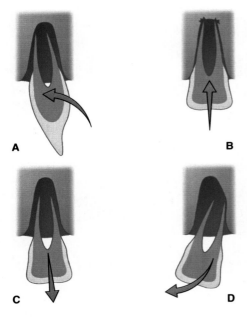

FIGURE 9.16 Loose teeth. Loose teeth may involve (**A**) partial displacement, (**B**) intrusion, (**C**) extrusion, or (**D**) avulsion.

A frequently used mouthguard is the thermal set, mouth-formed mouthguard, which consists of a firm outer shell fitted with a softer inner material. The softer material is thermally or chemically set after being molded to the player's teeth. When properly fitted, the mouth-formed guard can virtually match the efficacy and comfort of the custom-made guard. This type of guard is readily available, inexpensive, and has a loop strap for attachment to a face mask. The loop strap has two advantages: it prevents individuals from choking on the mouthguard, and it prevents the individual from losing the mouthguard.

Fractures

Any direct trauma to the upper or lower jaw can lead to fracture of one or more teeth. Fractures may occur through the enamel, dentin, pulp, or root of the tooth.

Signs and Symptoms

Fractures involving the enamel cause no symptoms and can be smoothed by the dentist to prevent further injury to the lips and inner lining of the oral cavity. Fractures extending into the dentin cause pain and increased sensitivity to cold and heat. Fractures exposing the pulp lead to severe pain and sensitivity.

Management

The individual should see a dentist within 24 hours of the incident.

Subluxated and Dislocated Teeth

The same mechanisms that cause tooth fractures can also lead to loosening (subluxation) or dislocation of a tooth.

Signs and Symptoms

A loosened tooth may be partially displaced, **intruded, extruded,** or avulsed (FIG. 9.16).

Management

If a tooth has been displaced outwardly or laterally, the coach can try to place the tooth back into its normal position without forcing it. Teeth that are intruded should be left alone; any attempt to move the tooth may result in permanent loss of the tooth or damage to any underlying permanent teeth. The individual should be referred to a dentist immediately.

A tooth that has been avulsed from its socket can sometimes be saved, but time is of the essence. When the tooth is located, it should be held by the crown to minimize damage to the ligament cells on the root surface. The tooth should be rinsed with saline, milk, or water. It is important not to rub the tooth or remove any dirt. If the individual or coach feels comfortable attempting to replant the tooth, such an attempt can be made. Otherwise, the tooth should be stored in saline, milk, or saliva for immediate transport with the individual to the dentist. If the tooth is replaced within 30 minutes, the prognosis for successful replanting is 90%. Implantation that occurs after 2 hours is usually unsuccessful. The product Save-A-Tooth® is an FDA-approved product that has produced positive outcomes in the management of dislocated teeth. The product provides an environment that can preserve and protect the tooth for several hours.

Ear Injuries

Several conditions can affect the ear. Except for boxing, wrestling, and water polo, specialized ear protection is uncommon. Box 9.7 identifies signs and symptoms of ear conditions that necessitate further examination by a physician.

Auricular Hematoma (Cauliflower Ear)

Auricular hematoma, or **"cauliflower ear,"** is a relatively minor injury caused when repeated blunt trauma pulls the cartilage away from the perichondrium (FIG. 9.17). A hematoma forms between the perichondrium and cartilage of the ear and compromises blood supply to

---

BOX 9.7 **Ear "Red Flags" Requiring Further Examination by a Physician**

- Bleeding or CSF from the ear canal
- Bleeding or swelling behind the ear (**Battle's sign**)
- Hematoma or swelling that removes the creases of the outer ear
- Tinnitus or hearing impairment
- Feeling of fullness in the ear; vertigo
- Foreign body in ear that cannot be easily removed
- "Popping" or itching in the ear
- Pain when the ear lobe is pulled

---

the cartilage. This condition, which is common in wrestling and rugby, can be prevented by wearing proper headgear.

Signs and Symptoms

Initially, pain, burning, or a throbbing sensation to the area may be reported subsequent to a single traumatic incidence or repeated trauma. Swelling to the area may also be evident. If left untreated, the condition results in a permanent deformity of the outer ear that resembles a cauliflower.

Management

Immediate treatment involves icing the region to reduce pain and swelling. An ice pack should be applied for 20 minutes. If the swelling is still present, the hematoma must be aspirated by a physician to avoid pressure and permanent cartilage damage. Protective headgear should be worn to prevent recurrence.

Internal Ear Injury

A blow to the ear, environmental events, pressure changes (seen in diving and scuba diving), and infection can injure the eardrum. Although typically seen in water sports, damage to the internal ear can occur in any sport, such as in soccer, when a player is hit on the ear by a ball.

Signs and Symptoms

When the injury is caused by a direct blow to the ear, symptoms include intense pain in the ear, a feeling of fullness in the ear, nausea, tinnitus, dizziness, and potential hearing loss.

Management

The presence of any of the noted symptoms warrants immediate referral to a physician. Ultimately, the cause of the injury will determine the appropriate treatment (e.g., antibiotic for infection; surgical repair for significant rupture of the eardrum). Most minor ruptures of the eardrum will heal spontaneously.

Swimmer's Ear

Swimmer's ear (**otitis externa**) is a bacterial infection involving the lining of the external auditory canal. It frequently occurs in individuals who do not dry the canal after being in water, resulting in a change of the pH of the ear canal's skin.

Signs and Symptoms

In acute conditions, pain is the predominant symptom. In chronic cases, itching is a more common symptom, and discomfort and pain are secondary. Gentle pressure around the external auditory

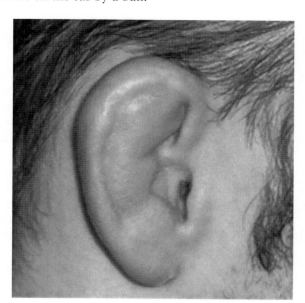

FIGURE 9.17 Cauliflower ear deformity. The hematoma results in the skin being pulled away from the ear cartilage.

opening and pulling on the pinna (outer ear) causes increased pain. If left untreated, the infection can spread to the middle ear, causing balance disturbances or hearing loss.

Management

While eardrops have been effective in treating this condition, physician referral is warranted to ensure accurate assessment of the condition. Eardrops should contain an acidifying agent, either aluminum acetate or vinegar. An effective home remedy is equal parts of white vinegar (acetic acid), 70% alcohol, and water. One or two drops after water exposure or after showering is the standard recommendation. Commercial earplugs do not always help prevent the condition. Custom earplugs from an audiologist or otolaryngologist may be necessary. The condition can also be prevented by using eardrops to dry the canal.

SUMMARY

1. Wearing protective equipment can significantly reduce the incidence and severity of head and facial injuries.

2. Signs that indicate a possible skull fracture include deformity; unequal pupils; discoloration around both eyes or behind the ears; bleeding or CSF leaking from the nose and/or ear; and any loss of sight or smell.

3. Cranial injuries are classified as focal (localized damage) (e.g., epidural hematoma; subdural hematoma; cerebral concussion) and diffuse (widespread damage) (e.g., concussion).

4. Signs or symptoms of increasing intracranial pressure following head trauma include severe headache; pupil irregularity or irregular eye tracking; confusion or progressive or sudden impairment of consciousness; rising blood pressure and falling pulse rate; and drastic changes in emotional control. These injuries require immediate physician referral by summoning EMS.

5. Signs and symptoms of a concussion include vacant stare; visual problems; headache or pressure in the head; delayed verbal and motor responses; confusion and inability to focus attention; disorientation; slurred or incoherent speech gross observable incoordination with balance; emotions out of proportion to circumstances; memory deficits; and any period of loss of consciousness.

6. Coaches, physical educators, and fitness specialists are often the first respondent in an injury situation. As such, these individuals must have a clear understanding of their roles and responsibilities in the prevention, assessment, and management of concussion.

7. A coach should not permit RTP following any signs or symptoms of a concussive injury. Rather, the coach should require the individual to be seen and released by an appropriate health care professional.

8. In addition to concussion, diffuse cerebral injuries include posttraumatic headaches, postconcussion syndrome, and second impact syndrome. These injuries should not be overlooked as each can have catastrophic consequences if unrecognized and mismanaged.

9. Direct trauma to the eye can lead to a corneal laceration, rupture of the globe, hemorrhage into the anterior chamber, detached retina, or an orbital fracture. Loss of visual acuity, abnormal eye movement, diplopia, numbness below the eye, or a downward displacement of the globe should signal a serious condition. The individual should be referred to an ophthalmologist immediately.

10. Fractures to the facial bones often result in malocclusion.

11. The nose is particularly susceptible to lateral displacement from trauma. Simultaneously, the trauma may also lead to a concussion.

12. Teeth that are intruded should be left alone; any attempt to move the tooth may result in permanent loss of the tooth. The individual should be referred to a dentist immediately.

13. A dislocated tooth should be located, held by the crown, rinsed in milk or a saline solution, and stored in saline, milk, or saliva for immediate transport with the individual to the dentist. The individual should be seen by a dentist within 30 minutes for replacement of the tooth.

14. Cauliflower ear, resulting from a hematoma between the perichondrium and cartilage of the ear, is completely preventable by wearing proper headgear.

15. Otitis externa is a bacterial infection involving the lining of the external auditory canal, commonly called "swimmer's ear." Otitis media is a localized infection of the middle ear.

APPLICATION QUESTIONS

1. A high school athletic director (AD) is faced with making budget cuts. The AD requests justification for purchasing mouthguards for teams other than football (i.e. soccer, basketball, lacrosse, field hockey). Provide rationale for ensuring that athletes in any sport which involves contact should be provided with mouthguards.

   _____

   _____

2. During a physical education class, a third-grade student using a scooter board accidently collides into the bleachers. In approaching the student, the physical education teacher notices bleeding from the scalp. Explain the immediate management of this injury.

   _____

   _____

3. While driving toward the basket, a basketball player is undercut. She falls sideways and strikes her head sharply on the floor. The individual complains of an intense headache, disorientation, and blurred vision. Do these signs and symptoms indicate that a skull fracture may be present? Explain your response.

   _____

   _____

4. After colliding with another player, a lacrosse player is lying down on the field complaining of a headache and dizziness. Following 15 minutes of ice application to the region, the individual complains of increasing headache, dizziness, and nausea. There is also increased mental confusion. What do these symptoms indicate? How should this injury be managed?

   _____

   _____

5. During a practice session, a high school rugby player comes off the field complaining of sustaining a blow to the head. The coach is the only adult available to assess the athlete. Explain an appropriate assessment by the coach in the evaluation of a potential concussion.

   _____

   _____

6. Following an assessment of a potential concussion sustained by a sixth-grade student during intramural basketball, the physical education teacher determines that the injury appears to be mild and there is no need for immediate referral to a physician. Does the physical education teacher need to take any additional action? Explain your response.

   _____

   _____

7. During a high school physical education class, two students inadvertently collide during a soccer activity. One of the students makes the statement that he "was momentarily stunned and saw stars." He also reports blurred vision that resolves in about 30 seconds. In order to monitor the student's condition, the physical education teacher instructs the students to remain next to him as the class continues. After 3 or 4 minutes, the individual reports feeling much better except for a slight headache. He indicates that he wants to participate in the activity. Can this individual return to activity?

   _____

   _____

8. A hockey player was taking a shot on goal when the stick hit the jaw of the player guarding him. The player comes off the ice bleeding from the mouth and unable to close the jaw. The player is having difficulty

articulating his words. Explain palpation of this condition. What type of injury should be suspected and why?

_____

_____

9. A basketball player received a lateral blow to the nose from an opposing player's elbow. The nose is bleeding and has a flattened appearance. What signs and symptoms indicate that this individual needs to be referred immediately to a physician?

_____

_____

10. Following a collision during a high school soccer game, an athlete complains of significant pain after being hit in the mouth. The inside of the upper lip is bleeding. One tooth is intruded. How should the coach manage this injury?

_____

_____

11. A wrestler was not wearing protective headgear during practice. He is now complaining about a burning, aching sensation on the outer ear. In inspecting the ear, the coach notices that the area is somewhat inflamed and sensitive to touch, but no swelling is apparent. How should the coach manage this situation? What signs might indicate a more serious problem?

_____

_____

12. While moving through the circuit training area in an exercise facility, an adult exerciser received a significant blow to the eye from another individual's elbow. What signs and symptoms indicate a serious condition?

_____

_____

REFERENCES

1. Ghiselli G, Schaadt G, and McAllister DR. 2003. On-the-field evaluation of an athlete with a head or neck injury. Clin Sports Med, 22(3):445–465.
2. Logan SM, Bell GW, and Leonard JC. 2001. Acute subdural hematoma in a high school football player after 2 unreported episodes of head trauma: A case report. J Ath Train, 36(4):433–436.
3. Putukian M, and Madden CC. Head injuries. In _The team physician's handbook_, edited by MB Mellion, et al. Philadelphia, PA: Hanley & Belfus, Inc., 2002.
4. Langlois JA, Rutland-Brown W, and Wald M. 2006. The epidemiology and impact of traumatic brain injury: A brief overview. J Head Trauma Rehabil, 21(5):375–378.
5. Gessel LM, et al. 2007. Concussions among United States high school and collegiate athletes. J Ath Train, 42(4):495–503.
6. Aubry M, Cantu RC, Dvorak J, et al. 2002. Summary and agreement statement of the First International Conference on Concussion in Sport, Vienna 2001: Recommendations for the improvement of safety and health of athletes who may suffer concussive injuries. Phys Sportsmed, 30(2):57–63.
7. McCrory P, Johnston K, Meeuwisse W, et al. 2005. Summary and agreement statement of the Second International Conference on Concussion in Sport, Prague 2004. Phys Sportsmed, 33(4):29–44.
8. Quality Standards Subcommittee of the American Academy of Neurology. 1997. Practice parameter: the management of concussion in sports. Neurology, 48(3): 581–585.
9. Cantu RC. 2001. Posttraumatic retrograde and anterograde amnesia: pathophysiology and implications in grading and safe return to play. J Ath Train, 36(3):244–248.
10. Bailes JE, and Hudson V. Classification of sport-related head trauma: a spectrum of mild to severe injury. J Ath Train, 36(3): 236–243.

CHAPTER

10

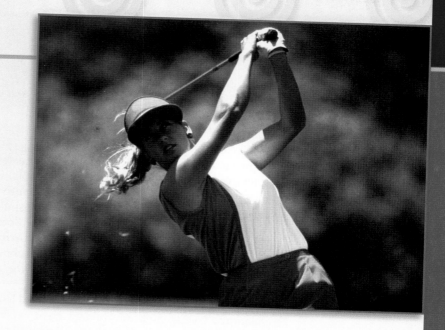

SPINAL CONDITIONS

LEARNING OUTCOMES

1. Explain the functional significance of the bony and soft tissue structures of the spine.

2. Describe the motion capabilities of the spine.

3. Identify the factors that contribute to mechanical loading on the spine.

4. Identify anatomical variations that can predispose individuals to cervical, thoracic, and lumbar injuries.

5. Explain general principles used to prevent injury to the spine.

6. Describe common injuries and conditions sustained by physically active individuals in the cervical, thoracic, and lumbar regions, including their sign, symptoms and immediate management.

7. Describe an on-site assessment of an acute spinal condition appropriate for use by a coach.

KEY TERMS (CONTINUED)

prolapsed disc	sciatica	spondylolisthesis
reflex	scoliosis	Valsalva maneuver

The spine is a complex linkage system that transfers loads between the upper and lower extremities, enables motion of the trunk in all three planes, and protects the delicate spinal cord. Most injuries to the neck and upper back are relatively minor, consisting of contusions, muscle strains, and ligament sprains. However, acute spinal fractures and dislocations in this region are extremely serious and can lead to paralysis or death. Sports-related cervical injuries account for 27% of all spinal cord injuries annually occurring in children, with the most common victim being an older adolescent male, and the most commonly involved sport being football.[1] Prompt and accurate on-site assessment is essential for optimizing the outcomes of these potentially devastating injuries.[2]

Low back pain (LBP) is a widespread problem that affects both the athletic and non-athletic populations. Nearly 30% of children have experienced LBP at some time, with the incidence increasing with age until about age 16, when the adult incidence of 75 to 80% is reached.[3] Low back pain is more common in boys than in girls, and is associated with increased physical activity and stronger back flexor muscles.[4,5] Although the main causes of LBP in athletes are musculotendinous strains and ligamentous sprains, chronic or recurring pain is often a symptom of degeneration of the lumbar discs or stress injuries to the bony articulations of the lumbar spine.[6] Pain emanating from the lumbar discs most commonly affects the low back, buttocks, and hips and may result from progressive damage to the annular fibers, and particularly the pain fibers that reside in the outer one third of the annulus.[7] Low back problems are especially common in equestrian sports, weightlifting, ice hockey, gymnastics, diving, football, wrestling, and aerobics.

This chapter begins with a review of the anatomy and the major actions of the spine. Identification of anatomical variations that may predispose individuals to cervical and thoracic spinal conditions leads into strategies used to prevent injury. Information, including signs, symptoms, and management, on common injuries sustained during participation in sport and physical activity is followed by a presentation of techniques than can be used by the coach in spinal injury assessment.

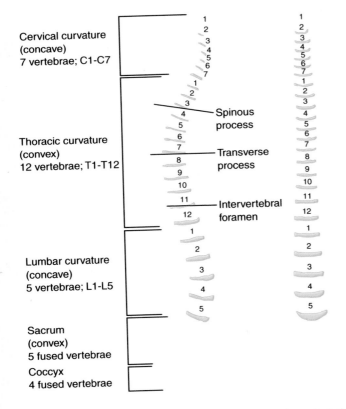

Cervical curvature
(concave)
7 vertebrae; C1-C7

Thoracic curvature
(convex)
12 vertebrae; T1-T12

Lumbar curvature
(concave)
5 vertebrae; L1-L5

Sacrum
(convex)
5 fused vertebrae

Coccyx
4 fused vertebrae

Spinous
process

Transverse
process

Intervertebral
foramen

FIGURE 10.1 The vertebral column. Four characteristic curves of the spine can be viewed from the lateral aspect.

ANATOMY OF THE SPINE

Vertebral Column

The five regions of the spine—namely, the cervical, thoracic, lumbar, sacral, and coccygeal regions—are structurally and functionally distinct. The spine includes four normal curves (FIG. 10.1). As viewed from the side, the thoracic and sacral curves are convex posteriorly, and the lumbar and cervical curves are concave posteriorly. These four curves constitute posture and can be modified by a host of factors, including heredity, disease, and forces acting on the spine.

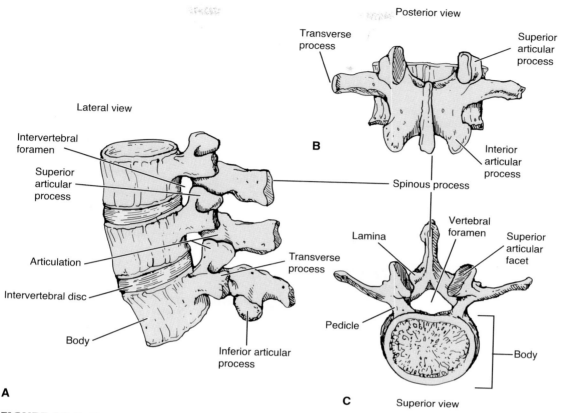

FIGURE 10.2 The structure of a typical vertebra. **A.** Lateral view. **B.** Posterior view. **C.** Superior view.

A typical vertebra consists of a body, a hollow ring known as the vertebral arch, and several bony processes (FIG. 10.2). The superior and inferior articular processes mate with the articular processes of adjacent vertebrae to form the **facet joints**. The right and left pedicles have notches on their superior and inferior borders that provide openings between adjacent pedicles and are called intervertebral foramina. The spinal nerves pass through these foramina. The spinous and transverse processes serve as handles for muscle attachments. Forming a stacked column, the neural arches, posterior sides of the bodies, and intervertebral discs form a protective passageway for the spinal cord and associated blood vessels. The thinnest part of the neural arch is called the pars interarticularis.

The cervical spine has seven vertebrae. The first cervical vertebra is called the atlas, because it bears the weight of the head. Articulating with the occipital condyles, the atlanto-occipital joint permits the nodding of the head (FIG. 10.3). The atlas does not have a body or a spinous process. Instead, it has anterior and posterior arches and a thick, lateral mass. The second cervical vertebra, or axis, is characterized by a tooth-like process called the dens or odontoid process, which projects upward from its body. This process is held in place against the inner surface of the atlas by the transverse ligament. This configuration allows the head to rotate and pivot on the neck. The transverse processes of the cervical vertebrae have a foramen (transverse foramen), through which the vertebral artery, vein, and a plexus of sympathetic nerves pass.

The thoracic spine includes 12 vertebrae. The thoracic vertebrae have extra facets (costal facets) on the transverse processes and the body for articulation with the ribs. The spinous processes of the thoracic vertebrae tend to be long and slender, and they direct markedly downward so that they overlap each other.

The lower spinal column includes five lumbar, five fused sacral, and four small, fused coccygeal vertebrae. The sacrum articulates with the ilium to form the sacroiliac (SI) joint.

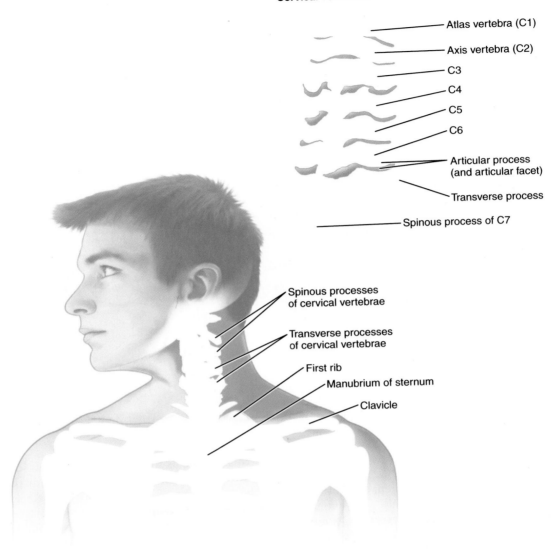

Cervical vertebrae

Atlas vertebra (C1)

Axis vertebra (C2)

C3

C4

C5

C6

Articular process
(and articular facet)

Transverse process

Spinous process of C7

Spinous processes
of cervical vertebrae

Transverse processes
of cervical vertebrae

First rib

Manubrium of sternum

Clavicle

FIGURE 10.3 Skeletal features of the cervical spine.

Vertebral size progressively increases from the cervical region down through the lumbar region. This serves a functional purpose, because when the body is in an upright position, each vertebra must support the weight of the trunk positioned above it as well as that of the arms and head. The size and angulation of the vertebral processes also vary throughout the spinal column. This changes the orientation of the facet joints, which limit range of motion (ROM) in the different spinal regions (FIG. 10.4).

Within the cervical, thoracic, and lumbar regions, any two adjacent vertebrae and the soft tissues between them are collectively referred to as a motion segment. The motion segment is referred to as the functional unit of the spine (FIG. 10.5).

Intervertebral Discs

Fibrocartilaginous discs provide cushioning between the articulating vertebral bodies. In the intervertebral disc, a thick ring of fibrous cartilage, the annulus fibrosus, surrounds a gelatinous material known as the nucleus pulposus. The discs have a dual function: they serve as shock absorbers

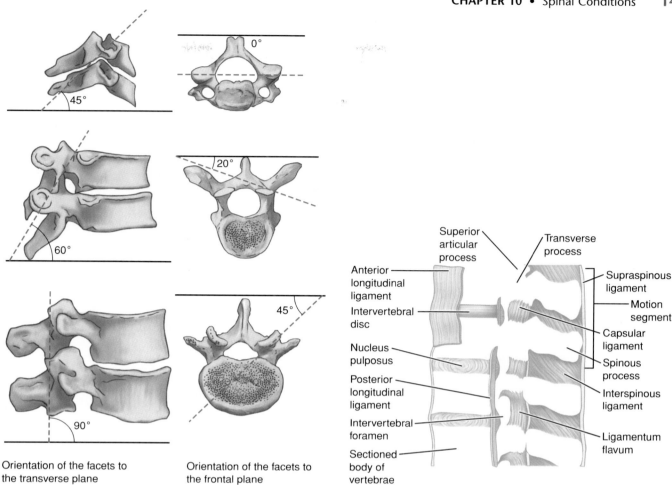

Orientation of the facets to the transverse plane

Orientation of the facets to the frontal plane

FIGURE 10.4 Approximate orientations of the facet joints. The facet joint orientation in both the sagittal plane (lateral view) and transverse plane (superior view) shifts progressively throughout the length of the spinal column. **A**. Cervical vertebrae (C3-C7). **B**. Thoracic vertebrae. **C**. Lumbar vertebrae.

FIGURE 10.5 Motion segment of the spine. A motion segment includes two adjacent vertebrae and the intervening soft tissues. It is considered the functional unit of the spine.

and allow the spine to bend. Because the discs receive no blood supply, they must rely on changes in posture and body position to produce a pumping action that brings in nutrients and flushes out metabolic waste products with an influx and outflux of fluid. Because maintaining a fixed body position curtails this pumping action, sitting in one position for a long period of time can negatively affect disc health.

Ligaments

Several strong ligaments support the spine and help stabilize the vertebrae (FIG. 10.6). Some ligaments (e.g., anterior and posterior longitudinal ligaments) connect the vertebral bodies of the motion segments; whereas, the supraspinous ligament attaches to the spinous processes throughout the length of the spine. The lumbar spine also contains several ligaments (e.g., iliolumbar ligaments, posterior SI ligament) that are responsible for maintaining its articulation with the sacrum.

Muscles

The muscles of the neck and trunk are paired, with one on the left and one on the right side of the body (FIG. 10.7). These muscles produce lateral flexion and/or rotation of the trunk when they act unilaterally and trunk flexion or extension when they act bilaterally.

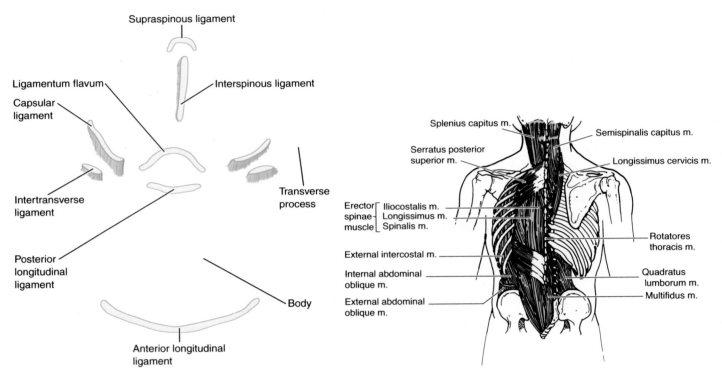

FIGURE 10.6 A superior view of the ligaments of the vertebral column.

FIGURE 10.7 Muscles of the spine.

Spinal Cord and Spinal Nerves

The brain and spinal cord make up the central nervous system. The spinal cord extends from the brain stem to the level of the first or second lumbar vertebrae. Like the brain, the spinal cord is encased in the three meninges. The spinal cord serves as the major neural pathway for conducting sensory impulses to the brain and motor impulses from the brain. It also provides direct connections between sensory and motor nerves inside the cord, enabling **reflex** activity. Reflex actions occur quickly, before the brain can process a sensory input and respond with an appropriate motor signal. An example of a reflex is removing a hand from a source of extreme heat through reflex action before the sensory information that the hand is being burned even reaches the brain.

Thirty-one pairs of spinal nerves emanate from the cord, including eight cervical, 12 thoracic, five lumbar, five sacral, and one coccygeal. A bundle of spinal nerves extends downward through the vertebral canal from the end of the spinal cord at the L1 to L2 level. This nerve bundle is known collectively as the **cauda equina**, after its resemblance to a horse's tail. Many of the spinal nerves converge (combine) and diverge (separate) to form a complex network of interjoining nerves, called a nerve plexus.

The Cervical Plexus

The cervical plexus consists of the spinal nerves C1 to C4. These nerves innervate muscles of the neck, shoulder, and the diaphragm (phrenic nerves C3 to C5) and supply sensation for the skin of the ear, neck, and upper chest.

The Brachial Plexus

The shoulder region and upper extremity receive sensory and motor innervation from the brachial plexus, which originates from the C5 through T1 nerve roots (FIG. 10.8). The nerve roots converge and diverge to form three trunks, followed by three divisions, then three cords. This complex structure terminates in distal branches that form the musculocutaneous, median, ulnar, axillary, and radial nerves, which innervate the arm, forearm, and hand.

The Lumbar Plexus

Supplying the anterior and medial muscles of the thigh region is the lumbar plexus, formed by the T12 through L5 nerve roots (FIG. 10.9). The posterior branches of the L2 through L4 nerve roots form the femoral nerve, innervating the quadriceps, whereas the anterior branches form the obturator nerve, innervating most of the adductor muscle group.

The Sacral Plexus

A portion of the lumbar plexus (L4, L5) forms the lumbosacral trunk and courses downward to form the upper portion of the sacral plexus. This plexus supplies the muscles of the buttock region and, through the sciatic nerve, the muscles of the posterior thigh and entire lower leg. The sciatic nerve is composed of two distinct nerves, the tibial nerve and common peroneal nerve.

Blood Vessels

The largest blood vessels coursing through the neck are the common carotid arteries. The common carotid arteries divide into external and internal carotid arteries, which provide the major blood supply to the brain, head, and face. The vertebral arteries, which are located in the posterior neck, are a source of blood supply for the spinal cord.

KINEMATICS AND MAJOR ACTIONS OF THE SPINE

Kinematics is the study of spatial and temporal aspects of motion, which translates to movement, form, or technique. Evaluation of the kinematics of a particular movement can provide information about timing and sequencing of movement, which can then yield important clues for injury prevention.

The vertebral joints enable motion in all planes of movement and also permit circumduction (FIGS. 10.10 and 10.11). The motion allowed between any two adjacent vertebrae is small. As such, spinal movements always involve a number of motion segments. The ROM allowed at each motion segment is governed by anatomical constraints that vary through the cervical, thoracic, and lumbar regions of the spine.

Flexion, Extension, and Hyperextension

Spinal flexion is anterior bending of the spine in the sagittal plane, with extension being the return to anatomical position from a position of flexion. The flexion/extension capability of the motion segments at different levels of the spine varies. When the spine is extended backward past anatomical position in the sagittal plane, the motion is termed hyperextension.

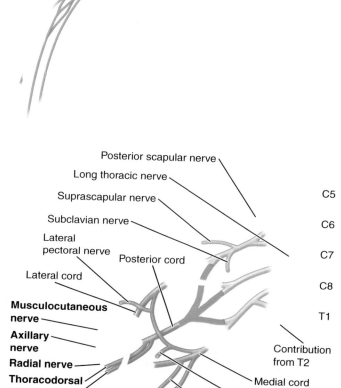

FIGURE 10.8 Brachial plexus. The brachial plexus is formed by the segmental nerves C₅ to T₁.

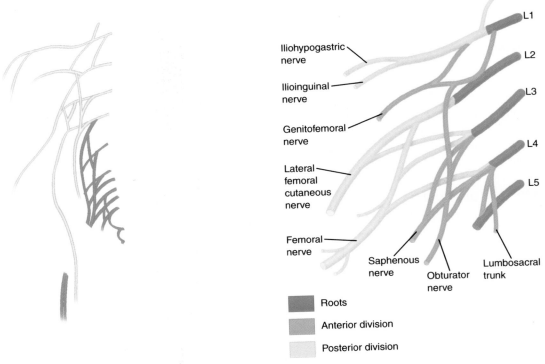

FIGURE 10.9 Lumbar plexus. The lumbar plexus is formed by the segmental nerves T$_{12}$ to L$_5$. The lower portion of the plexus merges with the upper portion of the sacral plexus to form the lumbosacral trunk.

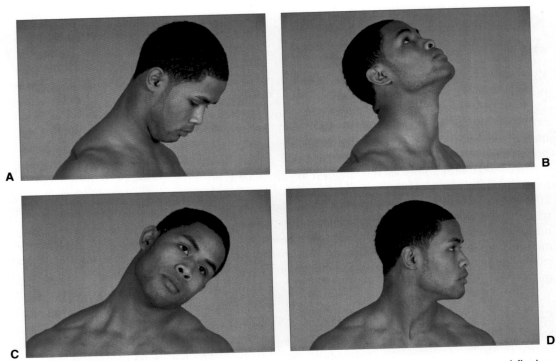

FIGURE 10.10 Active movements of the cervical spine. **A**. Flexion. **B**. Extension. **C**. Lateral flexion. **D**. Rotation.

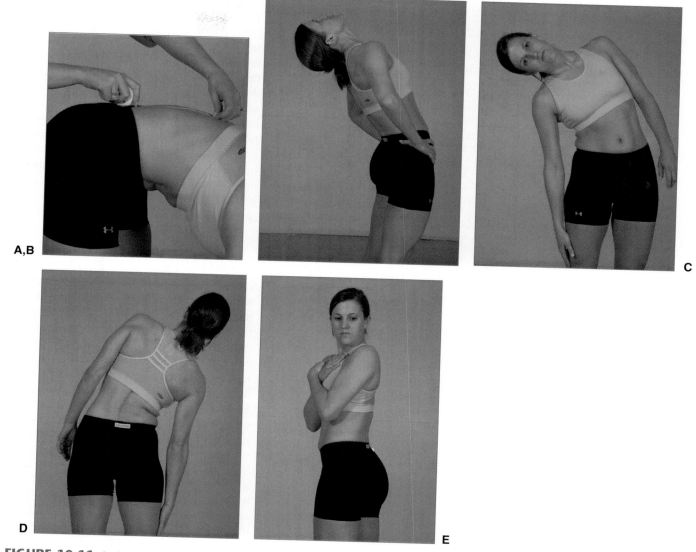

FIGURE 10.11 Active movements of the lumbar spine. **A**. Flexion. **B**. Extension. **C**. Lateral flexion. **D**. Rotation.

Lateral Flexion and Rotation

Movement of the spine away from anatomical position in a lateral direction in the frontal plane is termed lateral flexion. Rotation, which is movement around the longitudinal axis, produces a turning of the spine to the side (right or left).

ANATOMICAL VARIATIONS PREDISPOSING INDIVIDUALS TO SPINAL CONDITIONS

Excessive spinal **curvatures** can be congenital or acquired. Regardless of their cause, these conditions can be predisposing factors in the development of injuries or conditions related to the spine.

Kyphosis

Accentuation of the thoracic curve is called **kyphosis** (FIG. 10.12A) The cause of kyphosis can be congenital, **idiopathic** (unknown), or secondary to osteoporosis. Congenital kyphosis arises from deficits in the formation of either the vertebral bodies or the anterior and posterior vertebral elements. Idiopathic kyphosis, also known as Scheuermann's disease, or osteochondritis of the spine, is common among adolescents, and involves the development of one or more wedge-shaped vertebrae in the thoracic or lumbar regions through abnormal epiphyseal plate behavior. The individual typically has a round-shouldered appearance, with or without back pain. Weight lifters, gymnasts, swimmers, and football linemen, who overdevelop the pectoral muscles, are also prone to this condition.

Scoliosis

Lateral curvature of the spine is known as **scoliosis** (FIG. 10.12B). The lateral deformity, coupled with rotational deformity of the involved vertebrae, may range from mild to severe. Scoliosis may appear as either a "C" or an "S" curve involving the thoracic spine, lumbar spine, or both. Scoliosis can be structural or nonstructural. Structural scoliosis involves an inflexible curvature that persists with lateral bending of the spine. Nonstructural scoliosis curves are flexible and are corrected with lateral bending. Although congenital abnormalities, certain cancers, and leg length discrepancy may lead to scoliosis, approximately 70 to 90% of all cases are idiopathic. Idiopathic scoliosis is most commonly diagnosed between the ages of 10 and 13 years, but can be seen at any age, and is more common in females.

Symptoms associated with scoliosis vary with the severity of the condition. Mild cases are usually asymptomatic and self-limiting. Severe scoliosis, characterized by extreme lateral deviation and localized rotation of the spine, can be painful and deforming. In general, mild to moderate cases can be treated with strength, flexibility, and general fitness activities, while severe cases may require surgical intervention.

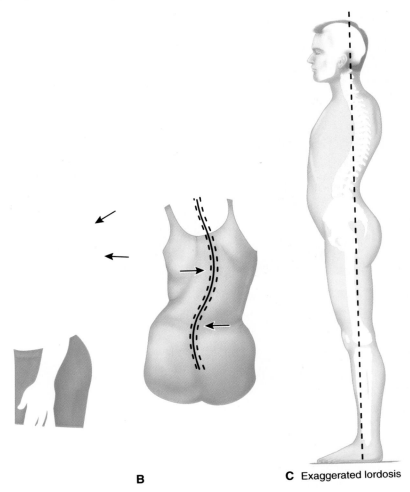

A   **B**   **C** Exaggerated lordosis

FIGURE 10.12 Spinal anomalies. **A.** Thoracic kyphosis. **B.** Scoliosis. **C.** Lordosis.

Lordosis

Abnormal exaggeration of the lumbar curve, or **lordosis**, is often associated with weakened abdominal muscles in combination with tight muscles, especially the hip flexors, tensor fasciae latae, and deep lumbar extensors (FIG. 10.12C). Other causes of lordosis include congenital spinal deformity, such as bilateral congenital hip dislocation; **spondylolisthesis**; compensatory action resulting from another deformity, such as kyphosis; hip flexion contractures; poor postural habits; and overtraining in sports requiring repeated lumbar hyperextension such as gymnastics, figure skating, and football (linemen). Because lordosis places added compressive stress on the posterior elements of the spine, LBP is a common symptom predisposing many individuals to low back injuries.

PREVENTION OF SPINAL CONDITIONS

Although most of the load on the spine is borne by the vertebral bodies and discs, the facet joints assist with some load bearing. Protective equipment can prevent some injuries to the cervical and thoracic regions. However, physical conditioning plays a more important role in preventing injuries to the overall region. In addition, because the low back is subjected to a variety of stresses as part of normal daily activities, an awareness of proper posture is essential to minimizing the risk of injury.

Physical Conditioning

Strengthening of the back muscles is imperative to stabilize the spinal column. Strengthening exercises for the cervical region may involve isometric contractions, manual resistance, or weight training with free weights or specialized machines. Exercises should include neck flexion, extension, lateral flexion, and rotation, as well as scapular elevation. Exercises to strengthen the thoracic region should involve back extension, lateral flexion, and rotation; abdominal strengthening; and exercises for the lower trapezius and latissimus dorsi. Exercises to strengthen the low back area should involve back extension, lateral flexion, and rotation. It is also important to strengthen the abdominal muscles in order to maintain appropriate postural alignment.

Normal ROM is also essential in stabilizing the spine and preventing injury. If warranted, stretching exercises should be used to promote and maintain normal ROM in the cervical, thoracic, and lumbar regions.

Protective Equipment

Several pieces of equipment can be used to protect the spine. In the cervical region, a neck roll or posterolateral pad made of a high, thick, and stiff material can be attached to shoulder pads to limit excessive motion of the cervical spine, and has been shown to reduce the incidence of repetitive burners and stingers. However, such restraints may also increase the risk of cervical spine injuries by limiting the natural flexibility of the neck. In the upper body, shoulder pads extend over and protect the upper thoracic region. Rib protectors composed of air-inflated, interconnected cylinders can protect a limited region of the thoracic spine.

Weight-training belts, abdominal binders, and other similar lumbar/sacral supportive devices support the abdominal contents, stabilize the trunk, and can potentially assist in preventing spinal deformity and damage. These devices place the low back in a more vertical lifting posture, decrease lumbar lordosis, limit pelvic torsion, and lessen axial loading on the spine by increasing intra-abdominal pressure, which, in turn, reduces compressive forces in the vertebral bodies.

Proper Skill Technique

Proper skill technique is vital in preventing spinal injuries. Helmets are designed to protect the cranial region from injury, but do not prevent axial loading on the cervical spine. It is critical that proper techniques be taught and reinforced in an effort to reduce the potential for injury.

Poor posture during walking, sitting, standing, lying down, and running may lead to chronic low back strain or sprains. Postural deformity cases should be assessed to determine the cause, and an appropriate exercise program should be developed to address the deficits.

Lifting technique can also affect spinal loading. It has been shown that executing a lift in a very rapid, jerking fashion dramatically increases compression and shear forces on the spine, as well as tension in the paraspinal muscles. For this reason, isotonic resistance exercises should always be performed in a slow, controlled fashion. Breathing technique should also be emphasized. Specifically, it is desirable to inhale deeply as a lift is initiated and exhale forcefully and smoothly at the end of the lift.

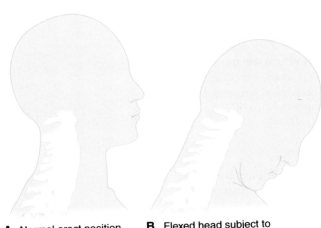

A Normal erect position

B Flexed head subject to compression forces (cervical vertebrae straightened)

FIGURE 10.13 Axial loading. **A**. In a normally erect position, the cervical spine is slightly extended. **B**. When a football tackle is executed with the head flexed at about 30°, the cervical vertebrae are aligned in a column and subjected to compressional forces, generated by the cervical muscles, and to axial loading.

CERVICAL SPINE CONDITIONS

The relatively small size of the cervical vertebrae, combined with the nearly horizontal orientation of the cervical facet joints, makes the cervical spine the most mobile region of the spinal column. As such, this area is especially vulnerable to injury. The major concern with cervical injuries is the potential involvement of the spinal cord and nerve roots.

Cervical flexion combined with axial compression loading is the leading mechanism of injury for severe cervical spine injuries. For example, when a football tackle is executed with the head in a flexed position, the cervical spine is aligned in a segmented column and subjected to both large compression forces, generated by the cervical muscles, and axial impact forces (FIG. 10.13). Impact causes loading along the longitudinal axis of the cervical vertebrae, leading to compression deformation. The intervertebral discs can initially absorb some energy; however, as continued force is exerted, further deformation and buckling occurs, leading to failure of the intervertebral discs, cervical vertebrae, or both (FIG. 10.14).

While a variety of injuries can be sustained to the cervical spine, the focus of this chapter will be acute injuries to the region. The coach must be prepared to make decisions concerning the nature and severity of acute injury to the cervical spine and, subsequently, determine the immediate management for the condition.

Acute Torticollis

Torticollis, or scoliosis of the cervical spine, is a deformity of the neck in which the head tilts toward one shoulder and simultaneously, the chin rotates toward the opposite shoulder. It is a symptom, as well as a disease, and has a host of underlying pathologies.

Acute torticollis, commonly referred to as "wry neck," as a result of a muscular strain often follows exposure to cold air currents or occasionally sleeping with the neck in an

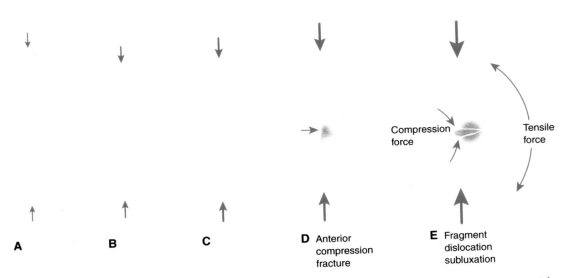

A   **B**   **C**   **D** Anterior compression fracture   **E** Fragment dislocation subluxation

Compression force   Tensile force

FIGURE 10.14 Results of cervical spine compression deformation. **A** and **B**. Axial loading on the vertebral column causes compressive deformation of the intervertebral discs. **C**. As load continues and maximum compression deformation is reached, angular deformation and buckling occurs. **D** and **E**. Continued force results in an anterior compression fracture, subluxation, or dislocation.

abnormal position, which leads to painful tender cervical muscles. However, any trauma involving the cervical spine can present with torticollis.

Signs and Symptoms

An individual will often awaken with acute torticollis. Due to painful muscle spasm, the individual presents with the head tilted to one side with the chin pointed to the opposite shoulder. If the head tilts right and the chin points left, the muscles on the right side are affected. Subsequently, ROM is limited. The condition can last for a couple of days or as long as 2 weeks.

Management

Treatment is symptomatic. It can include the use of heat or cold to reduce spasm as well as nonsteroidal analgesics for pain. Because the ROM of the cervical spine is compromised, the individual should not be permitted to engage in sport or physical activity. Regardless of the underlying cause, the criteria for return to activity should include normal ROM and strength. If the condition does not resolve in 2 to 3 days, the individual should not be permitted to return to activity until having been seen and released by an appropriate healthcare professional.

Cervical Strains

Cervical strains usually involve the sternocleidomastoid or upper trapezius, although other muscles may be involved. Strains can occur as a result of direct or indirect trauma associated with a tension force. For example, a wrestler's neck could be forced against the mat in a position of extreme lateral flexion. Another example is a player getting undercut while rebounding a basketball, resulting in a fall that propels the head forward (hyperflexion) and backward (hyperextension). Strains can also be associated with muscle weakness attributed to poor posture.

Signs and Symptoms

Signs and symptoms include pain, stiffness, muscle spasm, and restricted ROM. Increased pain occurs during active contraction or passive stretching of the involved muscle.

The initial management includes the application of cold to the involved area to help diminish pain and muscle spasm. Return to participation should not be permitted unless the individual is free of neck pain and ROM and neck strength is normal. If the signs and symptoms do not resolve within 24 to 48 hours, the coach should require the individual to obtain approval for return to participation from a qualified healthcare professional. It is important to rule out an underlying injury, such as a spinal fracture, dislocation, or disc injury. In addition, a healthcare professional could recommend additional treatment options, such as nonsteroidal anti-inflammatory drugs and/or use of a cervical collar for support.

Cervical Sprains

The same mechanisms that cause cervical strains also lead to cervical sprains. However, the mechanism for a sprain tends to be more violent in nature. Injury can occur to any of the major ligaments traversing the cervical spine, as well as to the capsular ligaments surrounding the facet joints. It should be noted that a cervical sprain and strain can occur simultaneously.

Signs and Symptoms

Pain, stiffness, and restricted ROM, but no neurologic or bony injury usually exists. Unlike cervical strains, the symptoms of a sprain can persist for several days.

Management

Initial management for a cervical sprain is the same as for a muscle strain. If the condition does not rapidly improve, referral to a physician is warranted to rule out a more serious underlying condition.

Cervical Fractures and Dislocations

Cervical fractures and dislocations can result from the axial loading and violent neck flexion (FIG. 10.15). This mechanism can be seen in unsafe practices, such as diving into shallow water, spearing in football, or landing on the posterior neck during gymnastics or trampoline activities. Some fractures, such as those to the spinous process or unilateral laminar fractures, may only require immobilization in a cervical collar. Others, such as a bilateral pars interarticularis fracture of C2 ("hangman's fracture"), may require a cervical collar or Halo vest immobilization.

Signs and Symptoms

Because neural damage can range from none to complete severance of the spinal cord, there is a range of accompanying symptoms (BOX 10.1). Painful palpation over the spinous processes, muscle spasm, or a palpable defect indicates a possible fracture or dislocation. Radiating pain, numbness, muscle weakness, paralysis, or loss of bladder or bowel control are all critical signs of neural damage. If a unilateral cervical dislocation is present, the neck is visibly tilted toward the dislocated side, with muscle tightness resulting from stretch on the convex side and muscle slack on the concave side.

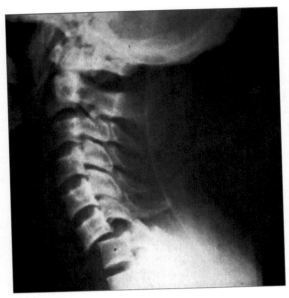

FIGURE 10.15 Cervical fracture/dislocation. The mechanism of axial loading and violent neck flexion can result in a cervical fracture/dislocation.

Management

Because spinal cord damage can lead to paralysis or death, a suspected unstable neck injury should be treated as a medical emergency. An unstable neck injury should be suspected in an unconscious individual, an individual who is awake but has numbness and/or paralysis, and in a neurologically intact individual who has neck pain or pain with neck movement. It is important that the coach understands that a cervical fracture or dislocation could be present even if there are no apparent neurological deficits. An individual with a cervical fracture or dislocation could still be able to walk off a playing field/court.

Immediate activation of the emergency plan, including summoning emergency medical services (EMS), is warranted. The individual should not be moved. While waiting for EMS to arrive, without moving the head or neck, the coach should stabilize the neck, assess the ABCs (airway, breathing, and circulation), and manage any life-threatening situations.

BRACHIAL PLEXUS INJURY

The brachial plexus is typically damaged in two ways (FIG. 10.16). A "stretch injury" can occur when the head is forced laterally away from the shoulder while the shoulder is simultaneously forced downward, such as when an individual is tackled and subsequently rolls onto the shoulder with the head turned to the opposite side. A stretch injury can also occur when the arm is forced into excessive external rotation, abduction, and extension. The other mechanism of injury involves a "pinching injury" when the head is rotated, laterally flexed, and compressed or extended to the same side of the shoulder, compressing the intervertebral foramen and impinging the nerve root.

RED FLAG 10.1 Indicating a Possible Cervical Spine Injury

- Pain over the spinous process, with or without deformity
- Unrelenting neck pain or muscle spasm
- Abnormal sensations in the head, neck, trunk, or extremities
- Muscular weakness in the extremities
- Loss of coordinated movement
- Paralysis or inability to move a body part
- Absent or weak reflexes
- Loss of bladder or bowel control
- Mechanism of injury involving violent axial loading, flexion, or rotation of the neck

Signs and Symptoms

This injury usually affects the upper trunk (C5, C6) of the brachial plexus and leads to a sensory loss or **paresthesia** in the appropriate dermatome: the lateral arm, or the thumb and index finger, respectively. Acute symptoms involve an immediate, severe, burning pain that radiates from the clavicular area down the arm into the hand, hence the nickname "burner" or "stinger." Pain is usually transient and subsides in 5 to 10 minutes, but tenderness over the supraclavicular area and shoulder weakness may persist for hours or days after the injury. The individual often tries to shake the arm to "get the feeling back." Muscle weakness is evident in shoulder abduction and external rotation. Symptoms from a brachial plexus injury are unilateral, meaning the symptoms only affect the involved side of the body.

Burners are graded in three levels (TABLE 10.1). Grade I burners represent **neurapraxia,** the mildest lesion, whereby only a temporary loss of sensation or loss of motor function occurs. Recovery usually occurs within days to a few weeks. Grade II burners are **axonotmesis** injuries that produce significant motor and mild sensory deficits that last at least 2 weeks, but full or normal function is usually restored. Grade III burners are **neurotmesis** injuries, which cause actual damage to the nerves. These severe injuries have a poor prognosis; motor and sensory deficits persist for up to 1 year.

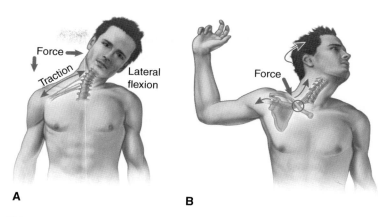

FIGURE 10.16 Common mechanisms of a brachial plexus stretch. **A.** A blow to the head causing lateral flexion and shoulder depression may lead to a traction injury to the upper trunk of the brachial plexus. **B.** An injury can also occur when a blow to supraclavicular region causes lateral flexion with rotation and extension of the cervical spine away from the blow.

Management

When weakness is present, the individual should be removed from activity. If strength and function return completely in 1 to 2 minutes, the individual can return to play. If any neurologic symptoms persist after this time, the individual should not be allowed to return to play until evaluated by a physician. Return to play should occur only when full strength, ROM, and sensation are restored in the cervical spine and extremity.

THORACIC SPINE INJURIES

The protective rib cage serves to limit movement in the thoracic motion segments. However, the thoracolumbar junction is a region of potentially high stress during flexion-extension movements of the trunk. Injuries to this area may include contusions, strains, sprains, fractures, and **apophysitis.**

TABLE 10.1	**Classifications of Burners**		
GRADE	INJURY	SIGNS	PROGNOSIS
I	Neurapraxia	Temporary loss of sensation and/or loss of motor function	Recovery within a few days to a few weeks
II	Axonotmesis	Significant motor and mild sensory deficits	Deficits last at least 2 weeks Regrowth is slow, but full or normal function is usually restored
III	Neurotmesis	Motor and sensory deficits persist for up to 1 year	Poor prognosis Surgical intervention is often necessary

Contusions

Direct blows to the back during contact sports frequently yield contusions to the muscles in the thoracic region. Contusions can range in severity but are generally characterized by pain, ecchymosis, spasm, and limited swelling.

Management

The initial management includes the application of cold to the involved area. If the signs and symptoms do not resolve within 2 to 3 days, the coach should require the individual to obtain approval for return to participation from a qualified healthcare professional.

Thoracic Strains and Sprains

Thoracic sprains and strains result from either overloading or overstretching muscles in the region through violent or sustained muscle contractions. Painful spasms of the back muscles serve as a protective mechanism to immobilize the injured area, and they may develop as a sympathetic response to a sprain. The presence of such spasms, however, makes it difficult to determine whether the injury is actually a strain or sprain.

Management

Cold should be applied to the involved area. The individual should be referred to a qualified healthcare practitioner for a definitive diagnosis and ongoing treatment options.

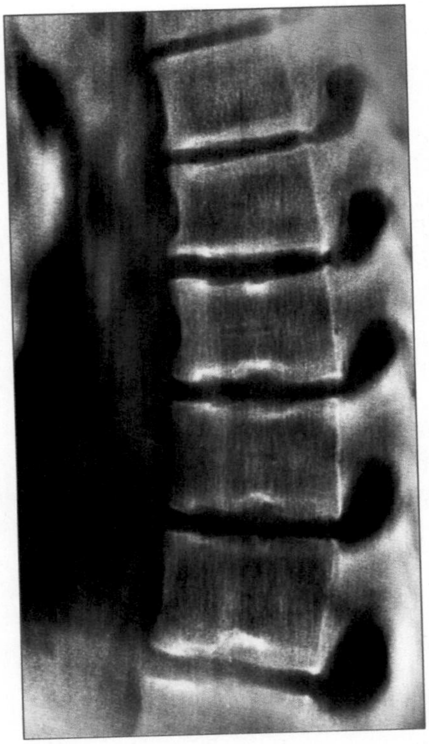

FIGURE 10.17 Thoracic fracture and apophysitis. Scheuermann's disease occurs when end plate changes lead to erosion in the anterior vertebral body, which drives a herniated disc forward into the body. In this radiograph, several end plate changes can be seen leading to erosion of the vertebral bodies.

Thoracic Spinal Fractures and Apophysitis

Thoracic fractures tend to be concentrated at the lower end of the thoracic spine in the transition region between the thoracic and lumbar curvatures. Large compressive loads, such as those sustained during heavy weight lifting, head-on contact in football or rugby, or landing on the buttock area during a fall, can fracture the vertebral end plates or lead to a wedge fracture, named after the shape of the deformed vertebral body. Females with **osteopenia**, a condition of reduced bone mineralization, are particularly susceptible to these fractures. More commonly, compressive stress during small, repetitive loads in an activity such as running leads to a progressive compression fracture of a weakened vertebral body. As with any fracture, pain and muscle guarding are present in the region of the fracture site.

Another leading cause of thoracic fractures among adolescents and young adults is Scheuermann's disease (FIG. 10.17). This condition, which appears to be related to mechanical stress, involves degeneration of the epiphyseal end plates of the vertebral bodies and typically includes at least three adjacent motion segments. Onset typically occurs in the late juvenile period from 8 to 12 years of age; more severe fixed deformities are seen in individuals 12 to 16 years of age. The condition is twice as common in girls as in boys. A high incidence of Scheuermann's disease has been documented among gymnasts, cyclists, wrestlers, and rowers. Repeated flexion-extension of the thoracic spine can cause inflammation of the apophyses, the growth centers of the vertebral bodies. Like Scheuermann's disease, **apophysitis** is a progressive condition characterized by local pain and tenderness.

Management

The presentation of any signs or symptoms that could be indicative of a fracture or apophysitis warrants immediate physician referral.

LUMBAR SPINE CONDITIONS

The lumbar spine must support the weight of the head, trunk, and arms, as well as any load held in the hands. In addition, the two lower lumbar motion

> ## BOX 10.2   Causes of Low Back Pain
>
> - Muscle strains and sprains
> - Sciatica
> - Protruded or herniated disc
> - Pathologic fracture
> - Disc space infections
> - Spinal infections (e.g., tuberculosis)
> - Neoplastic tumor (i.e., primary or metastatic)
> - Ankylosing spondylitis (arthritis of the spine)
> - Benign space-occupying lesions
> - Abdominal aortic aneurysm

segments (i.e., L4-L5, L5-S1) provide a large ROM in flexion-extension. As such, it is not surprising that mechanical abuse often results in episodes of LBP or that the lower lumbar discs are injured more frequently than any others in the spine.

Lumbar Strains and Sprains

An estimated 75 to 80% of the population experiences LBP stemming from mechanical injury to muscles, ligaments, or connective tissue (Box 10.2). Although LBP typically strikes adults, nearly 30% of children experience LBP up to the age of 16.[3] Although several known pathologies may cause LBP, reduced spinal flexibility, repeated stress, and activities that require maximal extension of the lumbar spine are most associated with chronic LBP.

Muscle strains may result from a sudden extension action with trunk rotation on an overtaxed, unprepared, or underdeveloped spine. Chronic strains may stem from improper posture, excessive lumbar lordosis, flat back or scoliosis.

Signs and Symptoms

Pain and discomfort can range from diffuse to localized. Pain does not radiate into the buttocks or posterior thigh, and there are no signs of neural involvement such as muscle weakness, sensory changes, or reflex inhibition. If a muscle strain is present, pain will increase with passive flexion and active or resisted extension.

Management

Acute protocol is followed to control pain and hemorrhage. Following cold treatment, passive stretching of the low back can help relieve muscle spasm. In moderate to severe cases, the individual should be referred to a physician.

Low Back Pain in Runners

Many runners develop muscle tightness in the hip flexors and hamstrings. Tight hip flexors tend to produce a forward body lean, leading to anterior pelvic tilt and hyperlordosis of the lumbar spine. Because the lumbar muscles develop tension to counteract the forward bending moment of the entire trunk when the trunk is in flexion, these muscles are particularly susceptible to strain. Coupled with tight hamstrings, a shorter stride often emerges.

In an effort to decrease the incidence of LBP, training techniques should allow for adequate progression of distance and intensity, and include extensive flexibility exercises for the hip and thigh region.

Signs and Symptoms

Symptoms include localized pain that increases with active and resisted back extension, but radiating pain and neurologic deficits are not present. Anterior pelvic tilt and hyperlordosis of the lumbar spine may also be present.

Management

Acute protocol is followed to control pain and muscle spasm. If symptoms become more pronounced or do not subside within a week, the individual should be referred to a physician to rule out a more serious underlying condition and additional treatment options (e.g., NSAIDs; muscle relaxants; electrical muscle stimulation; physical therapy).

Ultimately, the treatment focuses on avoiding excessive flexion activities and a sedentary posture. Flexion causes the mobile nucleus pulposus to shift posteriorly and press against the annulus fibrosus at its thinnest, least-buttressed place. In most cases, this just leads to pain, but in other cases, it may lead to a herniated disc. In addition, physical activity is necessary to pump fluid through the spinal discs to keep them properly hydrated; by interfering with that process, immobility can prolong pain.

Sciatica

Sciatica is not considered a condition in and of itself, but rather a set of symptoms attributed to a condition that compresses or irritates the sciatic nerve. Possible conditions include a herniated disc, annular tear, muscle-related disease, spinal stenosis, facet joint disease, and piriformis syndrome. Typically, sciatica affects only one side of the body.

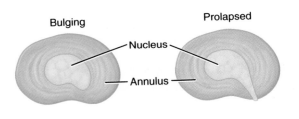

Signs and Symptoms

The symptoms of sciatica will ultimately depend on the actual cause or condition. As such, the following are general symptoms common to various causes of sciatica:

- Pain that follows a path from the low back, through the buttocks, through the posterior thigh and posterior lower leg
- Burning or tingling sensation that radiates down the leg
- Weakness of the muscles in the lower extremity
- Coughing, sneezing, straining, and prolonged sitting aggravate the symptoms
- Loss of bladder or bowel control

Management

Referral to a physician is necessary to check for a potentially serious underlying condition and treatment options. In some cases, sciatica will resolve with the use of heat or cold, over-the-counter anti-inflammatory medication, restricted activity, and time. In other cases, prescription medications, physical therapy, and/or surgical intervention may be the best course of action. Following return to activity, if symptoms resume, the activity should cease and the individual should be referred back to the physician.

FIGURE 10.18 Herniated discs. Herniated discs are categorized by severity as an eccentrically loaded nucleus progressively moves from (**A**) protruded through, (**B**) prolapsed, and (**C**) extruded, culminating in (**D**) sequestrated when the nuclear material moves into the canal to impinge on the adjacent spinal nerves.

Disc Injuries

Prolonged mechanical loading of the spine can lead to microruptures in the annulus fibrosus, resulting in degeneration of the disc (FIG. 10.18). Bulging or **protruded** discs refer to some eccentric accumulation of the nucleus with slight deformity of the annulus. When the eccentric nucleus produces a definite deformity as it works its way through the fibers of the annulus, it is called a **prolapsed disc**. It is called an **extruded disc** when the material moves into the spinal canal, where it runs the risk of impinging on adjacent nerve roots. Finally, with a **sequestrated disc**, the nuclear material has separated from the disc itself and potentially migrates. The most commonly herniated discs are the lower two lumbar discs at L4-L5 and L5-S1, followed by the two lower cervical discs. Most ruptures move in a posterior or posterolateral direction as a result of torsion and compression, not just compression.

Signs and Symptoms

Because the intervertebral discs are not innervated, the sensation of pain does not occur until the surrounding soft tissue structures are impinged. When compression is placed on a spinal nerve of the sciatic nerve complex (L4-S3), sensory and motor deficits are reflected in the myotome and dermatome patterns associated with the nerve root. In addition, alteration in tendon reflexes is apparent. A disc need not be completely herniated to give symptoms. Symptoms include sharp pain and muscle spasms at the site of the herniation that often shoot down the sciatic nerve into the lower extremity. The individual may walk in a slightly crouched position, leaning away from the side of the lesion. Forward trunk flexion may exacerbate pain and increase distal symptoms. Significant signs indicating the need for immediate referral to a physician include muscle weakness, sensory changes, and diminished reflexes in the lower extremity, and abnormal bladder or bowel function.

Management

This condition requires referral to a physician for accurate diagnosis and treatment options. The coach should not permit the individual to continue activity, as doing so could potentially exacerbate the condition. In addition, the coach could suggest the application of cold to the area to decrease pain and potential spasm.

Lumbar Fractures and Dislocations

Transverse or spinous process fractures result from extreme tension from the attached muscles or from a direct blow to the low back during participation in contact sports, such as football, rugby, soccer, basketball, hockey, and lacrosse. These fractures often lead to additional injury to surrounding soft tissues, but are not as serious as compression fractures.

Compression fractures more commonly involve the L1 vertebra at the thoracolumbar junction. Hyperflexion, or jack-knifing of the trunk, crushes the anterior aspect of the vertebral body. The primary danger with this injury is the possibility of bony fragments moving into the spinal canal and damaging the spinal cord or spinal nerves. Because of the facet joint orientation in the lumbar region, dislocations occur only when a fracture is present. Fracture dislocations resulting from sport participation are rare.

Signs and Symptoms

Symptoms include localized, palpable pain that may radiate down the nerve root if a bony fragment compresses a spinal nerve. Because the spinal cord ends at about L1 or L2 level, fractures of the lumbar vertebrae below this point do not pose a serious threat, but should be handled with care to minimize potential nerve damage to the cauda equina.

Management

If a fracture or dislocation is suspected, the emergency plan should be activated, including summoning of EMS for transport to the nearest medical facility.

SACRUM AND COCCYX CONDITIONS

Because the sacrum and coccyx are essentially immobile, the potential for mechanical injury to these regions is dramatically reduced. In many cases, injuries result from direct blows and stress on the SI joint.

Sacroiliac Joint Sprain

Sprains of the SI joint may result from a single traumatic episode involving bending and/or twisting, repetitive stress from lifting, a fall on the buttocks, excessive side-to-side or up-and-down motion during running and jogging, running on uneven terrain, suddenly slipping or stumbling forward, or wearing new shoes or orthoses. The injury may irritate or stretch the sacrotuberous or sacrospinous ligament, or may lead to an anterior or posterior rotation of one side of the pelvis relative to the other. Hypermobility results from rotation of the pelvis. During healing, the joint on the injured side may become hypermobile, allowing the joint to subluxate in either an anterior- or posterior-rotated position.

Signs and Symptoms

Symptoms may involve unilateral, dull pain in the sacral area that extends into the buttock and posterior thigh. Upon observation, the anterior superior iliac spine or posterior superior iliac spine may appear asymmetrical when compared bilaterally. A leg-length discrepancy may be present. Muscle spasm is not often seen. Standing on one leg and climbing stairs may increase the pain. Forward bending reveals a block to normal movement. Lateral flexion toward the injured side increases pain, as does straight leg raise beyond 45°.

Management

Immediate management includes the application of cold to control pain and spasm. Following the cold, gentle stretching may be performed to alleviate stiffness. If symptoms do not subside in 2 to 3 days, the individual should be referred to a physician for a definitive diagnosis and ongoing treatment options.

Coccygeal Conditions

Direct blows to the region can produce contusions and fractures of the coccyx.

Signs and Symptoms

Injury to the coccyx results in localized pain and tenderness to the area. The pain typically increases as a result of sitting, especially for prolonged periods of time, or when direct pressure is applied to the area. Pain resulting from a fracture may last for several months.

Management

Referral to a physician is appropriate to ensure an accurate diagnosis and rule out any underlying injuries. In general, treatment for coccygeal pain includes analgesics, use of padding for protection, and a ring seat to alleviate compression during sitting.

THE COACH AND ON-SITE ASSESSMENT OF AN ACUTE SPINAL CONDITION

Injury assessment of the spine is complex and should not be rushed. Given the potential for significant or catastrophic harm associated with a spinal injury, the coach must act in a very focused and deliberate manner in an effort to avoid any actions that could exacerbate an injury.

As with other on-site injury assessments, it begins as the coach is approaching the individual. The focus should be on observing the individual's overall presentation and attitude, with a particular focus on their willingness or ability to move. It may also be necessary for the coach to control any scene around the individual. For example, others around the injured individual should be instructed to step back and not touch the person.

Once the coach reaches the individual, it may become necessary to calm and reassure the individual. It will be extremely important to have the individual's attention as the assessment proceeds. As part of reassuring the individual, the coach should assess the individual's level of consciousness as it is possible for some mechanisms to produce trauma to both the head and the neck. If the individual loses consciousness or is not alert and attentive, the coach should activate the emergency plan, including summoning EMS. During this time, the individual should not be moved. Rather, the coach should stabilize the head and neck in the position in which it's found and advise the individual to remain still.

In most on-site assessments, the next step is to complete the history component of the exam. In the case of a potential spinal injury, the history should be delayed prior to the coach performing a brief neuromuscular assessment to detect any motor or sensory deficits that could be indicative of a spinal injury. As such, the coach should begin with the following questions:

- What happened? (An attempt to determine the mechanism of injury)
- Where is your pain?
- Are you experiencing any neck or back pain?
- Are you having any difficulty breathing or swallowing?
- Are you experiencing any unusual sensations in your arms or legs? (Unusual sensations would include numbing, tingling, and burning. If possible, the coach should initially avoid using descriptors and pose the question in an open-ended manner. However, if the coach is not satisfied that the individual understands the question, it may become necessary to specifically ask if there is any numbing, tingling, or burning.)
- Can you wiggle your fingers? Can you wiggle your toes? (The shoes do not need to be removed to perform this action.)
- (The coach should place two to three fingers in the individual's palm of the hand.) Can you gently squeeze my hand? (This should be performed on both hands.) (Next, the coach should place their hands in a position to resist ankle dorsiflexion.) Can you gently push your foot against my hand? (Again, this should be performed on both feet.) (The actions of squeezing the hand and pushing with the foot assess the cervical and lumber spinal nerve roots, respectively.)

In performing this initial assessment, the coach must be prepared to hear a positive response to a question and remain calm. It is essential that any on-going assessment and management be handled appropriately. In the absence of the coach and the injured participant remaining calm and focused, inappropriate judgment and actions could ensue.

Having asked the questions noted, the coach must make a decision on how to proceed. If the individual reports a mechanism which suggests severe injury, reports unusual sensations in the arms and/or legs, was unable to wiggle the fingers and/or toes, and/or was unable to squeeze the hand or push with the foot, the coach should manage the situation as a potentially serious spinal injury (APPLICATION STRATEGY 10.1).

APPLICATION STRATEGY 10.1
Management of a Potentially Serious Spinal Injury

- The individual should not be moved!
- If equipment is being worn, it should not be removed.
- The coach should stabilize the head and neck in the position in which they are found.
- The emergency plan should be activated, including summoning of EMS.
- The coach should monitor the vital signs while waiting for EMS to arrive.
- The coach should be prepared to manage any life-threatening conditions. (e.g., respiratory arrest; cardiac arrest; shock.)

APPLICATION STRATEGY 10.2

On-site Assessment of an Acute Spinal Injury: History, Observation, and Palpation

HISTORY
- Chief complaint
  - What's wrong?
- Mechanism of injury
  - What happened? What were you doing?
  - Are you able to demonstrate how it happened?
- Pain
  - Location
    - Where is the pain?
    - Can you point to a location where it hurts the most?
    - Do you have pain anywhere else in your body?
  - Type—Can you describe the pain (e.g., sharp, shooting, dull, achy, diffuse)?
  - Intensity—What is the level of pain on a scale from 1 to 10?
- Sounds
  - Did you hear anything?
- Feelings
  - Did you feel any unusual sensations (e.g., tearing, tingling, numbing, cracking)?

- Previous history
  - Have you ever injured this body part? (e.g., neck; back)
  - If so, what happened? What was the injury? Were you treated for it?
- Is there anything else you would like to tell me about your condition?

OBSERVATION
- General presentation—guarding; moving easily; postural appearance
- Injury site appearance—deformity; swelling; discoloration

PALPATION
- The coach should only perform palpation if there is a clear understanding of what is being palpated and why? A productive assessment appropriate to the standard of care of a coach does not necessitate palpation.

APPLICATION STRATEGY 10.3

On-site Assessment of an Acute Cervical Injury: Testing Component

TESTING
- Active range of motion (AROM)—bilateral comparison
  - As the patient performs the listed skills, observe for signs of pain, hesitation to move a body part, or abnormal movement.
  - Touch the chin to the chest (flexion)
  - Look up at the ceiling keeping the back straight (extension)
  - Turn the head sideways in both directions (lateral rotation)
  - Try to touch each ear to the shoulder in both directions (lateral flexion)
- Passive ROM should not be performed by the coach
- Resistive ROM

The coach should only perform resistive ROM for the muscles that govern the cervical spine if
- Instruction and approval for doing so has been obtained in advance from an appropriate healthcare practitioner
- AROM is normal and pain free as a way to assess strength.
- Activity/sport-specific functional testing
  - Performance of active movements typical of the movements executed by the individual during sport or activity participation (including weight training)
  - Should assess strength, agility, flexibility, joint stability, endurance, coordination, balance, and activity-specific skill performance

APPLICATION STRATEGY 10.4
On-site Assessment of an Acute Lumbar Injury: Testing Component

TESTING
- Active range of motion—bilateral comparison
  - Flexion
  - Extension
  - Lateral bending
  - Trunk rotation
- Activity/sport-specific functional testing
  - Performance of active movements typical of the movements executed by the individual during sport or activity participation (including weight training)
  - Should assess strength, agility, flexibility, joint stability, endurance, coordination, balance, and activity-specific skill performance

If the individual does not report any problems or demonstrate difficulties with these questions, the coach could proceed with the assessment by evaluating the individual's sensation as a means for obtaining additional information about the spinal nerve roots. Initially, the coach should assess upper body sensation. In visualizing the arm, the coach should divide it into right and left halves and proximal and distal halves. Next, alternating use of the pad of a finger and the edge of a finger nail, the coach should gently stroke a 1–2″ spot in each section. Following the strokes in each section, the coach should ask the individual if both sensations (i.e., pad of finger and fingernail) felt the same or different. This assessment should be performed on both arms. If the individual did not feel or could not distinguish the strokes in any section, the coach should manage the situation as a potentially serious spinal injury (APPLICATION STRATEGY 10.1). If the individual is able to distinguish the sensations, the coach should perform the same assessment on the lower extremities. Similarly, if the individual cannot distinguish sensations, the coach should manage the situation as a potentially serious spinal injury.

If the individual is able to distinguish the sensations, the coach should once again ask the individual about the location and intensity of their pain. If the individual reports that the neck or back pain (1) has not decreased, (2) has diminished, but is still significant, or (3) the pain has increased, the coach should manage the situation as a potentially serious spinal injury.

If the individual reports that the pain is diminished and not significant, the coach could proceed with an assessment in keeping with the adapted HOPS method (see Chapter 5). Specific guidelines for the coach to follow in assessing the cervical spine and the lumbar spine are provided in APPLICATION STRATEGIES 10.2, 10.3 and 10.4. In performing an assessment of a spinal condition, the coach should not hesitate to terminate the assessment and activate the emergency plan in the presence of any findings that suggest a serious injury (BOX 10.3). It is critical that the coach recognizes the potential consequences associated with a spinal injury and, as such, errs on the side of caution. An individual may be able to walk off a playing field or court, but that action does not rule out the potential for a serious spinal condition. When in doubt, it should always be assumed that a severe spinal injury is present and the emergency care plan should be activated.

► RED FLAG 10.3 Warrant Activation of the Emergency Plan
- Severe pain, point tenderness, or deformity along the vertebral column
- Loss or change in sensation anywhere in the body
- Paralysis or inability to move a body part
- Muscle weakness in a myotome
- Pain radiating into the extremities
- Any injury in which you are uncertain about the severity or nature

SUMMARY

1. The spine is a linkage system that transfers loads between the upper and lower extremities, enables motion in all three planes, and serves to protect the delicate spinal cord.

2. The spinal cord extends from the brain stem to the level of the first or second lumbar vertebrae. Thirty-one pairs of spinal nerves emanate from the cord, with the distal bundle of spinal nerves known as the cauda equine.

3. Anatomic variations that can predispose an individual to spinal injuries include kyphosis, scoliosis, lordosis, and par interarticularis fractures, which can lead to spondylolysis or spondylolisthesis.

4. Signs and symptoms that indicate a serious cervical spine injury include:
   • Pain over the spinous process, with or without deformity
   • Unrelenting neck pain or muscle spasm
   • Abnormal sensations on the head, neck, trunk, or extremities
   • Muscular weakness in the extremities
   • Paralysis or inability to move a body part
   • Absent or weak reflexes

5. A brachial plexus injury is a stretch injury commonly caused by tensile forces that lead to forceful downward traction of the clavicle while the head is distracted in the opposite direction. The injury usually affects the upper trunk (C5, C6) of the brachial plexus, leading to a sensory loss or paresthesia in the thumb and index finger.

6. Thoracic fractures tend to be concentrated at the lower end of the thoracic spine. Large compressive loads can lead to a wedge fracture.

7. Runners are particularly prone to LBP because of tight hip flexors and hamstrings. Symptoms include localized pain that increases with active and resisted back extension. Radiating pain and neurologic deficits are usually not present.

8. The most commonly herniated discs are between the L4-L5 and L5-S1 vertebrae. Most ruptures move in a posterior or posterolateral direction because of torsion and compression.

9. Significant signs that indicate a lumbar disc condition needing immediate referral to a physician include:
   • Muscle weakness
   • Sensory changes
   • Diminished reflexes in the lower extremity
   • Abnormal bladder or bowel function

10. In a traumatic spinal injury, a brief neuromuscular assessment should be performed to detect any motor or sensory deficits.

11. When assessing a nontraumatic spinal injury, the HOPS format should be adapted for use.

12. In performing an assessment of a spinal condition, the coach should not hesitate to terminate the assessment and activate the emergency plan in the presence of any findings that suggest a serious injury.

APPLICATION QUESTIONS

1. While throwing a two-handed overhead pass, a basketball player is hit on the anterior right arm. The arm is forced into excessive external rotation, abduction, and extension. The player experiences an immediate burning pain and prickly sensation that radiates down the arm and into the hand as well as an inability to raise the arm. What injury should be suspected? Is this a serious injury?

2. A high school field hockey coach notices during the practice warm-up that one of the players appears to have a "stiff neck." What questions should the coach ask as part of the history component of an assessment?

3. Following practice, a 15-year-old butterfly-stroke swimmer is complaining of localized pain and tenderness in the midback region over the thoracic spine. He reports that the pain came on gradually and only hurts during the execution of the stroke. How should the coach handle this situation? Why?

_____

_____

4. A middle school student reports to physical education class with a "wry neck." The activity for the day is basketball and the student is anxious to participate. Should the physical education teacher permit the student to participate in noncontact activities during the class? Why?

_____

_____

5. During a recreational football practice, a 16 year old executes a tackle on an opposing player. In making the contact, his head was in a slightly flexed position. The player walks off the field. He tells the coach that his neck hurts, but otherwise he feels fine. What actions should the coach take? Why?

_____

_____

6. A high school wrestler comes off the mat complaining of pain after having his neck twisted by an opponent. Following an assessment, the coach believes that the wrestler may have a cervical strain. How should the coach manage the condition?

_____

_____

7. A 40-year-old man initiated a training program to improve his cardiovascular fitness. His workout for the past month has consisted of running on a treadmill. Over the past week, he began to develop pain in the sacral region during his workout. The pain has now become so persistent and chronic that it hurts to sit for an extended time. What injury may be present? How should the fitness specialist handle this situation? Why?

_____

_____

8. A 17-year-old cheerleader reports to practice complaining of aching pain during trunk flexion aggravated with resisted hyperextension that produces sharp shooting pains into the low back and down the posterior leg. How should the coach handle this situation? Why?

_____

_____

9. During practice, a 16-year-old soccer player was undercut while heading the ball. The athlete is down on the field. When the coach reaches the athlete, he finds him conscious and alert, but obviously in pain. How should the coach proceed in assessing the individual?

_____

_____

10. Walking through a fitness facility, a 55-year-old man inadvertently trips over a piece of equipment that was lying on the floor. In assessing the individual, it becomes apparent to the fitness specialist that the individual has experienced trauma to the low back region. What signs and symptoms would suggest that EMS should be summoned? . . . that EMS does not need to be summoned, but that immediate referral to a physician is warranted?

_____

_____

REFERENCES

1. Brown RL, Brunn MA, and Garcia VF. 2001. Cervical spine injuries in children: A review of 103 patients treated consecutively at a level 1 pediatric trauma center. J Pediatr Surg, 36(8):1107–1114.
2. Banerjee R, Palumbo MA, and Fadale PD. 2004. Catastrophic cervical spine injuries in the collision sport athlete, part 1: Epidemiology, functional anatomy, and diagnosis. Am J Sports Med, 32(4):1077–1087.
3. Duggleby T, and Kumar S. 1997. Epidemiology of juvenile low back pain: A review. Disabil Rehabil, 19(12):505–512.
4. Burton AK. 1996. Low back pain in children and adolescents: To treat or not? Bull Hosp Jt Dis, 55(3):127–129.
5. Newcomer K, and Sinaki M. 1996. Low back pain and its relationship to back strength and physical activity in children. Acta Paediatr, 85(12):1433–1439.
6. Bono CM. 2004. Low-back pain in athletes. J Bone Joint Surg Am, 86-A:382–396.
7. Anderson MW. 2004. Lumbar discography: An update. Semin Roentgenol, 39:52–67.

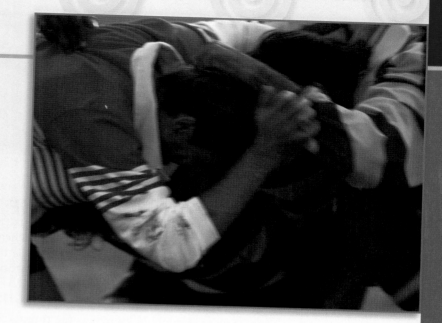

CHAPTER
11

THROAT, THORAX, AND VISCERAL CONDITIONS

KEY TERMS

appendicitis
cardiac tamponade
dyspnea
hematuria
hemothorax
hernias
hypoxia

(continued)

LEARNING OUTCOMES

1. Identify the important anatomic structures of the throat, thorax, and visceral regions.

2. Explain general principles to prevent injuries to the throat, thorax, and viscera.

3. Describe common injuries and conditions sustained by physically active individuals to the throat, thorax, and viscera, including their sign, symptoms, and immediate management.

4. Describe an on-site assessment of an acute throat, thorax, or visceral condition appropriate for use by a coach.

KEY TERMS (CONTINUED)

Kehr's sign	peritonitis	stitch in the side
Marfan's syndrome	pleura	sudden death
mitral valve prolapse	pneumothorax	tension pneumothorax
peristalsis	solar plexus punch	

ANATOMY REVIEW OF THE THROAT

The throat includes the pharynx, larynx, trachea, esophagus, a number of glands, and several major blood vessels (FIG. 11.1). Injuries to the throat are of particular concern because of the life-sustaining functions of the trachea and carotid arteries.

Pharynx, Larynx, and Esophagus

The pharynx, commonly known as the throat, connects the nasal cavity and mouth to the larynx and esophagus. The pharynx lies between the base of the skull and the sixth cervical vertebra. The laryngeal prominence on the thyroid cartilage that shields the front of the larynx is known as the "Adam's apple." A specialized spoon-shaped cartilage, the epiglottis, covers the superior opening of the larynx during swallowing to prevent food and liquids from entering. If a foreign body does slip past the epiglottis, the cough reflex is initiated, and the foreign body is normally ejected back into the pharynx. The larynx also contains the vocal cords, which are two bands of elastic connective tissue surrounded by mucosal folds. When expired air from the lungs passes over the vocal cords, sound is able to be produced.

The hyoid bone, the only bone of the body that does not articulate directly with any other bone, lies just inferior to the mandible in the anterior neck. It serves as an attachment point for neck muscles that raise and lower the larynx during swallowing and speech.

The esophagus carries food and liquids from the throat to the stomach. It is a muscle-walled tube that originates from the pharynx in the mid-neck and follows the anterior side of the spine. The coordinated action of the esophagus walls propels food into the stomach. When the esophagus is empty, the tube is collapsed.

Trachea

The trachea extends inferiorly from the larynx through the neck into the midthorax, where it divides into the two right and left bronchial tubes. The tracheal tube is formed by C-shaped rings of hyaline cartilage joined by fibroelastic connective tissue. Smooth muscle fibers of the trachealis muscle form the open side of the C and allow for expansion of the posteriorly adjacent esophagus as swallowed food passes. Contraction of the trachealis muscle during coughing can dramatically reduce the size of the airway, and, in doing so, increases the pressure inside the trachea to promote expulsion of mucus.

Blood Vessels of the Throat

The largest blood vessels coursing through the neck are the common carotid arteries (FIG. 11.2). The common carotid arteries, which provide the major blood supply to the brain, head, and face, divide into external and internal carotid arteries at the level of the "Adam's apple."

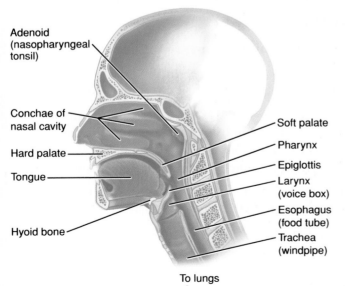

Adenoid (nasopharyngeal tonsil)

Conchae of nasal cavity

Hard palate

Tongue

Hyoid bone

Soft palate

Pharynx

Epiglottis

Larynx (voice box)

Esophagus (food tube)

Trachea (windpipe)

To lungs

FIGURE 11.1 Throat region. Lateral cross-sectional view.

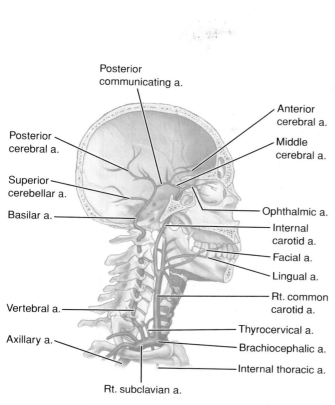

FIGURE 11.2 Arterial supply to the neck and throat region.

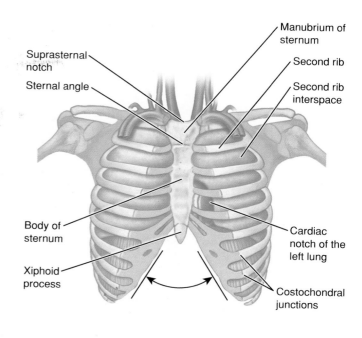

FIGURE 11.3 Thoracic cage. Note that only the first seven pairs of ribs articulate anteriorly with the sternum through the costal cartilages.

Branches from the carotid arteries include the superior thyroid arteries, facial artery, and lingual artery; these arteries supply the thyroid and larynx, the face and sinuses, and the mouth and tongue, respectively. Several arteries branch from the left and right subclavian arteries and course upward through the posterior side of the neck, including the costocervical trunk, thyrocervical trunk, and vertebral artery.

ANATOMY REVIEW OF THE THORAX

The thoracic cavity, or chest cavity, lies anterior to the spinal column and extends from the level of the clavicle down to the diaphragm. The bones of the thorax, including the sternum, ribs and costal cartilages, and thoracic vertebrae form a protective cage around the heart and lungs (FIG. 11.3). The costal cartilages of the first seven pairs of ribs attach directly to the sternum, and the costal cartilages of ribs 8 to 10 attach to the costal cartilages of the immediate superior ribs. The last two rib pairs are known as floating ribs because they do not attach anteriorly to any structure. The rib cage protects the heart and lungs.

The thoracic cavity is lined with a thin, double-layered membrane called the **pleura**. The pleural cavity, a narrow space between the pleural membranes, is filled with a pleural fluid secreted by the membranes, which enables the lungs to move against the thoracic wall with minimal friction during breathing. The primary bronchial tubes branch obliquely downward from the trachea, then branch into approximately 25 subsequent levels until the terminal bronchioles are reached (FIG. 11.4). These tiny air sacs, called alveoli, serve as diffusion chambers where oxygen from the lungs enters adjacent capillaries, and where carbon dioxide from the venous blood is returned to the lungs.

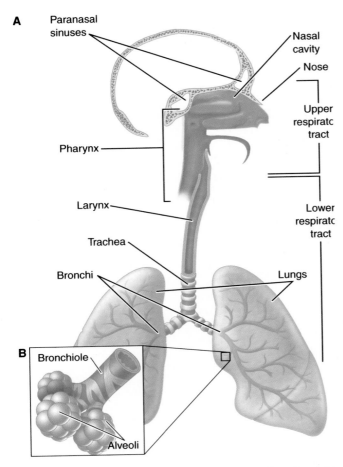

A

Paranasal sinuses

Nasal cavity

Nose

Upper respirato tract

Pharynx

Larynx

Lower respirato tract

Trachea

Bronchi

Lungs

B Bronchiole

Alveoli

FIGURE 11.4 Respiratory system. **A**. The trachea, bronchi, and lungs. **B**. The terminal ends of the bronchial tree are alveolar sacs, where oxygen and carbon dioxide are exchanged.

The major respiratory muscle is the diaphragm, a powerful sheet of muscle that separates the thoracic and abdominal cavities. During relaxation, the diaphragm is dome-shaped. During contraction, it flattens, thereby increasing the size of the thoracic cavity. This increase in cavity volume causes a decrease in intrathoracic pressure, resulting in inhalation of air into the lungs. The diaphragm is assisted by the intercostal muscles, both internal and external, which lift the rib cage and assist with breathing.

The heart and lungs have an intimate relationship, both physically and functionally. The right side of the heart pumps blood to the lungs, where it is oxygenated and where carbon dioxide is given off. The left side of the heart receives the freshly oxygenated blood from the lungs and pumps it out to the systemic circulation. The vessels interconnecting the heart and lungs are known as the pulmonary circuit, and the vessels that supply the body are known as the systemic circuit (FIG. 11.5).

ANATOMY REVIEW OF THE VISCERAL REGION

The visceral region includes the organs and vessels between the diaphragm and pelvic floor (FIG. 11.6). The region contains both solid and hollow organs. The solid organs include the spleen, liver, pancreas, kidneys, and adrenal glands. The hollow organs include the stomach, gall bladder, small and large intestines, bladder, and ureters. The pelvic girdle protects the lower abdominal organs.

Visceral Organs

The stomach is a J-shaped bag positioned between the esophagus and small intestine. Food is stored in the stomach for approximately 4 hours, during which time it is broken down by hydrochloric acid secreted in the stomach into a paste-like substance known as chyme. The chyme moves into the small intestine where it is progressively absorbed. A few substances, including water, electrolytes, aspirin, and alcohol, are absorbed into the bloodstream across the stomach lining without full digestion.

The small intestine, about 2 m (6 ft) in length, is responsible for most of the digestion and absorption of food as it is propelled through the organ in about 3 to 6 hours by waves of alternate circular contraction and relaxation by a process called **peristalsis**. Water and electrolytes are further absorbed from the stored material in the large intestine, or colon, during the next 12 to 24 hours.

The vermiform appendix protrudes from the large intestine in the right lower quadrant of the abdomen, and can become a protected environment for the accumulation of bacteria, leading to inflammation of the appendix, or **appendicitis**.

The liver, located in the upper right quadrant under the diaphragm, produces bile, a greenish liquid that helps break down fat in the small intestine. The liver also absorbs excess glucose from the bloodstream and stores it in the form of glycogen for later use. Additional functions of the liver include processing fats and amino acids, manufacturing blood proteins, and detoxifying certain poisons and drugs. The gallbladder functions as an accessory to the liver to store concentrated bile on its way to the small intestine.

The spleen, the largest of the lymphoid organs, is located in the upper left quadrant. It cleanses the blood of foreign matter, bacteria, viruses, and toxins; stores excess red blood cells for later reuse and releases others into the blood for processing by the liver; produces red blood cells in the fetus; and stores blood platelets. The pancreas secretes most of the digestive enzymes that break down food in the small intestine. It also secretes the hormones insulin and glucagon, which lower and elevate blood sugar levels, respectively.

The kidneys filter and cleanse the blood. They are vital for filtering out toxins, metabolic wastes, drugs, and excess ions and excreting them from the body in urine. The kidneys also return needed substances, such as water and electrolytes, to the blood. The ureters connect the kidneys to the urinary bladder, which is an expandable sac that stores urine.

Muscles of the Trunk

As is the case throughout the neck and trunk, muscles in the pelvic region are named in pairs, with one located on the left and the other on the right side of the body. These muscles cause lateral flexion or rotation when they contract unilaterally, but contribute to spinal flexion or extension when bilateral contractions occur (FIG. 11.7).

Blood Vessels of the Trunk

The major blood vessel of the trunk is the aorta, with its numerous branches (FIG. 11.8). The left and right coronary arteries branch from the ascending aorta to supply the heart muscle. The first arterial branch from the aortic arch is the brachiocephalic artery, which splits into the right common carotid artery and right subclavian artery. The second and third branches from the aortic arch are the left common carotid artery and left subclavian artery, respectively. The thoracic aorta yields 10 pairs of intercostal arteries to supply the muscles of the thorax, the bronchial arteries to the lungs, the esophageal artery to the esophagus, and the phrenic arteries to the diaphragm. The distal portion of the descending aorta becomes the abdominal aorta. The first branch of the abdominal aorta is the celiac trunk that forms the left gastric artery to the stomach, the splenic artery to the spleen, and the common hepatic artery to the liver.

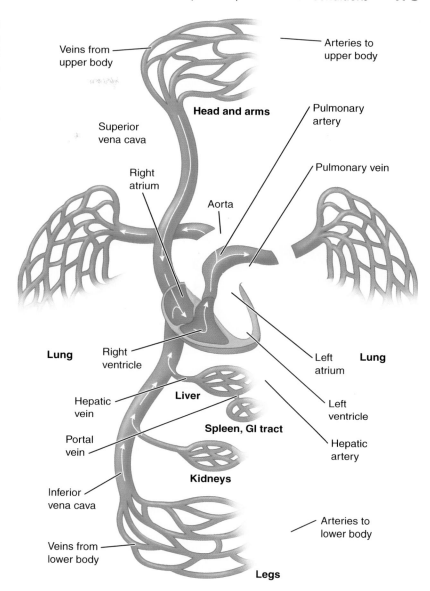

FIGURE 11.5 Pulmonary and systemic circulation in an adult.

PREVENTION OF INJURIES TO THE THROAT, THORAX, AND VISCERA

Injuries to the throat, thorax, and abdomen occur in nearly every sport, yet few sports require protective equipment for all players. In sports where high-velocity projectiles are present, throat and chest protectors are required only for specific players' positions (i.e., a catcher or goalie). As with other body regions, protective equipment, in combination with a well-rounded physical conditioning program, can reduce the risk of injury. Although proper skill technique can prevent some injuries, this is not a major factor in this region.

Protective Equipment

Face masks with throat protectors are required for participants in some sports (e.g., baseball/softball catchers, field hockey, ice hockey, and lacrosse goalies). In many cases, an extended pad is attached to the mask to protect the throat region.

Many participants in collision and contact sports wear full chest and abdominal protection. In young baseball and softball players (younger than 12 years), it has been suggested that all infield players wear chest protectors. Adolescent rib cages are less rigid, placing the heart at a greater risk from direct impact. In this age group, more baseball and softball deaths occur from impacts to the chest than to the head.

Shoulder pads can protect the upper thoracic region, and rib protectors can provide protection from rib, upper abdominal or low back contusions. Body suits made of mesh with pockets can hold rib and hip pads to protect the sides and back.

Physical Conditioning

Flexibility and strengthening of the torso muscles should not be an isolated program, but should include a well-rounded conditioning program for the back, shoulder, abdomen, and hip regions. Range of motion (ROM) and strengthening exercises should include both open and closed kinetic chain activities.

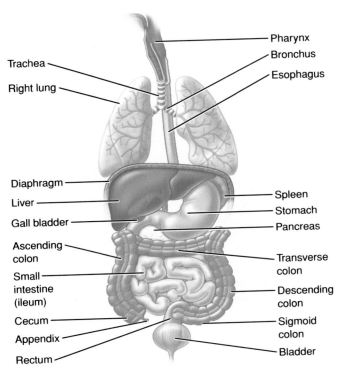

Trachea
Right lung
Diaphragm
Liver
Gall bladder
Ascending colon
Small intestine (ileum)
Cecum
Appendix
Rectum

Pharynx
Bronchus
Esophagus
Spleen
Stomach
Pancreas
Transverse colon
Descending colon
Sigmoid colon
Bladder

FIGURE 11.6 Anterior view of the visceral organs.

THROAT CONDITIONS

Neck Lacerations

Although uncommon, lacerations to the neck can occur. If the trauma is sufficiently deep, it can damage the jugular vein or carotid artery on the lateral side of the neck. Immediate control of hemorrhage is imperative. In addition to blood loss, air may be sucked into the vein and carried to the heart as an air embolism. Such an embolism can be fatal.

Management

Activation of the emergency plan, including summoning EMS, is warranted. While waiting for EMS to arrive, the coach should apply firm, direct pressure over the wound. The coach should also assess vital signs and treat for shock as necessary.

Contusions and Fractures

Contusions and fractures to the trachea, larynx, and hyoid bone can occur during hyperextension of the neck. In this position, the thyroid cartilage (Adam's apple) becomes prominent and vulnerable to direct impact forces. In rare instances, these injuries can be fatal as a result of the extravasation of blood into the laryngeal tissues leading to airway edema and asphyxia resulting from obstruction.

Signs and Symptoms

Immediate symptoms include hoarseness, **dyspnea** (difficulty breathing), coughing, difficulty swallowing, laryngeal tenderness, and an inability to make high-pitched "e" sounds. Significant trauma to the region can result in severe pain, laryngospasm, and acute respiratory distress

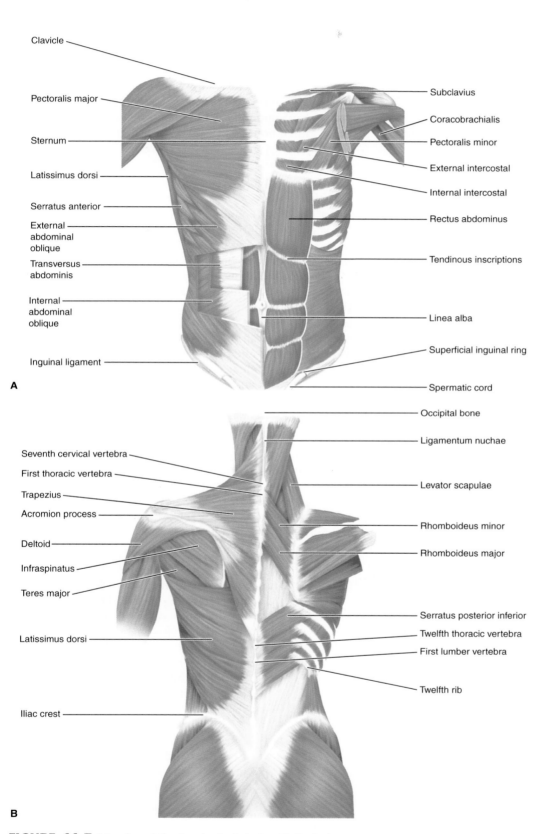

FIGURE 11.7 Muscles of the trunk. **A.** Anterior. **B.** Posterior.

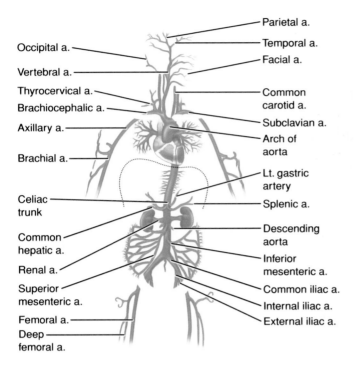

Occipital a.

Vertebral a.

Thyrocervical a.

Brachiocephalic a.

Axillary a.

Brachial a.

Celiac trunk

Common hepatic a.

Renal a.

Superior mesenteric a.

Femoral a.

Deep femoral a.

Parietal a.

Temporal a.

Facial a.

Common carotid a.

Subclavian a.

Arch of aorta

Lt. gastric artery

Splenic a.

Descending aorta

Inferior mesenteric a.

Common iliac a.

Internal iliac a.

External iliac a.

FIGURE 11.8 Arterial system of the trunk.

(BOX 11.1). Laryngospasm occurs when the adductor muscles of the vocal cords pull together in a shutter-like fashion, and the upper surface of the vocal cords closes over the top, causing complete obstruction. The individual may recover on-site and leave the area to return home, only to have increasing respiratory problems en route. As the internal hemorrhage and swelling increases, the occlusion becomes more complete, and breathing becomes more difficult. Panic and anxiety can increase respiration and, in doing so, compound the problem. Swelling is usually maximal within 6 hours, but may occur as late as 24 to 48 hours after injury. Cyanosis and loss of consciousness may occur with complete occlusion.

Management

In an effort to diminish panic and anxiety resulting from the sudden inability to breathe, the coach should immediately reassure the individual. The coach should also help the individual focus on their breathing rate.

If there is significant trauma, activation of the emergency plan, including summoning EMS is warranted. In these cases, it is important to consider an associated injury to the cervical spine. As such, the individual should not be moved. While waiting for EMS to arrive, the coach should assess vital signs and treat for shock as necessary.

If the individual recovers on-site, observation should continue throughout the day to note the presence of any delayed respiratory problems.

THORACIC CONDITIONS

Thoracic injuries are frequently caused by sudden deceleration and impact, which can lead to compression and subsequent deformation of the rib cage. The extent of damage depends on the direction, magnitude of force, and point of impact. For example, a glancing blow may contuse the chest wall, whereas a baseball that directly strikes the ribs may fracture a rib and drive the bony fragments internally, causing subsequent lung or cardiac damage. BOX 11.1 identifies signs and symptoms that indicate a serious thoracic condition.

► RED FLAG 11.1 Indicating a Serious Thoracic Condition

- Shortness of breath or difficulty in breathing
- Deviated trachea or trachea that moves during breathing
- Anxiety, fear, confusion, or restlessness
- Distended neck veins
- Bulging or bloodshot eyes
- Suspected rib or sternal fracture
- Severe chest pain aggravated by deep inspiration
- Abnormal chest movement on affected side
- Coughing up bright red or frothy blood
- Abnormal or absent breath sounds
- Rapid, weak pulse
- Low blood pressure
- Cyanosis

Stitch in the Side

A "**stitch in the side**" refers to a sharp pain or spasm in the chest wall, usually on the lower right side, during exertion. Potential causes include trapped colonic gas bubbles, localized diaphragmatic **hypoxia** with spasm, liver congestion with stretching of the liver capsule, and poor conditioning.

Management

The frequency of a stitch usually diminishes as an individual's aerobic conditioning level improves. Attempts can be made to run through the pain by:

- Forcibly exhaling through pursed lips
- Breathing deeply and regularly

- Leaning away from the affected side
- Stretching the arm on the affected side over the head as high as possible

Breast Conditions

Excessive breast motion during activity can lead to soreness, contusions, and nipple irritation. Although breast conditions are usually associated with females, men may also experience these conditions.

Contusions

Contusions to the breast may produce fat necrosis or hematoma formation, both of which are painful and may result in the formation of a localized breast mass. Appearance of these lesions on a mammogram may be indistinguishable from a malignant tumor. Direct trauma should be recorded on a female's permanent medical record to avoid any erroneous conclusions when reading a future mammogram.

Management

Immediate management for a breast contusion includes the application of ice and external support to the area.

Nipple Irritation

Nipple irritation is commonly seen in distance runners. Two commonly seen conditions are runner's nipples and cyclist's nipples.

Signs and Symptoms

Runner's nipples are associated with friction over the nipple area. As the shirt rubs over the nipples, friction is created that can lead to abrasions, blisters, or bleeding. Cyclist's nipples are caused by the combined effects of perspiration and wind-chill. In this condition, the nipples become cold and painful, and can persist for several days.

Management

For runner's nipples, the coach should advise the individual to cleanse the wound, apply an antibiotic ointment, and cover the wound with a nonadhering sterile gauze pad. Infection secondary to the injury may involve the entire nipple region or extend into the breast tissue, and may necessitate referral to a physician. This condition can be prevented by applying petroleum-based products and adhesive bandages over the nipples. Initial treatment for cyclist's nipples is to warm the nipples after completion of the event to prevent the irritation. This condition can be prevented by wearing a windproof jacket.

Strain of the Pectoralis Major Muscle

Pectoralis major muscle strains can occur in a variety of activities, including power lifting, particularly while bench pressing, boxing, wrestling. The mechanism of injury is usually indirect, resulting from extreme muscle tension. A pectoralis major strain can also result from direct trauma involving a sudden deceleration maneuver, such as when punching in boxing or blocking with an extended arm in football. A rupture results when the actively contracting muscle is overburdened by a load or extrinsic force that exceeds tissue tolerance. Ruptures are almost exclusively seen in males between 20 and 40 years of age.[1] A higher incidence of this injury is seen with anabolic steroid abuse.[2,3] Steroid use causes muscle hypertrophy and an increase in power secondary to rapid strength gain not accompanied by a concomitant increase in tendon size.

Signs and Symptoms

A mild muscle strain will produce some pain on resisted horizontal abduction. With a more severe strain or rupture, an audible pop, snap, or tearing sensation usually is accompanied by immediate, marked pain and weakness. The pain is often described as an aching or fatigue-like

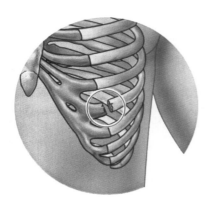

FIGURE 11.9 Undisplaced costochondral separation. The costal cartilage separates from the site at which the anterior margin of the rib attaches to the anterior end of the costal cartilage.

pain rather than a sharp pain. If the proximal attachment ruptures, the muscle retracts toward the axillary fold, causing it to appear enlarged. Swelling and ecchymosis are limited to the anterior chest wall. If the distal attachment is ruptured, the muscle bulges medially into the chest region, causing the axillary fold to appear thin. Swelling and ecchymosis occur on the anterior chest wall and upper arm. Shoulder motion is limited by pain.

Management

If a grade 1 injury is suspected, management involves standard acute care with cold and compression. If the signs and symptoms do not resolve within 2 to 3 days, the coach should require the individual to obtain approval for return to participation from a qualified healthcare professional. If a grade 2 or 3 injury is suspected, the individual should be referred to a qualified healthcare practitioner for a definitive diagnosis and ongoing treatment options.

Costochondral Injury

Costochondritis and costochondral sprains may occur during a collision with another object or as a result of a severe twisting motion of the thorax, such as during the sweep motion in rowing.[4] This action can sprain or separate the costal cartilage as it attaches to the sternum or where the anterior margin of the rib attaches to the anterior end of the costal cartilage, putting pressure on the intercostal nerve lying between it and the rib above (FIG. 11.9).

Signs and Symptoms

The individual may hear or feel a pop. The initial localized sharp pain may be followed by intermittent stabbing pain for several days. Pain may slowly decrease in intensity, but sharp clicks may occur during bending maneuvers as the displaced cartilage overrides the bone. A visible deformity and localized pain can be palpated at the involved joint. More severe sprains produce pain during deep inhalation.

Management

Standard acute protocol should be followed to reduce pain and inflammation. The individual should be referred to a physician for further assessment.

Sternal Fractures

The sternum is rarely fractured in sports, but may occur as a result of rapid deceleration and high impact into an object, or acute flexion that causes the upper fragment to displace anteriorly over the lower fragment. The fracture itself is not significant; however, the incidence of an associated intrathoracic injury is high.

Signs and Symptoms

The injury causes an immediate loss of breath. Localized pain is present with pressure over the sternum, and is aggravated by deep inspiration if the fracture is incomplete. If the fracture is complete, a palpable defect is present and pain occurs during normal respiration.

Management

If a sternal fracture is suspected, the emergency plan should be activated, including summoning EMS. Observation in the hospital with a cardiac monitor is often necessary because of the high incidence of associated intrathoracic trauma. While waiting for EMS to arrive, the coach should assess vital signs, and treat for shock as necessary.

Rib Fractures

Stress fractures to the ribs can result from an indirect force, such as a violent muscle contraction. They typically occur at the rib's weakest point (i.e., where it changes direction or has the smallest diameter).

Rib fractures are the most common thoracic injury as a result of blunt trauma.[5] Nondisplaced fractures are more common than displaced. If the fracture is displaced, internal injury should be suspected.

Signs and Symptoms

Intense localized pain over the fracture site is aggravated by deep inspiration, coughing, or chest movement. In many cases, the individual takes shallow breaths and leans toward the fracture site, stabilizing the area with a hand to prevent excessive movement of the chest to ease the pain. A visible contusion and palpable crepitus may be present at the impact site. Coughing up blood, especially bright red or frothy blood, should be noted.

Management

Treatment involves standard acute protocol. A 6-in elastic bandage can be wrapped around the thorax with circular motions distal to the injury site; or a sling and swathe may be used to immobilize the chest if pain is intense or multiple fractures are suspected. If one or two ribs are fractured, the individual should be referred immediately to an emergency care facility.

If signs and symptoms suggest an internal injury, the emergency plan should be activated, including summoning EMS. While waiting for EMS to arrive, the coach should assess vital signs and treat for shock as necessary.

INTERNAL COMPLICATIONS

Several conditions can alter breathing and cardiac function. Hyperventilation is associated with an inability to catch one's breath, and in most instances, is not a serious problem. Direct trauma to the thorax can lead to serious underlying problems, although these conditions are rare in sport participation. Among the more serious complications are pulmonary contusion, **pneumothorax, tension pneumothorax, hemothorax,** and heart contusions.

Hyperventilation

Hyperventilation is often linked to pain, stress, or trauma in sport participation. The respiratory rate increases during activity. Rapid, deep inhalations draw more oxygen into the lungs. Conversely, long exhalations result in too much carbon dioxide being exhaled.

Signs and Symptoms

Signs and symptoms include an inability to catch one's breath, numbness in the lips and hands, spasm of the hands, chest pain, dry mouth, dizziness, and occasionally, fainting.

Management

It is important to calm the individual, because panic and anxiety can complicate the condition. Treatment involves concentrating on slow inhalations through the nose and exhaling through the mouth until symptoms have stopped. Although breathing into a paper bag has proved to be quite successful in restoring the oxygen-carbon dioxide balance, many individuals find it embarrassing. Breathing into a paper bag is not needed except in severe cases.

Pneumothorax, Hemothorax, and Tension Pneumothorax

Three lung conditions—pneumothorax, hemothorax, and tension pneumothorax—can lead to a life-threatening situation (BOX 11.2). In **pneumothorax**, a fractured rib is the leading cause. When lung tissue is lacerated, air escapes into the pleural cavity with each inhalation and prevents the lung from fully expanding (FIG. 11.10). If the fractured rib tears lung tissue and blood vessels in the chest or chest cavity, it is called a **hemothorax**. In **tension pneumothorax**, air progressively accumulates in the pleural space around the injured lung during inspiration and cannot escape on expiration. The pleural space expands with each breath, resulting in the mediastinum (the partition in the thoracic cavity that separates the right and left lungs) being displaced to the opposite side, compressing the uninjured lung and thoracic aorta.

BOX 11.2	**Internal Lung Conditions**

- **Pneumothorax**—A condition whereby air is trapped in the pleural space, causing a portion of a lung to collapse.
- **Hemothorax**—An accumulation of blood, rather than air, into the pleural cavity.
- **Tension pneumothorax**—A situation in which air progressively accumulates in the pleural space during inspiration and cannot escape on expiration, resulting in a progressive increase in pressure in the pleural space that forces the mediastinum to be displaced to the opposite side, compressing the uninjured lung and thoracic aorta.

Signs and Symptoms

Severe pain during breathing, hypoxia, cyanosis, and signs of shock become immediately apparent. If a hemothorax is present, coughing up frothy blood may also be seen.

Management

Activation of the emergency plan, including summoning EMS, is warranted. While waiting for EMS to arrive, the coach should assess vital signs and treat for shock as necessary.

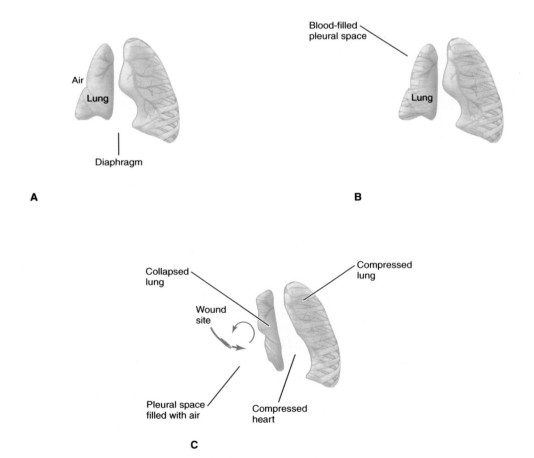

FIGURE 11.10 Internal complication to the lungs. **A.** Pneumothorax. **B.** Hemothorax. **C.** Tension pneumothorax. Each condition can become life-threatening if the lung collapses.

Heart Injuries

Blunt chest trauma can compress the heart between the sternum and spine, leading to blunt cardiac injury (formally called myocardial contusion). Red blood cells and fluid leak into the surrounding tissues and, in doing so, decreases circulation to the heart muscle. This action subsequently leads to localized cellular damage and necrosis of the heart tissue. Decreased cardiac output secondary to arrhythmias, or irregular heartbeats, are of major concern.

Blunt trauma may also lead to **cardiac tamponade**, the leading cause of traumatic death in youth baseball, and has also been reported in softball, ice hockey, and lacrosse.

Signs and Symptoms

Classic signs of cardiac tamponade include jugular venous distention (JVD) due to increased venous pressure or lack of cardiac filling. In nearly all cases, the individual collapses within seconds and goes into respiratory arrest.

Management

Resuscitation is unsuccessful in many cases, even when it is given immediately after injury. This may result from structural cardiac disruption caused by the trauma. Activation of the emergency plan, including summoning EMS, is warranted. While waiting for EMS to arrive, the coach should initiate breathing and chest compressions.

Sudden Death in Athletes

Sudden death is defined as an event that is nontraumatic, unexpected, and occurs instantaneously or within minutes of an abrupt change in an individual's previous clinical state. While hypertrophic cardiomyopathy is the most common cause of sudden cardiac death (refer to Chapter 8), other causes of sudden death include abnormalities in the coronary arteries, aortic rupture associated with **Marfan's syndrome**, and **mitral valve prolapse**. Marfan's syndrome is a genetic disorder of the connective tissue that can affect the skeleton, lungs, eyes, heart, and blood vessels. The hallmark characteristic is a weakened aorta that can rupture during exertion. Mitral valve prolapse occurs when redundant tissue is found on one or both leaflets of the mitral valve. During a ventricular contraction, a portion of the redundant tissue on the mitral valve pushes back beyond the normal limit. An abnormal sound results as blood is regurgitated back through the mitral valve into the left atrium. In an individual older than 35 years, the most common cause of sudden death is ischemic coronary artery disease.

Signs and Symptoms

Symptoms such as unexplained chest pain, sudden onset of fatigue, heartburn or indigestion, and excessive breathlessness during exercise signal a potential emergency.

Management

Activation of the emergency plan, including summoning EMS, is warranted. While waiting for EMS to arrive, the coach should initiate breathing and chest compressions.

ABDOMINAL WALL CONDITIONS

The muscles of the abdominal wall are strong and powerful, yet flexible enough to absorb impact. Consequently, injuries to the abdominal wall usually are minor. However, other conditions, such as a contusion to the solar plexus and **hernias**, can affect sport participation.

Muscle Strains

Muscle strains are caused by sudden twisting or sudden hyperextension of the spine. The rectus abdominis is the most commonly injured muscle. Complications arise when the epigastric artery or intramuscular vessels are damaged, leading to a rectus sheath hematoma.

Signs and Symptoms

Localized pain and spasm in the involved muscle may be present. Straight leg raising, performing a sit-up, or hyperextension of the back can increase the pain.

Management

If a grade 1 injury is suspected, management involves standard acute care with cold and compression. If the signs and symptoms do not resolve within 2 to 3 days, the coach should require the individual to obtain approval for return to participation from a qualified healthcare professional. If a grade 2 or 3 injury is suspected, the individual should be referred to a qualified healthcare practitioner for a definitive diagnosis and ongoing treatment options.

Solar Plexus Contusion ("Wind Knocked Out")

A blow to the abdomen with the muscles relaxed is referred to as a **"solar plexus punch."** Although the true cause of the breathing difficulty is unknown, it is thought to be caused by diaphragmatic spasm and transient contusion to the sympathetic celiac plexus.

Signs and Symptoms

The blow results in an immediate inability to catch one's breath (**dyspnea**). Fear and anxiety may complicate the condition.

Management

Any restrictive equipment and clothing around the abdomen should be loosened, and the individual instructed to flex the knees toward the chest. While it may seem paradoxic, the individual should be instructed to take a deep breath and hold it. This action should be repeated until normal breathing is restored. Another method for restoring normal breathing is to instruct the individual to whistle. This action forces the diaphragm to relax. Because a severe blow may lead to an intra-abdominal injury, assessment should be performed to rule out internal injury.

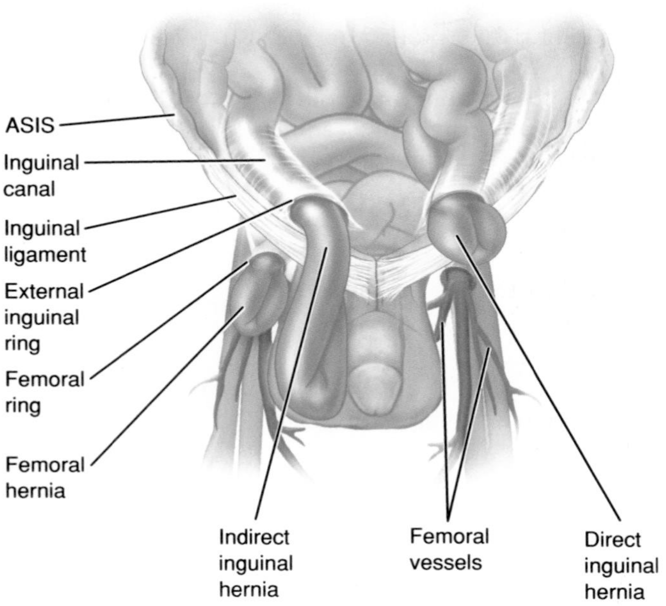

Hernia

A **hernia** is a protrusion of abdominal viscera through a weakened portion of the abdominal wall and typically occurs in or just above the groin (FIG. 11.11). Many hernias are asymptomatic until the preparticipation exam, when the physician palpates the protrusion by invaginating the scrotum with a finger. Protrusion of the hernia increases with coughing. The danger of a hernia lies in continued trauma to the weakened area during falls, blows, or increased intra-abdominal pressure exerted during activity. The hernia can twist on itself and produce a strangulated hernia, which can become gangrenous.

FIGURE 11.11 Hernias. A hernia may be classified as (**A**) indirect, in which the small intestine extends into the scrotum; (**B**) direction, in which the small intestine extends through a weakening in the internal inguinal ring; or (**C**) femoral, in which the small intestine protrudes posterior to the inguinal ligament and medial to the femoral artery.

Signs and symptoms

Symptoms vary, but for most hernias the first sign is a visible tender swelling and an aching feeling in the groin. If the hernia ruptures, symptoms may include a sharp, stinging pain or a feeling of something giving way at the site of the rupture, nausea, and vomiting.

Management

If a ruptured hernia is suspected, initiate the emergency care plan and position the individual on his or her back. Place a rolled blanket under the knees to reduce tension in the abdominal area, monitor the ABCs, and treat for possible shock until EMS arrives.

INTRA-ABDOMINAL CONDITIONS

Trauma to the abdomen can lead to severe internal hemorrhage if organs or major blood vessels are lacerated or ruptured. Injuries can be open or closed, with closed injuries typically caused by blunt trauma. If damaged, hollow viscera can leak their contents into the abdominal cavity, causing severe hemorrhage, **peritonitis**, and shock. Many signs and symptoms indicating intra-abdominal injuries are similar in nature, regardless of the organ involved (BOX 11.3). Variations arise in the area of palpable pain and the site of referred pain.

Acute management of suspected intra-abdominal injuries is also very similar, regardless of the injured organ. Initially, the coach should keep the individual relaxed while assessing airway, breathing, and circulation. If necessary, the emergency medical plan should be activated, including summoning of EMS. While waiting for EMS to arrive, the individual should be placed in a supine position with the knees flexed to relax the low back and abdominal muscles. The vital signs should be monitored regularly, and the individual should be treated for shock.

> ## ► RED FLAG 11.3 Indicating a Serious Intra-abdominal Condition
>
> - Rapid, weak pulse, low blood pressure, or cyanosis (shock)
> - Abdominal pain, often starting as mild, then rapidly increasing in severity
> - Coughing up or vomiting blood that looks like used coffee grounds
> - Localized tenderness and rigidity over the injured organ
> - Referred pain to the shoulder tip, back, or groin
> - Diffuse hemorrhage or distention of the abdomen
> - Nausea
> - Weakness
> - Individual may lean forward and bring the knees to the chest to reduce tension in the abdominal muscles
> - Cramps or muscle guarding (splinting)
> - Shallow breathing. Abdominal respiratory motion may be absent
> - Blood in the urine or stool

Splenic Rupture

Although rarely injured in sport participation, certain systemic disorders, such as infectious mononucleosis, can enlarge the spleen, making it vulnerable to injury. The spleen is the most commonly injured abdominal organ and is the most frequent cause of death from abdominal blunt trauma in sport.[3] Subsequent to trauma, the spleen can lose blood very rapidly because of its vascularity. However, the spleen can splint itself and stop hemorrhaging. While this may appear advantageous, it is actually problematic because the splinting is not sufficient and delayed hemorrhage can be produced days, weeks, or months later after a seemingly minor jarring motion.

An individual who has infectious mononucleosis should be disqualified from contact and strenuous noncontact sports and physical activity for at least 3 weeks. After 3 weeks, return to strenuous noncontact sports and physical activity is acceptable if the individual feels up to activity, the spleen is nonpalpable, and liver function tests are normal. If the spleen remains palpable or liver function tests are abnormal, contact sports and activities are contraindicated for an additional week or longer.[5]

Signs and Symptoms

Indications of a splenic rupture include a history of blunt trauma to the left upper quadrant, and a persistent dull pain in the upper left quadrant, left lower chest, and left shoulder, referred to as **Kehr's sign**. Symptoms at the time of injury include nausea, cold and clammy skin, and signs of shock.

Liver Contusion and Rupture

A direct blow to the upper right quadrant can contuse the liver. As with the spleen, systemic diseases, such as hepatitis, can enlarge the liver, making it more susceptible to injury. An individual with an enlarged liver (i.e., hepatomegaly) should avoid contact sports until the liver has returned to its normal size or is nonpalpable.

Signs and Symptoms

Significant palpable pain, point tenderness, hypotension, and shock are indicative of liver trauma. In addition, pain may be referred to the inferior angle of the right scapula.

Kidney Contusion

The kidney may be injured as a result of a direct blow or a contrecoup injury from a high-speed collision. Because the kidney is normally distended by blood, an external force can cause abnormal extension of the engorged kidney. The degree of renal injury depends on the extent of the distention, and the angle and magnitude of the blow.

Signs and Symptoms

The individual may complain of pain, tenderness, and **hematuria**. Pain can be referred posteriorly to the low back region, sides of the buttocks, and anteriorly to the lower abdomen. Hypovolemic shock may result from extensive bleeding.

THE COACH AND ON-SITE ASSESSMENT OF THE THROAT, THORAX, AND ABDOMINAL REGIONS

Injury assessment should focus on the primary survey, history of the injury, and assessment of vital signs. Chest or abdominal trauma, although initially appearing superficial and minor, can mask internal hemorrhage and swelling that can seriously compromise function of the vital organs. In addition, the individual's condition can slowly deteriorate, leading to a life-threatening condition. Although general observation can confirm the possibility of a serious underlying condition, a good history of the injury and constant monitoring of vital signs are stronger assessment tools.

As with other on-site injury assessments, it begins as the coach is approaching the individual. The focus should be on observing the individual's overall presentation and attitude as well as their willingness and ability to move. Observation of body position can indicate the site, nature, and severity of injury. For example, in an acute thoracic injury, the individual may lean toward the injured side, using an arm or hand to stabilize the region. In an acute abdominal injury, the individual may lie on the injured side and bring the knees toward the chest to relax the abdominal muscles.

Once the coach reaches the individual, a primary survey should be performed. If there is any reason to suspect a spinal injury, the coach should complete a spinal injury assessment (refer to Chapter 10). If the individual is having difficulty breathing, anxiety and panic may exacerbate the condition. As such, prior to initiating any assessment, it may become necessary for the coach to calm and reassure the individual. Following the completion of the primary survey and having ruled out a spinal injury, it may be appropriate to delay the history component of the examination and initiate the secondary survey with a focus on the assessment of vital signs. If at any point during the secondary survey, signs and symptoms suggest a potentially serious of life-threatening injury (BOX 11.4), the coach should activate the emergency plan, including activation of EMS.

The history component of the examination can provide extremely valuable information in the assessment of a throat, thorax, or visceral condition (APPLICATION STRATEGY 11.1). In particular, the mechanism of injury as well as the location and extent of pain are critical to determining injury to a specific organ (BOX 11.5). If the history of the injury includes trauma involving force (e.g., compression; tension), the coach should inspect the site of the actual injury for any deformity, swelling, or discoloration. While a qualified healthcare practitioner could obtain important information in the palpation component of an assessment, the skills required in the palpation of conditions involving the throat, thorax, and abdominal regions are not within the standard of care of a coach and, as such, should not be attempted. In a similar manner, the few tests that exist for assessing the thorax and visceral area are too advanced for use by the coach. APPLICATION STRATEGY 11.1 provides a framework for the on-site assessment of a conscious individual with a potential nonorthopedic injury (e.g., thoracic or abdominal injury).

► RED FLAG 11.4 Indicating When to Activate EMS

- Rapid, weak pulse
- Cyanotic
- Sudden, sharp chest pain aggravated with deep inspiration
- Shortness of breath, shallow breathing, or difficulty in breathing
- Deviated trachea or trachea that moves during breathing
- Abnormal chest movement on affected side
- Coughing up bright red or frothy blood
- Coughing up or vomiting blood that looks like used coffee grounds
- Localized abdominal pain or rigidity, often starting as mild, then rapidly increasing in severity

BOX 11.5 Common Sites of Referred Pain

ORGAN	LOCATION OF PAIN
Appendicitis	Lower right quadrant
Bladder	Lower pelvic region over pubic bone
Heart	Left shoulder, down medial left arm, or it can extend into neck and jaw
Kidneys	Posterior lumbar region radiating to flanks and groin
Liver and gallbladder	Upper right quadrant or right shoulder
Lung and diaphragm	Upper shoulders and neck
Spleen	Left shoulder or proximal third of left arm (Kehr's sign)

APPLICATION STRATEGY 11.1

Assessment of Throat, Thorax, or Visceral Conditions—History Component

HISTORY
- Chief complaint
  - What's wrong?
  - What happened?
  - What were you doing?
  - What position were you in and from what direction was the force (e.g., glancing, direct, or violent muscle contraction)?
- Pain
  - Are you experiencing any pain? If so, where? (Consider the potential for referred pain.) Are you experiencing any pain other than the site of the trauma?
  - Can you describe the pain (sharp, aching, burning, radiating)?
  - Did the pain disappear, and then gradually increase (spontaneous pneumothorax, ruptured spleen)?
- Does it hurt to take a deep breath?
- What motions aggravate the symptoms? In what position are you most comfortable?
- Sounds/feelings
  - Did you hear anything?
  - Did you feel any unusual sensations (e.g., tearing, tingling, numbing, cracking)?
  - Are you nauseous?
  - Are you dizzy or lightheaded?
- Have you had any medical problems recently? (e.g., mononucleosis)
- Previous history
  - Has this ever happened to you before? If so, what happened? Were you treated for it

SUMMARY

1. The throat includes the pharynx, larynx, trachea, esophagus, a number of glands, and several major blood vessels. Injuries to the throat are of particular concern because of the life-sustaining functions of the trachea and carotid arteries.

2. The diaphragm is a sheet of muscle that separates the thoracic cavity (heart, lungs, and ribs) from the abdominal cavity. It plays a critical role in respiration.

3. The visceral region includes both solid (i.e., spleen, liver, pancreas, kidneys, and adrenal glands) and hollow organs (i.e., stomach, gall bladder, small and large intestines, bladder, and ureters).

4. Blows to the throat may result in severe pain, laryngospasm, and acute respiratory distress.

5. A "stitch in the side" is a sharp pain or spasm in the chest wall, usually on the lower right side. Several strategies can be used to enable an individual to address the pain.

6. A pectoralis major muscle strain involves an actively contracting muscle overburdened by a load or extrinsic force that exceeds tissue tolerance. If muscle fibers have been ruptured, resisted horizontal adduction and internal rotation of the shoulder are weak and accentuate the deformity.

7. Signs and symptoms indicating a possible internal thoracic condition include:
   - Shortness of breath or difficulty in breathing
   - Severe chest pain aggravated by deep inspiration
   - Abnormal chest movement
   - Abnormal or absent breath sounds

8. Signs and symptoms indicating a possible intra-abdominal condition include:
   - Severe abdominal pain
   - Nausea or vomiting
   - Distended abdomen
   - Tenderness, rigidity, or muscle spasm
   - Blood in the urine or stool

9. Certain injuries may not develop until hours, days, or weeks later. As such, the presumption of possible intrathoracic or intra-abdominal injuries with any blunt trauma necessitates referral to a qualified healthcare practitioner.

10. Injury assessment for the thorax and visceral region should focus on the vital signs and history of the injury.

11. If at any time, signs and symptoms indicate an intrathoracic or intra-abdominal injury, the emergency medical plan should be activated, including summoning of EMS. While waiting for EMS to arrive, the coach should continue to monitor vital signs and treat for shock as necessary.

12. If on-site recovery occurs, the individual should still be provided with information identifying signs and symptoms that could develop later and indicate that the condition is getting worse. The individual should also be provided with instructions for seeking medical assistance.

APPLICATION QUESTIONS

1. During a rebound attempt, a high school basketball player is struck in the anterior neck with an elbow. The player is coughing and having difficulty swallowing. What injury should be suspected? How should the coach manage the situation?

2. In an effort to improve his cardiovascular fitness, one of your clients, a healthy 35-year-old male, began a supervised running program. He has been running for 3 weeks. He occasionally experiences a stitch in the side while running. A physician has advised him that the condition is not serious and suggested that he may attempt to run though the pain. What strategies would you recommend as ways to alleviate the pain while running?

3. One of the eight grade students in your physical education class experiences hyperventilation during an activity. What is the management for this condition?

_____

_____

4. In attempting an overhead hit in volleyball, a high school volleyball player experiences pain in the abdominal region. There is no visible swelling or discoloration. There is no radiating pain. The athlete is unable to do a sit-up due to pain. How should the coach manage this condition?

_____

_____

5. Following a blow to the abdomen, a high school ice hockey player experiences dyspnea. A solar plexus contusion is suspected. How should the coach mange the situation? Why?

_____

_____

6. During a lacrosse scrimmage in a physical education class, a 16-year-old female student was inadvertently struck in the abdomen with another student's stick. She experienced a sudden onset of abdominal pain in the upper right quadrant. She also reported pain to the inferior angle of the right scapula. What injury should be suspected? How should the physical education teacher manage this condition? Why?

_____

_____

7. During practice, a 16-year-old football player was struck in the abdomen with a helmet and experienced a sudden onset of abdominal pain in the upper left quadrant. How should the coach proceed with the assessment of this injury to determine the extent and severity of injury? What signs and symptoms would suggest an internal injury?

_____

_____

8. A 35-year-old male client at a fitness facility is performing bench press when he suddenly experiences significant pain in the belly of the pectoralis major. He reports that he heard an audible pop and felt a tearing sensation. In observing the involved area, the fitness specialist notes the muscle is bulging medially into the chest region. The individual is hesitant to move the shoulder. What condition should be suspected? How should the fitness specialist manage the condition?

_____

_____

REFERENCES

1. Beloosesky Y, Grinblat J, Hendell D, and Sommer R. 2002. Pectoralis major rupture in a 97-year old woman. J Am Geriatr Soc, 50(8):1465–1468.
2. Dodds SD, and Wolfe SW. 2002. Injuries to the pectoralis major. Sports Med, 32(14):945–952.
3. Chang CJ, and Graves DW. Athletic injuries of the thorax and abdomen. In *The team physician's handbook*, edited by MB Mellion, WM Walsh, C Madden, M Putukian, and GL Shelton. Philadelphia, PA: Hanley & Belfus, 2002.
4. Moeller JL. 1996. Contraindications to athletic participation. Spinal, systemic, dermatologic, paired-organ, and other issues. Phys Sportsmed, 24(9):57–70.
5. Golden PA. 2000. Thoracic trauma. Orthop Nurs, 19(5):37–46.

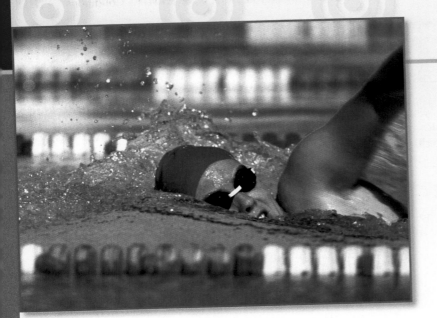

SHOULDER CONDITIONS

KEY TERMS

brachial plexus

dead arm syndrome

glenoid labrum

impingement
   syndrome

little league shoulder

rotator cuff

thoracic outlet
   compression
   syndrome

LEARNING OUTCOMES

1. Describe the major articulations that comprise the shoulder complex.

2. Identify the major motions available at the shoulder.

3. Explain general principles used to prevent injuries to the shoulder.

4. Describe common injuries and conditions sustained by physically active individuals to the shoulder complex, including their sign, symptoms, and immediate management.

5. Describe an on-site assessment of an acute shoulder injury appropriate for use by a coach.

The loose structure of the shoulder complex enables extreme mobility, but provides little stability. As a result, the shoulder is much more prone to injury than the hip. Common injuries include dislocations, clavicular fractures, muscle and tendon strains, **rotator cuff** tears, acromioclavicular (AC) sprains, bursitis, bicipital tendonitis, and **impingement syndrome**.[1,2] Shoulder injuries commonly occur in activities involving an overhead motion, such as baseball, swimming, tennis, volleyball, and weightlifting. In fact, shoulder pain is the most common musculoskeletal complaint among competitive swimmers, with 40 to 70% reporting a history of shoulder pain.[3] Dislocations of the shoulder articulations are not uncommon in contact sports, such as wrestling and football.[4]

This chapter begins with a general anatomy review of the shoulder region, followed by an overview of common injuries to the shoulder complex. Information pertaining to mechanism of injury, signs and symptoms, and management by the coach will be provided. Finally, a basic assessment of the region is presented.

SHOULDER ANATOMY

The arm articulates with the trunk at the shoulder, or pectoral girdle, comprised of the scapula and clavicle (FIG. 12.1). The shoulder region has five separate articulations: the sternoclavicular (SC) joint, AC joint, coracoclavicular joint, glenohumeral (GH) joint, and scapulothoracic joint. The articulation referred to specifically as the shoulder joint is the GH joint; the remaining articulations are collectively referred to as the shoulder girdle. The SC and AC joints enhance motion of the clavicle and scapula, enabling the GH joint to provide a greater range of motion (ROM).

Sternoclavicular Joint

As the name suggests, the SC joint consists of the articulation of the superior sternum, or manubrium, with the proximal clavicle. The SC joint is surrounded by a joint capsule that is thickened anteriorly and posteriorly by four ligaments, including the interclavicular, costoclavicular, and anterior and posterior SC ligaments.

The SC joint enables rotation of the clavicle with respect to the sternum. The joint allows motion of the distal clavicle in superior, inferior, anterior, and posterior directions, along with some forward and backward rotation of the clavicle. As such, rotation occurs at the SC joint during motions, such as shrugging the shoulders, reaching above the head, and in most throwing-type activities. Because the first rib is joined by its cartilage to the manubrium just inferior to the joint, motion of the clavicle in the inferior direction is restricted. The close-packed position for the SC joint occurs with maximal shoulder elevation.

Acromioclavicular Joint

The AC joint consists of the articulation of the medial facet of the acromion process of the scapula with the distal clavicle (see FIG. 12.1). As an irregular, diarthrodial joint, limited motion is permitted in all three planes.

The joint is enclosed by a capsule, although the capsule is thinner than that of the SC joint. The strong superior and inferior AC ligaments cross the joint, providing stability. The coracoacromial ligament, sometimes referred to as the "arch" ligament, also attaches to the inferior lip of the AC joint to serve as a buffer between the rotator cuff muscles and the bony acromion process.

The close-packed position of the AC joint occurs when the humerus is abducted at 90°. Injuries to the AC joint are common in athletes involved in throwing and other overhead activities.[5]

Coracoclavicular Joint

The coracoclavicular joint is a syndesmosis in which the coracoid process of the scapula and the inferior surface of the clavicle are joined by the coracoclavicular ligament (see FIG. 12.1). This ligament resists independent upward movement of the clavicle, downward movement of the scapula, and anteroposterior movement of the clavicle or scapula. Minimal movement is permitted at this joint. The coracoclavicular ligaments are frequently ruptured during contact sports, such as football, hockey, and rugby.[6]

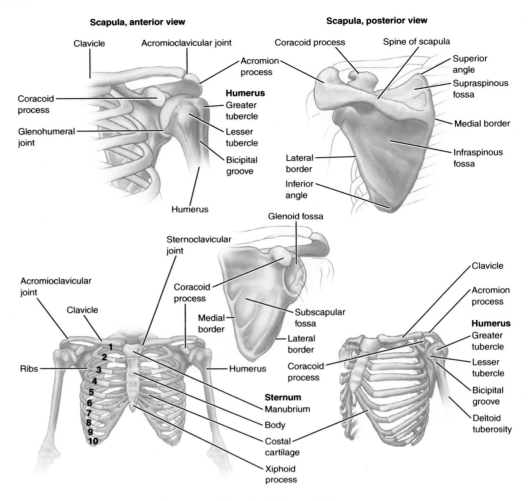

FIGURE 12.1 Skeletal features of the shoulder and chest.

Glenohumeral Joint

The GH joint is the articulation between the glenoid fossa of the scapula and the head of the humerus. Although the joint enables a greater total ROM than any other joint in the human body, it is lacking in bony stability. This partially results from the hemispheric head of the humerus, which has three to four times the amount of surface area as compared with the shallow glenoid fossa. Because the glenoid fossa is also less curved than the humeral head, the humerus not only rotates, but moves linearly across the surface of the glenoid fossa when humeral motion occurs, an action that predisposes the joint to impingement injuries.

The tendons of four muscles, including the supraspinatus, infraspinatus, teres minor, and subscapularis, also join the joint capsule (FIGS. 12.2 and 12.3). These muscles are referred to as the SITS muscles, after the first letter of each muscle's name. They are also known as the **rotator cuff** muscles because they all act to rotate the humerus and because their tendons merge to form a collagenous cuff around the joint. Tension in the rotator cuff muscles helps to hold the head of the humerus against the glenoid fossa, further contributing to joint stability. The joint is most stable in its close-packed position when the humerus is abducted and laterally rotated.

Scapulothoracic Joint

Because muscles attaching to the scapula permit its motion with respect to the trunk or thorax, this region is sometimes described as the scapulothoracic joint (FIGS. 12.2 and 12.3). The scapular muscles perform two functions. The first is stabilization of the shoulder region. For example, when a barbell is lifted from the floor, the levator scapula, trapezius, and rhomboids develop tension to support the scapula and, in turn, the entire shoulder through the AC joint. The second

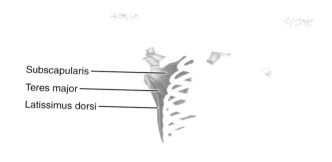

Subscapularis
Teres major
Latissimus dorsi

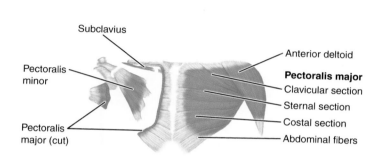
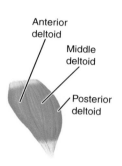

Subclavius

Pectoralis minor

Pectoralis major (cut)

Anterior deltoid

Pectoralis major
Clavicular section
Sternal section
Costal section
Abdominal fibers

Anterior deltoid
Middle deltoid
Posterior deltoid

FIGURE 12.2 Muscles of the shoulder and chest.

function is to facilitate movements of the upper extremity through appropriate positioning of the GH joint. During an overhand throw, for example, the rhomboids contract to move the entire shoulder posteriorly as the arm and hand move backward during the preparatory phase. As the arm and hand then move forward to execute the throw, tension in the rhomboids is released to permit forward movement of the shoulder, enabling medial rotation of the humerus.

Bursae

The shoulder is surrounded by several bursae, including the subcoracoid, subscapularis, and the most important, the subacromial. The subacromial bursa lies in the subacromial space where it is surrounded by the acromion process of the scapula and the coracoacromial ligament above and the GH joint below. The bursa cushions the rotator cuff muscles, particularly the supraspinatus, from the overlying bony acromion and provides the major component of the subacromial gliding mechanism. The bursa can become irritated when repeatedly compressed during overhead arm action.

Nerves and Blood Vessels of the Shoulder

Innervation of the upper extremity arises from the **brachial plexus**, a combination of nerves branching primarily from the lower four cervical (C5 to C8) and the first thoracic (T1) spinal nerves (see FIG. 10.8). The branches from these nerves extend from the neck anteriorly and laterally, passing between the clavicle and first rib. Injuries to the clavicle in this region can damage the brachial plexus.

The subclavian artery passes beneath the clavicle to become the axillary artery, providing the major blood supply to the shoulder (FIG. 12.4). Branches of the axillary artery include the thoracoacromial trunk, lateral thoracic artery, subscapular artery, and thoracodorsal artery, as well as the anterior and posterior humeral circumflex arteries that supply the head of the humerus.

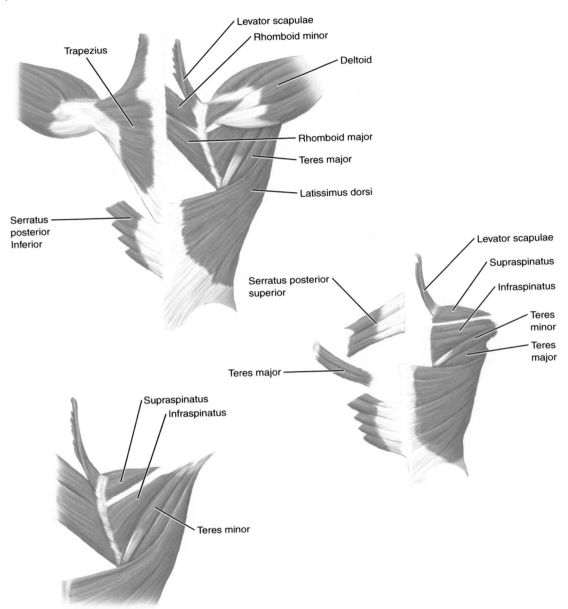

FIGURE 12.3 Muscles of the shoulder and upper back.

KINEMATICS AND MAJOR MUSCLE ACTIONS OF THE SHOULDER COMPLEX

The shoulder is the most freely moveable joint in the body, with motion capability in all three planes (FIG. 12.5). Sagittal plane movements at the shoulder include flexion (i.e., elevation of the arm in an anterior direction), extension (i.e., return of the arm from a position of flexion to the side of the body), and hyperextension (i.e., elevation of the arm in a posterior direction). Frontal plane movements include abduction (i.e., elevation of the arm in a lateral direction) and adduction (i.e., return of the arm from a position of abduction to the side of the body). Transverse plane movements include horizontal adduction (i.e., horizontally extended arm is moved medially) and horizontal abduction (i.e., horizontally extended arm is moved laterally). The humerus can also rotate medially (i.e., anterior face of

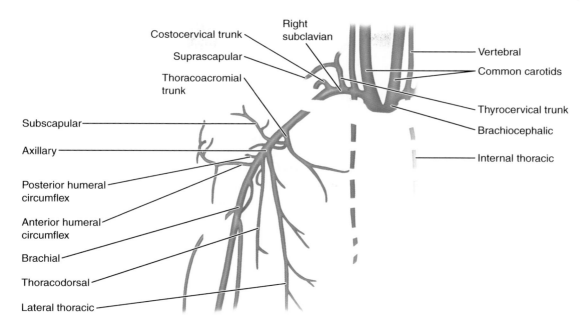

FIGURE 12.4 Blood supply to the shoulder.

humerus is moved medially) and laterally (i.e., anterior face of humerus is moved laterally). Elevation of the humerus in all planes is accompanied by about 55° of external rotation.[7]

Coordination of Shoulder Movements

The extensive ROM afforded by the shoulder partially results from the loose structure of the GH joint, and partially from the proximity of the other shoulder articulations and the movement capabilities they provide. Movement at the shoulder typically involves some rotation at the SC, AC, and GH joints. For example, as the arm is elevated past 30° of abduction, or the first 45° to 60° of flexion, the scapula also rotates, contributing approximately one-third of the total rotational movement of the humerus. This important coordination of scapular and humeral movements, known as scapulohumeral rhythm, enables a much greater ROM at the shoulder than if the scapula were fixed (FIG. 12.6). Also contributing to the first 90° of humeral elevation is the elevation of the clavicle through approximately 35° to 45° of motion at the SC joint. The AC joint contributes to overall movement capability as well, with rotation occurring during the first 30° of humeral elevation, and then again as the arm is moved past 135°.[8]

Glenohumeral Flexion

The muscles that cross the GH joint anteriorly are positioned to contribute to flexion (see FIGS. 12.2 and 12.3). The anterior deltoid and clavicular pectoralis major are the primary shoulder flexors, with assistance provided by the coracobrachialis and short head of the biceps brachii. Because the biceps brachii also crosses the elbow joint, it is capable of exerting more force at the shoulder when the elbow is in full extension.

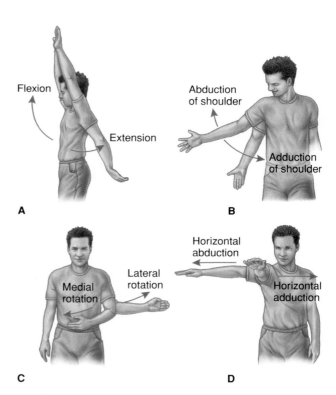

FIGURE 12.5 Movements of the arm at the shoulder. **A.** Flexion and extension. **B.** Abduction and adduction. **C.** Medial and lateral rotation. **D.** Horizontal abduction and adduction. Combined movements are called circumduction.

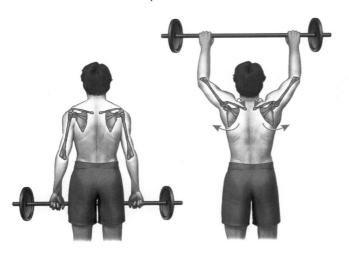

FIGURE 12.6 Scapulohumeral rhythm. The coordinated movement of the scapula needed to facilitate motion of the humerus is known as scapulohumeral rhythm. The arrows indicate the direction the scapulae must rotate to raise the arms.

Glenohumeral Extension

When extension is not resisted, the action is caused by gravity. Eccentric contraction of the flexor muscles serves as a controlling or braking mechanism. When resistance to extension is offered, the posterior GH muscles act, including the sternocostal pectoralis, latissimus dorsi, and teres major, with assistance provided by the posterior deltoid and long head of the triceps brachii (see FIGS. 12.2 and 12.3).

Glenohumeral Abduction

The muscles superior to the GH joint produce abduction and include the middle deltoid and supraspinatus (see FIGS. 12.2 and 12.3). During the contribution of the middle deltoid, from approximately 90° through 180° of abduction, the infraspinatus, subscapularis, and teres minor produce inferiorly directed force to neutralize the superiorly directed dislocating force produced by the middle deltoid. This action serves an important function in preventing impingement of the supraspinatus and subacromial bursa. The long head of the biceps brachii provides GH stability during abduction.

Glenohumeral Adduction

As with extension, adduction in the absence of resistance results from gravitational force, with the abductors controlling the speed of motion. When resistance is present, adduction is accomplished through the action of the muscles positioned on the inferior side of the GH joint, including the latissimus dorsi, teres major, and sternocostal pectoralis (see FIGS. 12.2 and 12.3). The short head of the biceps and long head of the triceps contribute minor assistance. When the arm is elevated above 90°, the coracobrachialis and subscapularis also assist.

Lateral and Medial Rotation of the Humerus

Lateral rotators of the humerus lie on the posterior aspect of the humerus, including the infraspinatus and teres minor, with assistance provided by the posterior deltoid. Muscles on the anterior side of the humerus contribute to medial rotation. These include the subscapularis and teres major, with assistance from the pectoralis major, anterior deltoid, latissimus dorsi, and short head of the biceps (see FIGS. 12.2 and 12.3).

PREVENTION OF SHOULDER CONDITIONS

Acute and chronic injuries to the shoulder complex are common in sport participation. Many contact and collision sports do require some protective equipment, but in most cases, flexibility, physical conditioning, and proper technique are the primary factors that can reduce the risk of injury to this vulnerable area.

Physical Conditioning

Lack of flexibility can predispose an individual to joint sprains and muscular strains. Warm-up exercises should focus on general joint flexibility, and may be performed alone or with a partner using proprioceptive neuromuscular facilitation (PNF) stretching techniques. Individuals using the throwing motion in their sport should increase ROM in external rotation, as this has been shown to increase the velocity of the throwing arm and decrease shearing forces on the GH joint. Several flexibility exercises for the shoulder complex are demonstrated in APPLICATION STRATEGY 12.1.

Strengthening programs should focus on muscles acting on both the GH and scapulothoracic region. Strength in the infraspinatus, teres minor, and posterior shoulder musculature is necessary to:

- Begin the cocking phase of throwing.
- Fix the shoulder girdle during the acceleration phase.

APPLICATION STRATEGY 12.1

Flexibility Exercises for the Shoulder Region

- Posterior capsular stretch. Horizontally adduct the arm across the chest while the opposite hand assists the stretch.

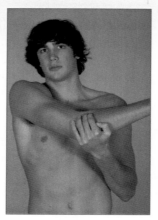

- Anterior and posterior capsular stretch. Hold onto both sides of a doorway with the hands behind the back. Straighten the arms while leaning forward. Repeat with the hand in front while leaning backward.

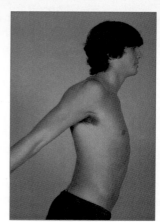

- Inferior capsular stretch. Hold the involved arm over the head with the elbow flexed. Use the opposite hand to assist in the stretching. Add a side stretch.

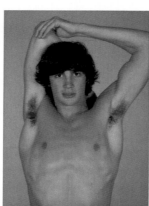

- Medial and lateral rotators. Using a towel, bat, or racquet, pull the arm to stretch it into lateral rotation. Repeat in medial rotation.

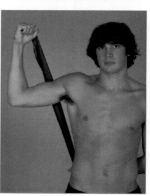

- Provide adequate muscle tension, with eccentric contractions, for smooth deceleration through the follow-through phase

A weakened supraspinatus is present in many chronic shoulder problems, particularly among throwers. Concentric and eccentric contractions with light resistance in the first 30° of abduction can strengthen this muscle. Strengthening the scapular stabilizers can be accomplished by doing push-ups or moving the arm through a resisted diagonal pattern of external rotation and horizontal abduction. Other strengthening exercises are provided in APPLICATION STRATEGY 12.2.

Protective Equipment

Contact and collision sports, such as football, lacrosse, and ice hockey, require shoulder pads to protect exposed bony protuberances from impact. Although shoulder pads do prevent some soft tissue injuries in this region, they do not protect the GH joint from excessive motion.

Proper Skill Technique

Coordinated muscle contractions are necessary for the smooth execution of the throwing motion. Any disruption in the sequencing of integrated movements can lead to additional stress on the GH joint and surrounding soft tissue structures. High-speed photography, often used to record the mechanics of the throwing motion, can lead to early detection of improper technique. In addition to proper throwing technique, participants in contact and collision sports should be

APPLICATION STRATEGY 12.2

Strengthening Exercises for the Shoulder Complex

A. Shoulder shrugs. Elevate the shoulders toward the ears and hold. Pull the shoulders back, pinch the shoulder blades together, and hold. Relax and repeat.

B. Scapular abduction (protraction). Lift the weight directly upward, lifting the posterior shoulder from the table. Relax and repeat.

C. Scapular adduction (retraction). Perform bent-over rowing while flexing the elbows. When the end of the motion is reached, pinch the shoulder blades together and hold.

D. Bench press or incline press. Place the hands shoulder-width apart and push the barbell directly above the shoulder joint. This exercise should be performed with a spotter.

E. Bent arm lateral flies, supine position. Keeping the elbows slightly flexed, lift the dumbbells directly over the shoulders. Lower the dumbbells until they are parallel to the floor, then repeat. An alternative method is to move the dumbbells in a diagonal pattern. In the prone position, the exercise strengthens the trapezius.

F. Lateral pull-downs. In a seated position, grasp the handle and pull the bar behind the head. An alternative method is to pull the bar in front of the body.

G. Surgical tubing. Secure the tubing. Work in diagonal functional patterns similar to those skills experienced in a specific sport/ activity.

taught the shoulder-roll method of falling, rather than falling on an outstretched arm. This technique reduces direct compression of the articular joints and disperses the force over a wider area.

SPRAINS TO THE SHOULDER COMPLEX

Ligamentous injuries to the SC joint, AC joint, and GH joint can result from compression, tension, and shearing forces occurring in a single episode, or from repetitive overload. A common method of injury is a fall or direct hit on the lateral aspect of the acromion. The force is first transmitted to the site of impact, then to the AC joint and the clavicle, and finally to the SC joint. Failure can occur at any one of these sites. Acute sprains are common in hockey, rugby, football, soccer, equestrian sports, and the martial arts.

Sternoclavicular Joint Sprain—Anterior Displacement

The SC joint is the main axis of rotation for movements of the clavicle and scapula. The majority of injuries result from compression related to a direct blow, as when a supine individual is landed on by another participant, or more commonly, by indirect forces transmitted from a blow to the shoulder or a fall on an outstretched arm. The disruption typically drives the proximal clavicle superior, medial, and anterior, disrupting the costoclavicular and SC ligaments and leading to anterior displacement.

Signs and Symptoms

First-degree injuries are characterized by point tenderness and mild pain over the SC joint, with no visible deformity. Characteristics of second-degree injuries include:

- A joint subluxation leading to bruising, swelling, and pain
- Inability to horizontally adduct the arm without considerable pain
- Holding the arm forward and close to the body, supporting it across the chest
- Pain with scapular protraction and retraction can reproduce pain

Third-degree sprains involve a prominent displacement of the sternal end of the clavicle and may involve a fracture. There is a complete rupture of the SC and costoclavicular ligaments. In a third-degree sprain, the movement limitations present in a second-degree sprain are greater and produce more pain. Pain is severe when the shoulders are brought together by a lateral force.

Management

The immediate management includes the application of cold to the area. The individual should also be placed in a sling. This injury requires physician referral. If a grade II or grade III injury is suspected, the individual should be referred to an emergency medical facility.

Sternoclavicular Joint Sprain—Posterior Displacement

Although rare, posterior, or retrosternal, displacement is more serious because of the potential injury to the esophagus, trachea, internal thoracic artery and vein, and the brachiocephalic and subclavian artery and vein. The most common mechanism of injury is a blow to the posterolateral aspect of the shoulder with the arm adducted and flexed, such as a fall on the shoulder displacing the distal clavicle posteriorly.[9] This action may occur during a piling-on injury in football. Less commonly, the injury may be caused by a direct blow to the anteromedial end of the clavicle.

Signs and Symptoms

The individual has a palpable depression between the sternal end of the clavicle and manubrium, is unable to perform shoulder protraction, and may have difficulty swallowing and breathing. The individual may also complain of numbness and weakness of the upper extremity secondary to the compression of structures in the thoracic inlet. If the venous vascular vessels are impinged, the patient may have venous congestion or engorgement in the ipsilateral arm and a diminished radial pulse.[9]

Management

Posterior displacement can become life-threatening. The emergency plan should be activated, including summoning of EMS.

Acromioclavicular Joint Sprain

The AC joint is weak and easily injured by a direct blow, fall on the point of the shoulder (called a shoulder pointer), or force transmitted up the long axis of the humerus during a fall with the humerus in an adducted position.[10] In these cases, the acromion is driven away from the clavicle or vice versa. Although often referred to as a "separated shoulder," ruptures of the AC and/or coracoclavicular ligaments can result in an AC dislocation; therefore, they are more correctly referred to as sprains.

Classification of Injury

Like other joint injuries, AC sprains may be classified as first-degree (i.e., mild), second-degree (i.e., moderate), or third-degree (i.e., severe). However, because of the complexity of the joint, AC sprains are often classified as Types I to VI based on the extent of ligamentous damage, degree of instability, and the direction in which the clavicle displaces relative to the acromion and coracoid process (BOX 12.1).

BOX 12.1	Classification of Acromioclavicular Joint Sprains	
GRADE	**DEGREE**	**INJURED STRUCTURES**
Type I	First	Stretch or partial damage of the AC ligament and capsule
Type II	Second	Rupture of AC ligament and partial strain of coracoclavicular ligament
Type III	Second	Rupture of AC ligament and coracoclavicular ligament
Type IV to VI	Third	Rupture of AC ligament and coracoclavicular ligament, and tearing of deltoid and trapezius fascia

Signs and Symptoms

Type I injuries have no disruption of the AC or coracoclavicular ligaments. Minimal swelling and pain are present over the joint line, and increase with abduction past 90°. The injury is inherently stable and pain is self-limiting.

Type II injuries result from a more severe blow to the shoulder. The AC ligaments are torn, but the coracoclavicular ligament, only minimally sprained, is intact. Vertical stability is maintained, but sagittal plane stability is compromised. The clavicle rides above the level of the acromion, and a minor step or gap is present at the joint line. Pain increases when the distal clavicle is depressed or moved in an anterior-posterior direction, and during passive horizontal adduction.

Type III injuries have complete disruption of the AC and coracoclavicular ligaments, resulting in visible prominence of the distal clavicle. There will be obvious swelling and bruising and, more significantly, depression or drooping of the shoulder girdle.

Higher-grade injuries (IV to VI) are caused by more violent forces. Extensive mobility and pain in the area may signify tearing of the deltoid and trapezius muscle attachments at the distal clavicle. These rare injuries must be carefully evaluated for associated neurologic injuries.

Management

The immediate management includes the application of cold to the area. The individual should also be placed in a sling. This injury requires physician referral. If a type II or higher is suspected, the individual should be referred to an emergency medical facility.

Glenohumeral Joint Sprain

Damage to the GH joint can occur when the arm is forcefully abducted (e.g., when making an arm tackle in football), but more commonly is caused by excessive shoulder external rotation and extension (i.e., arm in the overhead position). When the arm rotates externally, the anterior capsule and GH ligaments are stretched or torn, causing the humeral head to slip out of the glenoid fossa in an anterior-inferior direction (FIG. 12.7). A direct blow or forceful movement that pushes the humerus posteriorly can also result in damage to the joint capsule.

Signs and Symptoms

In a first-degree injury, the anterior shoulder is particularly painful to palpation and movement, especially when the mechanism of injury is reproduced. Active ROM may be slightly limited, but pain does not occur on adduction or internal rotation, such as occurs with a muscular strain. A second-degree sprain produces some joint laxity. In addition, pain, swelling, and bruising are usually significant, and ROM, particularly abduction, is limited. A third-degree injury is considered a dislocation and is discussed in the next section.

Management

The immediate management includes the application of cold to the area. The individual should also be placed in a sling. This injury requires physician referral to ensure accurate assessment and appropriate treatment.

Glenohumeral Dislocations

The GH joint is the most frequently dislocated major joint in the body. Ninety percent of shoulder dislocations are

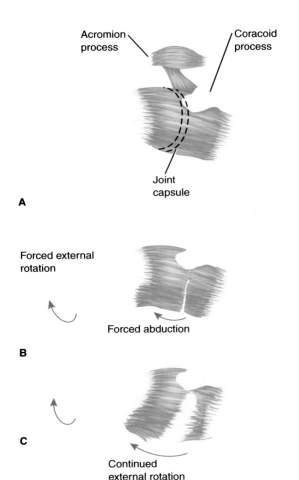

FIGURE 12.7 GH sprains. **A**. Normal abduction with some stretching of the fibers. **B**. Forced external rotation and abduction with minimal tears to the joint capsule leading to a moderate or second-degree sprain. **C**. Continuation of the forced movement causes a third-degree sprain or shoulder dislocation.

anterior; posterior dislocations rank second in occurrence. Inferior dislocations are rare and often accompanied by neurovascular injury and facture.[11] Dislocations can be acute or chronic.

Acute Dislocations

Anterior

Many acute dislocations have an associated fracture or nerve damage. Therefore, this injury is considered serious, and necessitates immediate transportation to the nearest medical facility for reduction.

Signs and Symptoms. An initial dislocation presents with intense pain. Tingling and numbness may extend down the arm into the hand. In a first-time anterior dislocation, the injured arm is often held in slight abduction (20° to 30°) and external rotation, and is stabilized against the body by the opposite hand. Visually, a sharp contour on the affected shoulder, with a prominent acromion process, can be seen when compared with the smooth deltoid outline on the unaffected shoulder. The individual will not allow the arm to be brought across the chest.

Posterior

Posterior dislocations occur from a fall on or a blow to the anterior surface of the shoulder which drives the head of the humerus posteriorly.

Signs and Symptoms. The arm is carried tightly against the chest and across the front of the trunk in rigid adduction and internal rotation. The anterior shoulder appears flat, the coracoid process is prominent, and a corresponding bulge may be seen posteriorly, if not masked by a heavy deltoid musculature. Any attempt to move the arm into external rotation and abduction produces severe pain. Because the biceps brachii is unable to function in this position, the individual is unable to supinate the forearm with the shoulder flexed.

Management. Muscle spasm sets in very quickly following dislocation and makes reduction more difficult. Management of a first-time dislocation requires immediate referral to a physician. As such, in some settings, it may be necessary to activate the emergency plan. The injury should be treated as a fracture. The arm should be immobilized in a comfortable position. In order to prevent unnecessary movement of the humerus, a rolled towel or thin pillow can be placed between the thoracic wall and humerus prior to applying a sling. Ice should be applied to control hemorrhage and muscle spasm.

In evaluating this injury, if possible, the coach should assess both the axillary nerve and artery, because both structures can be damaged in a dislocation. A pulse may be taken on the medial proximal humerus over the brachial artery or on the radial pulse at the wrist. The axillary nerve can be assessed by stroking the skin on the upper lateral arm to assess sensation. Deficits with pulse or sensation definitely warrant activation of the emergency plan, including summoning of EMS.

Chronic Dislocations

Recurrent dislocations, or "trick shoulders," tend to be anterior dislocations that are intracapsular. The mechanism of injury is the same as acute dislocations. However, as the number of occurrences increases, the forces needed to produce the injury decrease, as do the associated muscle spasm, pain, and swelling. The individual is aware of the shoulder displacing because the arm gives the sensation of "going dead," referred to as the **dead arm syndrome**. Activities in which recurrent posterior subluxations are common include the follow-through of a throwing motion or a racquet swing, the ascent phase of a push-up or a bench press, the recoil following a block in football, and certain swimming strokes.

Signs and Symptoms. Pain is the major complaint, with crepitation and/or clicking after the arm shifts back into the appropriate position. However, recurrent dislocations may be less painful than an initial dislocation. Many individuals voluntarily reduce the injury by positioning the arm in flexion, adduction, and internal rotation.

Management. If the injury does not reduce, the individual should be placed in a sling and swathe, or the arm may be stabilized next to the body with an elastic wrap. Ice should be applied to control pain and inflammation. The individual should be referred immediately to a physician for reduction of the injury and further care.

OVERUSE CONDITIONS

During abduction, the strong deltoid muscle pulls the humeral head superiorly, relative to the glenoid fossa. The rotator cuff muscles are critical in counteracting this migration. If the tendons are weak, they are incapable of depressing the humeral head in the glenoid fossa during overhead motions. This can lead to impingement of the supraspinatus tendon and subacromial bursa between the acromion, the coracoacromial ligament, and the greater tubercle of the humerus. This compressive action can lead to a rotator cuff strain, impingement syndrome, bursitis, or bicipital tendinitis, or a combination of these injuries.

Rotator Cuff and Impingement Injuries

Chronic rotator cuff tears to the SITS muscles result from repetitive microtraumatic episodes that primarily impinge on the supraspinatus tendon just proximal to the greater tubercle of the humerus (FIG. 12.8). Partial tears are usually seen in young individuals, with total tears typically seen in adults older than 30 years. In older age groups, chronic tears can lead to cuff thinning, degeneration, and total rupture of the supraspinatus tendon.

Impingement syndrome implies an actual mechanical abutment of the rotator cuff and the subacromial bursa against the coracoacromial ligament and acromion. This injury is caused from the force overload to the rotator cuff and bursa that occurs during the abduction, forward flexion, and medial rotation cycle of shoulder movements. In addition to injury to the supraspinatus tendon and subacromial bursa, the **glenoid labrum** and long head of the biceps brachii may also be injured. The condition is also sometimes called "painful arc" syndrome or "swimmer's shoulder." BOX 12.2 lists several factors that can increase the risk for an impingement syndrome.

Signs and Symptoms

Initially, pain is described as deep in the shoulder and present at night. Activity increases the pain, but only in the impingement position. As repetitive trauma continues, pain becomes progressively worse, particularly between 70° and 120° (i.e., "painful arc") of active and resisted abduction. Because forced scapular protraction leads to further impingement and pain, the

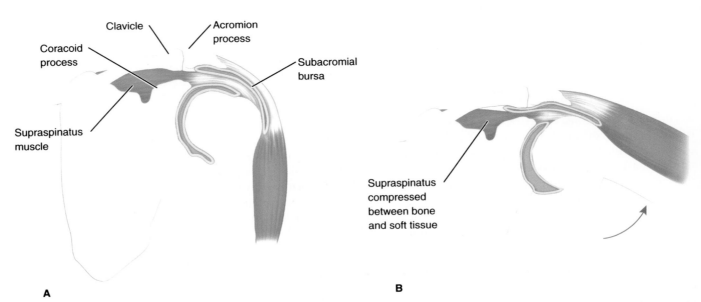

FIGURE 12.8 Supraspinatus tendon during abduction. **A.** Normal position. **B.** Abducted position. Repetitive overhead motions can impinge the muscle or tendon between the acromion process and coracoacromial ligament, resulting in a chronic rotator cuff injury.

> ### BOX 12.2 Factors Contributing to Impingement Syndrome
>
> - **Excessive amount of overhead movement (i.e., overuse)**
> - **Limited subacromial space under coracoacromial arch and limited flexibility of coracoacromial ligament**
> - **Thickness of the supraspinatus and biceps brachii tendon**
> - **Lack of flexibility and strength of the supraspinatus and biceps brachii**
> - **Weakness of the posterior cuff muscles (e.g., infraspinatus or teres minor)**
> - **Tightness of the posterior cuff muscles**
> - **Hypermobility of the shoulder joints**
> - **Imbalance in muscle strength, coordination, and endurance of the scapular muscles (e.g., serratus anterior or rhomboids)**
> - **Shape of the acromion**
> - **Training devices (e.g., use of hand paddles or tubing)**

individual may be unable to sleep on the involved side. If a full thickness tear has been sustained, atrophy may be apparent in the supraspinatus or infraspinatus fossa.

Management

In assessing this condition, it should become apparent to the coach during the history component that the injury is overuse in nature and, as such, the coach should refrain from continuing assessment. Rather, the coach should refer this individual to a physician for accurate diagnosis and treatment options. The coach should not permit the individual to continue activity, as doing so could potentially exacerbate the condition. In addition, the coach could suggest the application of cold to the area to decrease pain and potential spasm.

Bursitis

Bursitis is not generally an isolated condition, but rather is associated with other injuries, such as an impingement syndrome and pre-existing degenerative changes in the rotator cuff. The large subacromial bursa is commonly injured in swimmers, baseball, softball, and tennis players. Located between the coracoacromial ligament and the underlying supraspinatus muscle, this bursa provides the shoulder with some inherent gliding ability. During an overhead throwing motion, this bursa can become impinged in the subacromial space.

Signs and Symptoms

Frequently, sudden shoulder pain is reported during the initiation and acceleration of the throwing motion. Point tenderness can be elicited on the anterior and lateral edges of the acromion process. A painful arc exists between 70° and 120° of passive abduction. Inability to sleep, especially on the affected side, occurs because of forced scapular protraction that leads to further impingement of the bursa. Pain is often referred to the distal deltoid attachment.

Management

Management is the same as for a rotator cuff strain or impingement syndrome.

Bicipital Tendinitis

Injury to the biceps brachii tendon often occurs from repetitive overuse during rapid overhead movements involving excessive elbow flexion and supination activities, such as those performed by racquet sport players, shot-putters, baseball/softball pitchers, football quarterbacks, swimmers, and javelin throwers. Irritation of the tendon occurs as it passes back and forth in the intertubercular (bicipital) groove of the humerus. The tendon may partially sublux because of laxity of the traverse humeral ligament, a poorly developed lesser tubercle, or both. A direct blow to the tendon or tendon sheath can lead to bicipital tenosynovitis. Anterior impingement syndrome associated with overhead rotational activity may also damage the tendon.

Signs and Symptoms

Pain and tenderness is present over the bicipital groove when the shoulder is internally and externally rotated. In internal rotation, the pain stays medial; in external rotation, the pain is located in the midline or just lateral to the groove. Pain may also be elicited when the tendon is passively stretched in extreme shoulder extension with the elbow extended and forearm pronated. Pain could also be present with resisted supination and elbow flexion.

Management

Management is the same as for a rotator cuff strain or impingement syndrome.

Biceps Tendon Rupture

Prolonged tendinitis can make the tendon vulnerable to forceful rupture during repetitive overhead motions, commonly seen in swimmers, or in forceful flexion activities against excessive resistance, as seen in weight lifters or gymnasts. The rupture occurs as a result of the avascular portion of the proximal long head of the biceps tendon constantly passing over the head of the humerus during arm motion. This condition is often seen in degenerative tendons in older individuals and in individuals who have had corticosteroid injections into the tendon.

Signs and Symptoms

The individual often hears and feels a snapping sensation, and experiences intense pain. Ecchymosis and a visible, palpable defect can be seen in the muscle belly when the individual flexes the biceps. If the muscle mass moves distally as a result of a proximal long-head rupture, a "Popeye" appearance is clearly visible. Partial ruptures may produce only slight muscular deformity but are still associated with pain and weakness in elbow flexion and supination. Distal biceps rupture results in marked weakness with flexion and supination of the forearm.

Management

The immediate management includes placing the individual in a sling and applying cold to the area. This action should be followed by immediate referral to a physician or emergency medical care facility.

Thoracic Outlet Compression Syndrome

Thoracic outlet compression syndrome is a condition in which nerves and/or vessels become compressed in the proximal neck or axilla (FIG. 12.9). There are two clearly defined forms of this condition. One is a neurologic syndrome, accounting for about 90% of all cases, that involves the lower trunk of the brachial plexus and is caused by abnormal nerve stretch or compression. Another is a vascular form that involves the subclavian artery and vein, and is more common in men than women.[12] Thoracic outlet compression syndrome often is aggravated in activities that require overhead rotational stresses while muscles are loaded, such as weight lifting and swimming. Disorders associated with thoracic outlet syndrome include

- Compression of the medial cord of the brachial plexus
- Compression of the subclavian artery and vein
- Cervical rib syndrome
- Scalenus-anterior syndrome
- Hyperabduction syndrome
- Costoclavicular space syndrome
- Poor posture with drooping shoulders

Signs and Symptoms

If a nerve is compressed, an aching pain, pins-and-needles sensation, or numbness in the side or back of the neck extends across the shoulder down the medial arm to the ulnar aspect of the hand.

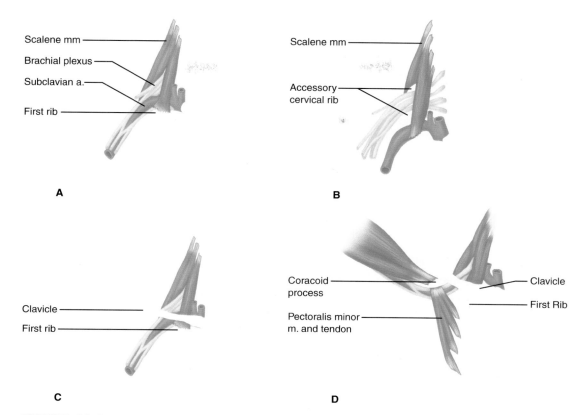

FIGURE 12.9 Location and etiology of thoracic outlet syndrome. **A.** Scalenus anterior syndrome. **B.** Cervical rib syndrome. **C.** Costoclavicular space syndrome. **D.** Hyperabduction syndrome.

Weakness in grasp and atrophy of the hand muscles may also be present. If arterial or venous vessels are compressed, signs and symptoms vary depending on the specific structure being obstructed. Blockage of the subclavian vein produces edema, stiffness (especially in the hand), and venous engorgement of the arm with cyanosis. If untreated, this may result in thrombophlebitis. The individual may present these signs and symptoms several hours after a bout of intense exercise. Occlusion of the subclavian artery results in a rapid onset of coolness, numbness in the entire arm, and fatigue after exertional overhead activity. A detailed history is needed, and it is essential to evaluate the cervical spine, shoulder, elbow, and hand for evidence of neurovascular compression.

Management

Immediate referral to a physician is necessary for more extensive assessment to rule out serious vascular involvement.

FRACTURES

Most fractures to the shoulder region result from a fall on the point of the shoulder, rolling over onto the top of the shoulder, or indirect forces caused by falling on an outstretched arm. Clavicular fractures are more common than fractures to the scapula and proximal humerus, with nearly 80% occurring in the midclavicular region.

Clavicular Fractures

Because of the S-shaped configuration of the clavicle, it is highly susceptible to compressive forces caused by a blow or fall on the point of the shoulder, a direct blow to the bone by an opponent or object, or falling on an outstretched arm. Activities that have a high incidence of clavicular injury include ice hockey, football, martial arts, lacrosse, gymnastics, weight lifting, wrestling, racquetball, squash, and bicycling.

Nearly 80% of traumatic fractures occur in the middle one-third of the clavicle.[11] The sternocleidomastoid muscle pulls the proximal bone fragment upward, allowing the distal shoulder to collapse downward and medially from the force of gravity and the pull of the pectoralis major muscle.

Signs and Symptoms

Swelling, ecchymosis, and a deformity may be visible and palpable at the fracture site. Greenstick fractures, typically seen in adolescents, also produce a noticeable deformity. Pain occurs with any shoulder motion, and may radiate into the trapezius area. In older adults, fractures of the distal clavicle may involve tears of the coracoclavicular ligament, resulting in an increased deformity. Complications, although rare, may arise if bony fragments penetrate local arteries or nerves.

Management

The immediate management includes placing the individual in a sling and swathe. This action should be followed by immediate referral to a physician or emergency medical care facility.

Scapular Fractures

Scapular fractures may involve the body of the scapula, spine of the scapula, acromion process, coracoid process, or GH joint. Avulsion fractures to the coracoid process result from direct trauma, or forceful contraction of the pectoralis minor or short head of the biceps brachii. Fractures to the glenoid area are associated with shoulder subluxations and dislocations. In this case, treatment is dictated by the shoulder dislocation rather than the fracture, and often requires open reduction and internal fixation or shoulder reconstruction.

Signs and Symptoms

Most fractures result in minimal displacement and exhibit localized hemorrhage, pain, and tenderness. The individual is reluctant to move the injured arm and prefers to maintain it in adduction. Arm abduction is painful. It is critical to note any signs or symptoms that would suggest underlying pulmonary injury (e.g., pneumothorax or hemothorax).

Management

The arm should be immobilized immediately in a sling and swathe. Application of ice should be used to minimize hematoma formation. The individual should be immediately referred to a physician or emergency medical care facility.

Epiphyseal and Avulsion Fractures

Epiphyseal centers around the shoulder region remain unfused for a longer span of time than is typically seen at other epiphyseal sites. For example, the medial clavicular growth plate does not close until approximately age 25 years, and is often misdiagnosed as a SC subluxation/dislocation. The proximal humeral epiphysis does not close until 18 to 21 years of age. An epiphyseal fracture at this site, called **little league shoulder**, is often caused by repetitive medial rotation and adduction traction forces placed on the shoulder during pitching (FIG. 12.10). Catchers may also sustain this fracture because they throw the ball as hard and often as pitchers, but with less of a windup. The injury usually occurs during the deceleration and follow-through phases of throwing or pitching.

Avulsion fractures to the coracoid process can be seen in a young individual when forceful, repetitive throwing places too much stress on the growth plate. Fractures of the greater and lesser tubercle are often associated with anterior and posterior GH dislocations, respectively. When the tubercle cannot be maintained in a stable position, open reduction and internal fixation is often required.

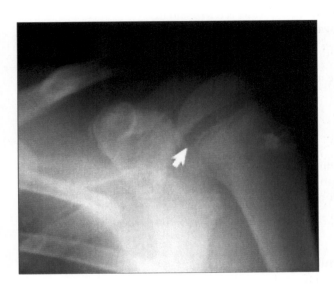

FIGURE 12.10 Epiphyseal fracture to the proximal humeral growth center. The arrow indicates the fracture site.

Signs and Symptoms

In an epiphyseal fracture, the individual complains of acute shoulder pain when attempting to throw hard, which, if ignored, may result in an acute displacement of the weakened physis. Pain may be elicited with deep palpation in the axilla. In an avulsion fracture, pain can be elicited by deep palpation over the specific bony landmark.

Management

The arm should be immobilized in a sling and swathe. Ice should be applied to control pain and swelling, and immediate referral to a physician or emergency medical care facility is warranted for further care.

Humeral Fractures

Humeral fractures result from violent compressive forces from a direct blow, a fall on the upper arm, or a fall on an outstretched hand with the elbow extended. The surgical neck is the most common site for proximal humeral fractures, and may display an appearance similar to a dislocation (Fig. 12.11).

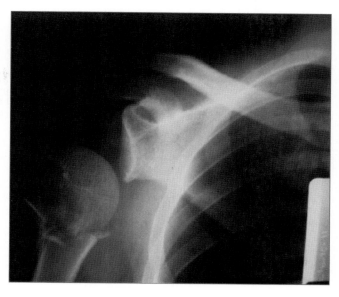

FIGURE 12.11 Fracture to the surgical neck of the humerus. The arrow indicates the fracture site.

Signs and Symptoms

Pain, swelling, hemorrhage, discoloration, an inability to move the arm, an inability to supinate the forearm, and possible paralysis may be present. The arm is often held splinted against the body.

Management

The arm should be immobilized in a sling and swathe. Ice should be applied to control pain and swelling, and immediate referral to a physician or emergency medical care facility is warranted for further care. In some settings, this injury may warrant activation of the emergency action plan.

THE COACH AND ON-SITE ASSESSMENT OF AN ACUTE SHOULDER CONDITION

The shoulder complex is a complicated region to assess because of the many important structures located in such a small area. While most injuries involving the shoulder complex will require physician referral, they are not typically life-threatening conditions. Even still, the coach should be aware that some conditions will require activation of the emergency plan, including summoning of EMS (Box 12.3).

As with other on-site injury assessments, it begins as the coach is approaching the individual. The focus should be on observing the individual's overall presentation, attitude, and general

---

BOX 12.3	**Signs and Symptoms That Necessitate Immediate Referral to a Physician or an Emergency Medical Facility**

- **Obvious deformity suggesting a suspected fracture, separation, or dislocation**
- **Significant loss of motion or weakness in the myotomes**
- **Joint instability**
- **Abnormal sensation in the shoulder, arm, or hand**
- **Absent or weak pulse distal to the injury**
- **Any significant, unexplained pain**

APPLICATION STRATEGY 12.3

On-site Assessment of a Shoulder: History, Observation, and Palpation

HISTORY
- Chief complaint
  - What's wrong?
- Mechanism of injury
  - What happened? What were you doing? Was there a direct blow? Did you fall? How (outstretched arm; flexed arm; outstretched hand)? Are you able to demonstrate how it happened?
- Acute or chronic injury (Onset)
  - Do you remember when it started hurting?
  - How long has this been bothering you?
- Pain
  - Location
  - Where is the pain?
  - Can you point to a location where it hurts the most?
  - Type—Can you describe the pain (e.g., sharp, shooting, dull, achy, diffuse)?
  - Intensity—What is the level of pain on a scale from 1-10?
- Sounds/Feelings
  - Did you hear anything when the injury happened (e.g., pop; snap; crack)?
  - Did you feel any unusual sensations (e.g., tearing; tingling; numbing; cracking) when the injury happened?
- Previous history
  - Have you ever injured your shoulder before? If so, what happened? What was the injury? Were you treated for it?
- OTHER important/helpful information
  - Have you made any changes in performance technique (e.g., throwing style; swimming strokes)?
  - Are you able to perform activity-specific skills (e.g., throw, swimming strokes)?
  - Have you changed your weight training workouts (e.g., increased weight or number of repetitions; added new exercises)?
  - Are you able to perform normal motions/ADLs?
  - Is there anything else you would like to tell me about your condition?

OBSERVATION
- General presentation
  - Guarding
  - Moving easily; hesitant to move

- Specific to shoulder
  - The manner in which the individual is holding their arm
  - Resting position—swelling in the joint may prevent full shoulder adduction
  - Soft tissue symmetry (i.e., muscle atrophy, hypertrophy)
  - Shape and contour of the bony and soft tissue structures (scapula and muscle atrophy)
  - Injury site appearance – deformity; swelling; discoloration

PALPATION
The coach should only perform palpation if there is a clear understanding of what is being palpated and why? A productive assessment appropriate to the standard of care of a coach does not necessitate palpation.

TESTING
- Active Range of Motion (AROM) – bilateral comparison
  - Shoulder abduction with the hand supinated
  - Shoulder adduction to the side of the body
  - Humeral internal and external rotation
  - Shoulder flexion and extension
  - Elbow flexion and extension
- Passive range of motion should not be performed by the coach

Resistive range of motion
- The coach should only perform resistive range of motion for the muscles that govern the shoulder if instruction and approval for doing so has been obtained in advance from an appropriate healthcare practitioner
- AROM is normal and pain free as a way to assess strength.

ACTIVITY/SPORT-SPECIFIC FUNCTIONAL TESTING
- Performance of active movements typical of the movements executed by the individual during sport or activity participation (including weight training)
- Should assess strength, agility, flexibility, joint stability, endurance, coordination, balance, and activity-specific skill performance

posture, with a particular focus on their willingness or ability to move and their apparent pain level. Subsequent to the history and observation components of an assessment, the coach should have established a strong suspicion of the structures that may be damaged. As such, during the physical examination component, only tests that are absolutely necessary, if any, should be performed (see APPLICATION STRATEGY 12.3).

If the coach elects to perform the testing component of the assessment, it should begin with active ROM of the neck. Because pain is frequently referred from the cervical region into the shoulder, neck flexion, extension, rotation, and lateral flexion should be assessed for fluid motion and presence of pain. If pain is present at the neck, the coach should consider the possibility of a neck injury and refer the individual to a physician or emergency medical facility.

If no problems are noted during neck movement, the coach could continue with assessing the ROM of the shoulder.

Finally, while it is not per se a part of a shoulder assessment, there may be times when an individual reports pain to the shoulder in the absence of any trauma involving the shoulder. The coach should keep in mind that the shoulder is a common site for referred pain from orthopedic or visceral origins. As such, the possibility of an internal injury (i.e., involving the thorax or abdomen) should be considered particularly when the individual presents a vague history of injury to the shoulder girdle.

SUMMARY

1. The shoulder complex does not function in an isolated fashion; rather, a series of joints work together in a coordinated manner to allow complicated patterns of motion. Subsequently, injury to one structure can affect other structures.

2. A moderate SC sprain is characterized by pain and swelling over the joint and an inability to horizontally adduct the arm without increased pain. The arm is typically held forward and close to the body.

3. A moderate AC sprain is characterized by an elevated distal clavicle, indicating that the coracoclavicular ligament and the AC ligaments have been torn. The individual typically has a depressed or drooping shoulder.

4. Anterior GH dislocations are more common than posterior dislocations. The injured arm is often stabilized against the body as it is held in slight abduction and external rotation.

5. Impingement syndromes involve an abutment of the supraspinatus tendon and subacromial bursa under the coracoacromial ligament and acromion process. The glenoid labrum and long head of the biceps brachii may also be injured.

6. Thoracic outlet compression syndrome may involve compression of the lower trunk of the brachial plexus or the subclavian artery and vein. If a nerve is compressed, an aching pain or numbness may extend across the shoulder to the ulnar aspect of the hand. If arterial or venous vessels are compressed, coolness, numbness in the entire arm, and fatigue occur after exertional, overhead activity.

7. The surgical neck is the most common site for proximal humeral fractures in adults. However,

adolescents have a high degree of proximal humeral epiphyseal fractures due to repetitive medial rotation and adduction traction forces placed on the shoulder during pitching motions.

8. Pain may be referred to the shoulder from other areas of the body, particularly the heart, lungs, visceral organs, and cervical spine region.

9. Injuries that should be immediately referred to a physician include
   • Obvious deformity suggesting a suspected fracture, separation, or dislocation
   • Significant loss of motion or weakness in the myotomes
   • Joint instability
   • Abnormal sensations in either the segmental dermatomes or peripheral cutaneous patterns
   • Absent or weak pulse distal to the injury
   • Any significant, unexplained pain

10. Subsequent to the history and observation components of an assessment, the coach should have established a strong suspicion of the structures that may be damaged. As such, during the physical examination component, only those tests that are absolutely necessary, if any, should be performed.

11. The management for a majority of shoulder injuries involves immobilizing the arm in a sling, swathe, or another commercial product that adequately pads and supports the limb, applying cold to reduce swelling, and referring the individual to a physician or emergency care facility. There are conditions which could require summoning of EMS (e.g. posterior SC sprain).

APPLICATION QUESTIONS

1. During a recreation league soccer game, a 14-year-old player comes to the sideline complaining of pain. He states that he fell on the point of his shoulder. How should the coach perform the observation component of an assessment for this injury?

2. Why is impingement syndrome a problem for swimmers in particular? What limitations in ROM would be present if a swimmer has a shoulder impingement problem?

3. A wrestler falls on an outstretched arm. In assessing the injury, it immediately becomes apparent to the coach that the GH joint is anteriorly displaced. How should the coach manage this situation?

4. During a physical education class, a third-grade student fell on an outstretched arm, and is complaining of pain on the top of the shoulder. Following completion of the history and observation components of an assessment, the coach notes that the distal clavicle appears somewhat elevated and that there is increased pain with horizontal adduction of the arm across the chest and shoulder flexion. What structures may be involved in this injury? How should the physical education teacher manage this situation?

5. A 10-year-old gymnast lost her balance on a dismount and fell on an outstretched arm. She immediately felt intense pain in the shoulder region and is now unable to move the arm. The shoulder appears to sag down and forward, and there is a noticeable bump in the midclavicular region. What possible condition might be suspected? How should the coach manage the injury?

6. A 35-year-old female comes to your exercise facility indicating a desire to increase upper body strength and flexibility. The individual has no history of shoulder injury and has not engaged in a regular exercise regime since college. Demonstrate exercises used to increase flexibility and strength of the shoulder complex.

7. Following the first inning, a Little League pitcher complains of shoulder pain. He does not recall an acute injury, but reports intermittent pain and soreness with activity for the past week. How should the coach handle this situation?

8. A 16-year-old basketball player sustains his second GH dislocation in 2 years. Is the individual likely to sustain another dislocation to that joint? Why or why not?

9. What is the mechanism of injury (MOI) for a posterior GH dislocation? Describe a real-life situation (in a physical education class, a sport setting, or a weight training session) that could result in this injury. What tissues become damaged as a result of a posterior GH dislocation? What is the management for a posterior GH dislocation?

10. What is the MOI of a biceps tendon rupture? Describe a real-life example that could result in this injury. What are the signs and symptoms of a biceps tendon rupture?

11. If thoracic outlet syndrome is suspected, why is it important to assess for signs of neurovascular compression?

12. A 30-year-old male accidently trips and falls on a piece of equipment lying on the floor of the fitness facility. In falling, he landed on an outstretched arm. What questions should the fitness specialist responding to the on-site injury ask as part of the history component of an assessment of the injury?

REFERENCES

1. Nadler SF, Sherman AL, and Malanga GA. 2004. Sport-specific shoulder injuries. Phys Med Rehabil Clin N Am, 15(vi):607–626.
2. Quillen DM, Wuchner M, and Hatch RL. 2004. Acute shoulder injuries. Am Fam Physician, 70:1947–1954.
3. Yanai T, Hay JG, and Miller GF. 2000. Shoulder impingement in front-crawl swimming: I. A method to identify impingement. Med Sci Sports Exerc, 32(1):21–29.
4. Kelly BT, Barnes RP, Powell JW, and Warren RF. 2004. Shoulder injuries to quarterbacks in the national football league. Am J Sports Med, 32:328–331.
5. Buss DD, and Watts JD. 2003. Acromioclavicular injuries in the throwing athlete. Clin Sports Med, 22:327–341, vii.
6. Costic RS, et al. 2003. Viscoelastic behavior and structural properties of the coracoclavicular ligaments. Scand J Med Sci Sports, 13:305–310.
7. Stokdijk M, Eilers PH, Nagels J, and Rozing PM. 2003. External rotation in the glenohumeral joint during elevation of the arm. Clin Biomech (Bristol, Avon), 18:296–302.
8. Hall SJ. Basic Biomechanics. Dubuque, IA: McGraw-Hill, 2007.
9. Asplund C. 2004. Posterior sternoclavicular joint dislocation in a wrestler. Mil Med, 169 (2):134–136.
10. Quillen DM, Wuchner M, and Hatch RL. 2004. Acute shoulder injuries. Am Fam Physician, 70(10):1947–1955.
11. Bicos J, and Nicholson GP. 2003. Treatment and results of sternoclavicular joint injuries. Clin Sports Med, 22(2):359–370.
12. Samarasam I, Sadhu D, Agarwal S, and Nayak S. 2004. Surgical management of thoracic outlet syndrome: a 10-year experience. ANZ J Surg, 74(6):450–454.

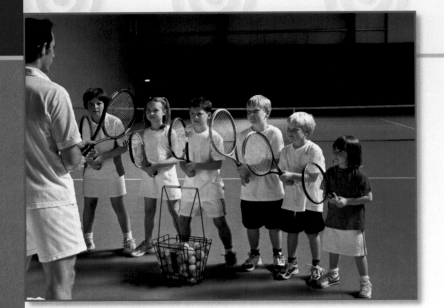

ELBOW, WRIST, AND HAND CONDITIONS

KEY TERMS

anatomical snuff box

aseptic necrosis

Bennett's fracture

carpal tunnel syndrome

circumduction

Colles' fracture

cyclist's palsy

de Quervain's tenosynovitis

epicondylitis

gamekeeper's thumb

hypothenar

(continued)

LEARNING OUTCOMES

1. Describe the major articulations that comprise the elbow, wrist, and hand.

2. Identify the major motions available at the elbow, wrist, and hand.

3. Explain general principles used to prevent injuries to the elbow, wrist, and hand.

4. Describe common injuries and conditions sustained by physically active individuals to the elbow, wrist, and hand including their sign, symptoms, and immediate management.

5. Describe an on-site assessment of an acute injury to the elbow, wrist, and hand appropriate for use by a coach.

KEY TERMS (CONTINUED)

ischemic necrosis	Mallet finger	stenosing
jersey finger	saddle joint	thenar
little league elbow	Smith's fracture	Volkmann's contracture

The arms perform lifting and carrying tasks, cushion the body during collisions, and lessen body momentum during falls. Acute injuries to the elbow, wrist, and hand often result from the natural tendency to sustain the force of a fall on the hyperextended wrist, which can sprain or dislocate the wrist or elbow. Performance in many sports is also contingent on the ability of the arms to effectively swing a racquet or club, or to position the hands for throwing and catching a ball. This can lead to overuse injuries, such as medial or lateral **epicondylitis**. In addition, sports such as wrestling, football, hockey, and skiing place undue stress on the thumb and fingers, leading to finger sprains and strains.

This chapter begins with a review of the anatomy of the elbow, wrist, and hand, followed by an overview of common injuries to the shoulder complex. Information pertaining to mechanism of injury, signs and symptoms, and management by the coach will be provided. Finally, a basic assessment of the region appropriate for coaches is presented.

ANATOMY REVIEW OF THE ELBOW, WRIST, AND HAND

The Elbow

Although the elbow may be generally thought of as a simple hinge joint, the elbow actually encompasses three articulations—the humeroulnar, humeroradial, and proximal radioulnar joints. The bony structure of the elbow and forearm is displayed in Fig. 13.1. The muscles of the anterior and posterior arm and forearm are shown in Figs. 13.2 and 13.3.

The largest joint at the elbow, the humeroulnar joint, is a hinge joint with motion capabilities of primarily flexion and extension. In some individuals, particularly women, a small amount of overextension (5° to 15°) is allowed. The humeroradial joint is a gliding joint, with motion restricted to the sagittal plane by the adjacent humeroulnar joint. The annular ligament binds the proximal head of the radius to the radial notch of the ulna forming the proximal radioulnar joint. This is a pivot joint with forearm pronation and supination occurring as the radius rolls medially and laterally over the ulna.

Several strong ligaments, primarily the ulnar (medial) and radial (lateral) collateral ligaments, bind the three articulations together and a single joint capsule surrounds all three joints (Fig. 13.4). The two collateral ligaments are strong and fan-shaped.

The Wrist

The wrist and hand are composed of numerous small bones and articulations. These function effectively to enable the dexterous movements performed by the hands during both daily living and sport activities.

The wrist consists of a series of radiocarpal and intercarpal articulations (Fig. 13.5). Most wrist motion, however, occurs at the radiocarpal joint, a condyloid joint where the radius articulates with the scaphoid, lunate, and triquetrum. The joint allows sagittal plane motion (flexion, extension, and hyperextension) and frontal plane motion (radial deviation

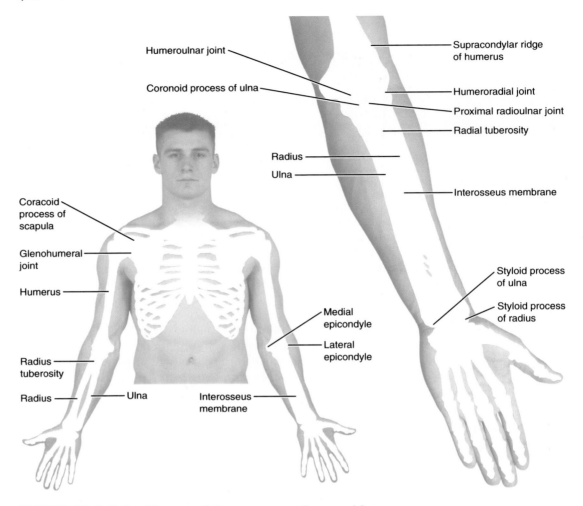

FIGURE 13.1 Skeletal features of the upper arm, elbow, and forearm.

and ulnar deviation), as well as **circumduction**. The muscles of the wrist and hand are provided in FIG. 13.5.

The Hand

In the hand, several joints are required to provide the extensive motion capabilities needed for sports participation. Included are the carpometacarpal (CM), intermetacarpal (IM), metacarpophalangeal (MCP), and interphalangeal (IP) joints (FIG. 13.5). The fingers are numbered digits one through five, with the first digit being the thumb.

The CM joint of the thumb is a classic **saddle joint** that allows rotation along its long axis to perform flexion, extension, abduction, adduction, and opposition. The CM joints of the four fingers are essentially gliding joints. The CM and IM joints of the fingers are mutually surrounded by joint capsules that are reinforced by the dorsal, volar, and interosseous CM ligaments.

The knuckles of the hand are formed by the MCP joints, which are each enclosed in a capsule that is reinforced by strong collateral ligaments. The MCP joints of the fingers allow flexion, extension, abduction, adduction, and circumduction. Among the fingers, abduction is defined as movement away from the middle finger, and adduction is movement toward the middle finger. The MCP joint of the thumb functions more as a hinge joint, and the primary movements are flexion and extension.

The proximal interphalangeal (PIP) and distal interphalangeal (DIP) joints of the fingers, and the single IP joint of the thumb, are all hinge joints. An articular capsule joined by volar

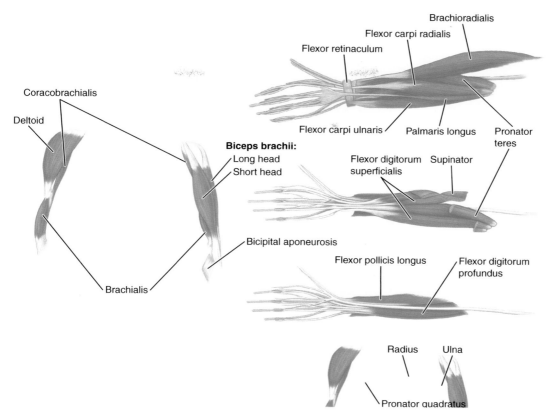

FIGURE 13.2 Muscles of the anterior arm and forearm.

and collateral ligaments surround each IP joint. The IP joints permit flexion, extension, and, in some individuals, slight hyperextension.

Bursae of the Elbow

Although there are several small bursae about the elbow, the most clinically relevant is the subcutaneous olecranon bursa located between the olecranon and skin surface. The lubricating function of the bursa facilitates smooth gliding of the skin over the olecranon process during elbow flexion and extension.

Nerves and Blood Vessels to the Elbow, Wrist, and Hand

The major nerves of the elbow region (median, ulnar, and radial) descend from the brachial plexus and extend into the forearm and hand. (FIGS. 13.6 and 13.7). The major arteries of the elbow and forearm region are the brachial, ulnar, and radial arteries (FIG. 13.8). The brachial artery supplies blood to the elbow joint and the flexor muscles of the arm and can be easily palpated in the anterior elbow. Distal to the elbow, the brachial artery splits into the ulnar and radial arteries.

The radial artery supplies the muscles on the radial side of the forearm, as well as the thumb and index finger (FIG. 13.9). The ulnar artery divides into anterior and posterior interosseous arteries to supply the deep flexor muscles and extensor muscles of the forearm, respectively. In the palm, the radial and ulnar arteries merge to form the superficial and deep palmar arches. Digital arteries branch from the palmar arches to supply the fingers, and branches from the carpal arch run distally along the metacarpal bones.

The radial artery is superficial on the anterior aspect of the wrist. The pulse is readily palpable at this site. Pulses can be taken for both arteries on the anterior aspect of the wrist.

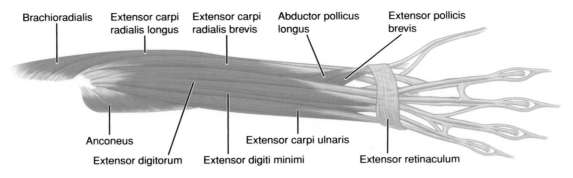

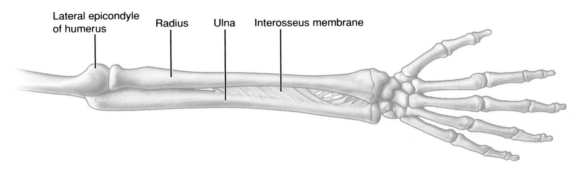

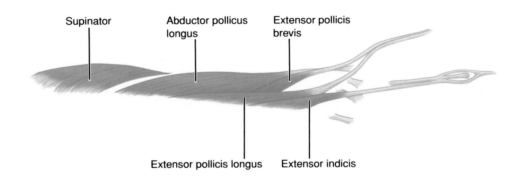

FIGURE 13.3 Muscles of the posterior forearm.

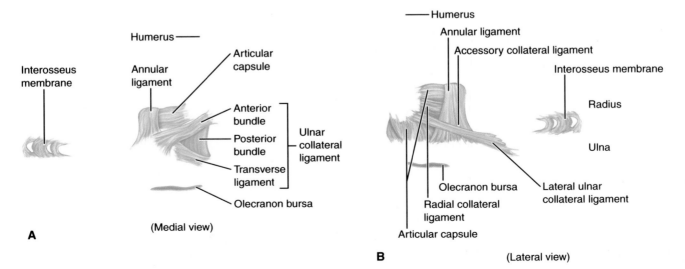

FIGURE 13.4 Major ligaments and the olecranon bursa of the elbow. **A.** Medial view. **B.** Lateral view.

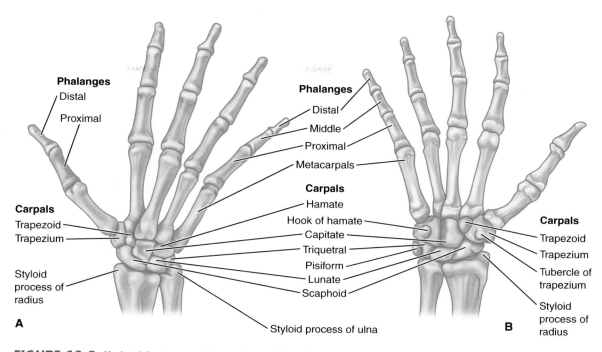

FIGURE 13.5 Skeletal features of the wrist and hand. **A.** Anterior view. **B.** Posterior view.

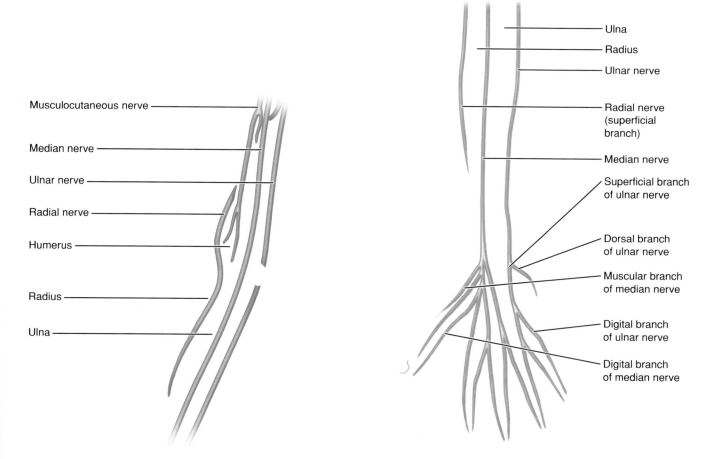

FIGURE 13.6 Nerves of the elbow region.

FIGURE 13.7 Nerves of the wrist and hand.

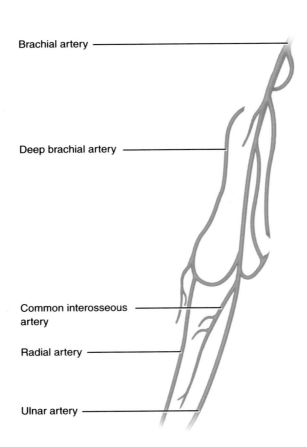

FIGURE 13.8 Blood supply to the elbow region.

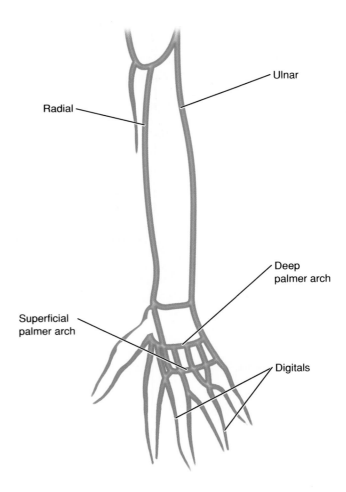

FIGURE 13.9 Blood supply to the wrist and hand.

KINEMATICS AND MAJOR MUSCLE ACTIONS OF THE ELBOW, WRIST, AND HAND

The Elbow

The three associated joints at the elbow allow motion in two planes. Flexion and extension are sagittal plane movements that occur at the humeroulnar and humeroradial joints; pronation and supination are longitudinal rotational movements that take place at the proximal radioulnar joint.

Flexion and Extension

The elbow flexors include those muscles crossing the anterior side of the joint. The primary elbow flexor is the brachialis. Because the distal attachment of the brachialis is the coronoid process of the ulna, the muscle is equally effective when the forearm is in supination and pronation. Another elbow flexor, the biceps brachii, has both long and short heads attached to the radial tuberosity via a single common tendon. When the forearm is supinated, the biceps contributes effectively to flexion because it is slightly stretched. When the forearm is pronated, the muscle is less taut and consequently less effective. The brachioradialis, which is also an elbow flexor, is most effective when the forearm is in a neutral position (i.e., midway between full pronation and full supination). Other flexor muscles that cross the elbow are important dynamic stabilizers of the joint. In particular, the flexor carpi ulnaris and flexor digitorum superficialis provide significant stability to the medial elbow during a variety of activities, including throwing.

The triceps is the major elbow extensor. Although the three heads have separate origins, they attach to the olecranon process of the ulna through a common distal tendon. The small anconeus muscle also assists with extension at the elbow.

Pronation and Supination

Pronation and supination of the forearm occur when the radius rotates around the ulna (Fig. 13.10). There are three radioulnar articulations: the proximal, middle, and distal radioulnar joints. The primary pronator muscle is the pronator quadratus, which attaches to the distal ulna and radius. The pronator teres, which crosses the proximal radioulnar joint, assists with pronation. As the name suggests, the supinator is the muscle primarily responsible for supination. During resistance or elbow flexion, the biceps also participates in supination.

The Wrist and Hand

The wrist is capable of sagittal and frontal plane movements (Fig. 13.11). Flexion occurs when the palmar surface of the hand is moved toward the anterior forearm. Extension involves the return of the hand to anatomical position from a position of flexion, and hyperextension occurs when the dorsal surface of the hand is brought toward the posterior forearm. Movement of the hand toward the radial side of the arm is radial deviation; movement in the opposite direction is known as ulnar deviation. Movement of the hand through all four directions is termed circumduction.

FIGURE 13.10 Forearm movements. **A.** Supination occurs when the radius and ulna are parallel to each other. **B.** Pronation involves the rotation of the radius over the ulna.

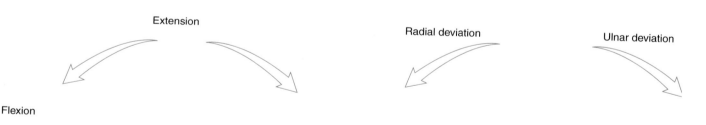

FIGURE 13.11 Directional movement capabilities at the wrist. **A.** Sagittal plane movements. **B.** Frontal plane movements.

Flexion

The major flexor muscles of the wrist are the flexor carpi radialis and flexor carpi ulnaris. The palmaris longus, which is often absent in one or both forearms, contributes to flexion. The flexor digitorum superficialis and flexor digitorum profundus assist with flexion at the wrist when the fingers are completely extended, but when the fingers are in flexion, these muscles cannot develop sufficient tension to assist.

Extension and Hyperextension

The extensor carpi radialis longus, extensor carpi radialis brevis, and extensor carpi ulnaris produce extension and hyperextension at the wrist. The other posterior wrist muscles may also assist with extension movements, particularly when the fingers are in flexion. Included are the extensor pollicis longus, extensor indicis, extensor digiti minimi, and extensor digitorum.

Radial and Ulnar Deviation

The flexor and extensor muscles of the wrist cooperatively develop tension to produce radial and ulnar deviation of the hand at the wrist. The flexor carpi radialis and extensor carpi radialis act to produce radial deviation, and the flexor carpi ulnaris and extensor carpi ulnaris cause ulnar deviation.

Carpometacarpal Joint Motion

The CM joint of the thumb allows a large range of movement, comparable to that of a ball-and-socket joint. However, the fifth CM joint permits significantly less range of motion and only a very small amount of motion is allowed at the second through fourth CM joints, because of the presence of restrictive ligaments.

Metacarpophalangeal Joint Motion

The MCP joints of the fingers allow flexion, extension, abduction, adduction, and circumduction (FIG. 13.12). Among the fingers, abduction is defined as movement away from the middle finger and adduction is movement toward the middle finger. The MCP joint of the thumb functions more as a hinge joint, with the primary movements being flexion and extension.

Interphalangeal Joint Motion

The IP joints permit flexion and extension, and in some individuals, slight hyperextension. These are classic hinge joints.

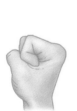 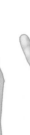 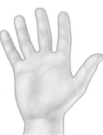 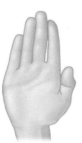 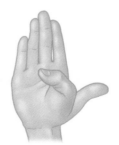 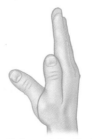 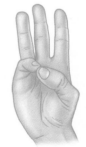

Flexion   Extension   Abduction   Adduction   Thumb flexion and extension   Palmar abduction/ adduction of thumb   Opposition of the thumb and fingertips

FIGURE 13.12 Directional movement capabilities at the fingers and thumb. **A.** Flexion. **B.** Extension. **C.** Abduction. **D.** Adduction. **E.** Thumb flexion and extension. **F.** Palmar abduction/adduction of the thumb. **G.** Opposition of the thumb and fingertips.

PREVENTION OF INJURIES

The very nature of many contact and collision sports places the wrist and hand in an extremely vulnerable position for injury. The elbow, wrist, and hand are often subjected to compressive forces. The hand, in particular, is usually the first point of contact to cushion the body during collisions, to deflect flying objects, or to lessen body impact during a fall.

Physical Conditioning

Many of the muscles that move the elbow also move the shoulder or wrist. Therefore, flexibility and strength exercises must focus on the entire arm. Exercises illustrated in APPLICATION STRATEGY 13.1 improve general strength at the elbow and wrist and can be combined with strengthening exercises for the shoulder complex (see Chapter 12). Other exercises, such as squeezing a tennis ball or a spring-loaded grip device, can be used to strengthen the finger flexors.

Protective Equipment

Although ice hockey and men's lacrosse do have specific pads to protect the upper arm, elbow, and forearm, most sports do not require any protection for the elbow region. Goalies, baseball and softball catchers, and field players in many sports, such as hockey and lacrosse, are required to wear wrist and hand protection. The padded gloves prevent direct compression from a stick, puck, or ball. Several other gloves have extra padding on high-impact areas, aid in gripping, and protect the hand from abrasions.

Proper Technique

Nearly all overuse injuries are directly related to repetitive throwing-type motions that produce microtraumatic tensile forces on the surrounding soft tissue structures. Children who use a sidearm throwing motion are three times more likely to develop problems than those who use a more traditional overhead technique. Movement analysis can detect improper technique in the acceleration and follow-through phase that contribute to these excessive tensile forces.

An important skill technique that can prevent injury of the wrist and hand is proper instruction on the shoulder-roll method of falling. In this technique, the force of impact is dispersed over a wider area, lessening the risk for injury from direct axial loading on the extended wrist.

CONTUSIONS

Direct blows to arm and forearm are frequently associated with contact and collision sports. Contusions result from a compressive force sustained from a direct blow. Such injuries vary in severity in accordance with the area and depth over which blood vessels are ruptured.

Signs and Symptoms

Ecchymosis may be present if the hemorrhage is superficial. Significant trauma can lead to internal hemorrhage, rapid swelling, and hematoma formation that can limit ROM.

Chronic blows to the anterior arm can result in the development of ectopic bone in either the belly of the muscle (i.e., myositis ossificans) or as a bony outgrowth (i.e., exostosis) of the underlying bone. The deltoid and brachialis muscle belly are common sites for the development of myositis ossificans after trauma. A particularly vulnerable site is just proximal to the deltoid's insertion on the lateral aspect of the humerus where the bone is least padded by muscle tissue. Standard shoulder pads do not extend far enough to protect the area, and the edge of the pad itself may contribute to the injury. The developing mass can become painful and disabling if the radial nerve is contused, leading to transitory paralysis of the extensor forearm muscles.

"Tackler's exostosis," also known as blocker's spur, commonly seen in football linemen, is not a true myositis ossificans, because the ectopic formation is not infiltrated into the muscle, but rather is an irritative exostosis arising from the bone. A painful bony mass, usually in the form of a spur with a sharp edge, can be palpated on the anterolateral aspect of the humerus.

APPLICATION STRATEGY 13.1

Exercises to Prevent Injury to the Elbow Region

Begin all exercises with light resistance using dumbbells or surgical tubing.

1. Biceps curl—Support the involved arm on the leg, and fully flex the elbow. This can also be performed bilaterally in a standing position with a barbell.

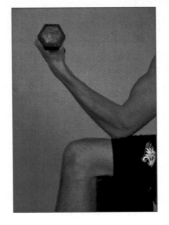

2. Triceps curl—Raise the involved arm over the head. Extend the involved arm at the elbow. This can also be performed bilaterally in a supine or standing position with a barbell.

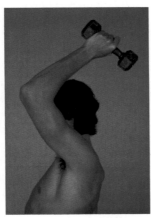

3. Wrist flexion—Support the involved forearm on a table or your leg with the hand off the edge. With the palm facing up, slowly perform a full wrist curl and return to the starting position.

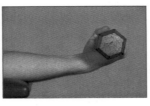

4. Wrist extension—Support the involved forearm on a table or your leg with the hand off the edge. With the palm facing down, slowly perform a full reverse wrist curl and return to the starting position.

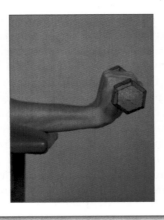

5. Forearm pronation/supination—Support the involved forearm on a table or your leg with the hand over the edge. With surgical tubing or a hand dumbbell, roll the forearm into pronation, then return to supination. Adjust the surgical tubing and reverse the exercise, stressing the supinators. The elbow remain stationary.

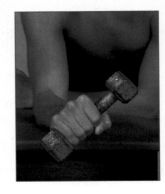

6. Ulnar/radial deviation—Support the involved forearm on a table or your leg with the hand over the edge. With surgical tubing or a hand dumbbell, perform ulnar deviation. Reverse directions and perform radial deviation. An alternate method is to stand with the arm at the side holding a hammer or weighted bar. Raise the wrist in ulnar deviation. Repeat in radial deviation.

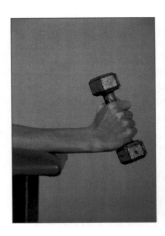

7. Wrist curl-ups—Exercising the wrist extensors is performed by gripping the bar with both palms facing down. Slowly wind the cord onto the bar until the weight reaches the top; then slowly unwind the cord. Reverse hand position to work the wrist flexors.

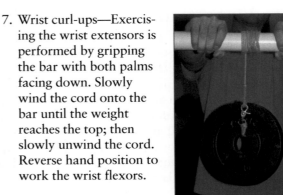

Management

Although many contusions are minor, it is always important to be alert for an underlying fracture. Initial treatment involves ice, compression, elevation, and rest. Symptoms usually disappear in 2 to 3 days. If not, the individual should be referred to a physician for follow-up care.

OLECRANON BURSITIS

The subcutaneous olecranon bursa is the largest bursa in the elbow region. The superficial location predisposes the bursa to either direct macrotrauma or cumulative microtrauma by repetitive elbow flexion and extension. The bursitis can be acute or chronic, aseptic or septic. Common mechanisms of olecranon bursa injury include

- A fall on a flexed elbow
- Constantly leaning on one's elbow ("student's elbow")
- Repetitive pressure and friction
- Repetitive flexion and extension
- Infection

Acute and Chronic Bursitis

A fall on a flexed elbow can lead to an acutely inflamed bursa. Constantly leaning on one's elbow, repetitive pressure, and friction can lead to a chronic inflamed bursa.

Signs and Symptoms

The acutely inflamed bursa presents with an immediate tender, swollen area of redness in the posterior elbow. The swelling is relatively painless. If the bursa ruptures, a discrete, sharply demarcated goose egg is visible directly over the olecranon process. Motion is limited at the extreme of flexion as tension increases over the bursa.

Management

Acute management involves ice, rest, and a compressive wrap applied for the first 24 hours. If there is significant distention, the individual should be referred to a physician as the condition may necessitate aspiration to relive the swelling.

Chronic bursitis is managed with application of cold to the area, nonsteroidal anti-inflammatory medications, and the use of elbow cushions to protect the area from further insult.

Septic Bursitis

Occasionally, the bursa can become infected, regardless of acute trauma to the area. This may result from skin breakdown and a poor blood supply to the area.

Signs and Symptoms

The area is hot to the touch and inflamed. The individual shows traditional signs of infection, including malaise (feeling lousy), fever, pain, restricted motion, tenderness, and swelling at the elbow.

Management

An individual with an infected bursa should be referred to a physician. The physician usually aspirates the bursa and takes a culture of the fluid to determine the presence of septic bursitis.

SPRAINS AND DISLOCATIONS

Most common ligament tears in the elbow result from repetitive tensile forces that irritate and tear the ligaments, particularly the ulnar collateral ligament. Traumatic elbow sprains are usually caused by hyperextension or a sudden, violent, unidirectional valgus force that drives the ulna in a posterior or posterolateral direction. In the wrist and hand, hyperextension is also the leading mechanism of injury, although hyperflexion or rotation may also lead to injury. When caused by a single episode, the severity of the injury depends on characteristics of the injury force (its point of application, magnitude, rate, and direction); position of the hand or elbow at impact; and relative strength of the bones and supporting ligaments.

Unfortunately, most individuals do not allow ample time for healing because they need to perform simple daily activities. Consequently, many sprains are neglected, leading to chronic instability.

Elbow Sprain

Repetitive tensile forces irritate and tear the ligaments, particularly the ulnar collateral ligament. When this occurs, pain can be palpated directly over the involved ligament. When forces are excessive, the resulting injury may be an elbow dislocation.

Signs and Symptoms

If the ulnar collateral ligament is injured, a history of pain localized on the medial aspect of the elbow during the late cocking and acceleration phases of throwing is common. Point tenderness can be palpated directly over the ligament and increases if a valgus force or stress is applied. If the radial collateral ligament is injured, pain is localized on the lateral aspect of the elbow and increases with varus stress.

Management

Treatment involves standard acute care with ice, compression, and use of a sling. This injury requires physician referral for accurate diagnosis and treatment options.

Dislocations

In adolescents, the most common traumatic injury to the elbow is subluxation or dislocation of the proximal radial head, often associated with an immature annular ligament. Referred to as "nursemaid's elbow" or "pulled-elbow syndrome," the condition results from longitudinal traction of an extended and pronated upper extremity, such as when a young child is swung by the arms. A small tear in the annular ligament allows the radial head to migrate out from under the annular ligament. If an individual is unable to pronate and supinate the forearm without pain, immediate referral to a physician is warranted.

Most ulnar dislocations occur in individuals younger than 20 years, with a peak incidence in the teenage years.[1] The mechanism of injury is usually hyperextension or a sudden, violent unidirectional valgus force that drives the ulna posterior or posterolateral. Approximately 60% of patients have associated fractures of the medial epicondyle, radial head, coronoid process, or olecranon process.[2] When the dislocation is associated with both radial head and coronoid fractures, it has been termed the "terrible triad of the elbow" because of the difficulties inherent in treatment and the consistently poor reported outcomes as compared to a simple elbow dislocation.[3] The injury may also involve disruption of the anterior capsule, tearing of the brachialis muscle, injury to the ulnar collateral ligament, and, rarely, brachial artery compromise or nerve injury to the median or ulnar nerves.[1]

Signs and Symptoms

A snapping or cracking sensation is experienced on impact. It is followed by severe pain, rapid swelling, total loss of function, and an obvious deformity (FIG. 13.13). The arm is frequently held in flexion, with the forearm appearing shortened. The olecranon and radial head are palpable posteriorly, and a slight indentation in the triceps is visible just proximal to the olecranon.

Management

This injury should be considered a medical emergency. As such, activation of the emergency action plan is warranted, including summoning of EMS. Because of the risk of neurovascular injury, the coach should not make any attempt to change the position of the arm. If tolerable,

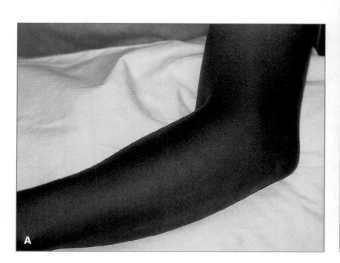

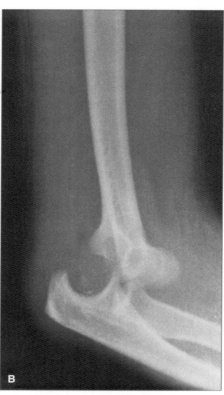

FIGURE 13.13 Elbow dislocation. **A.** Clinical view of a posterior dislocation. **B.** Radiograph of a typical posterior dislocation. Note the coronoid process is adjacent to the olecranon fossa.

application of cold to the area will help to manage swelling and inflammation while EMS is en route. Reduction of a dislocated elbow is usually performed under general or regional anesthesia.

Wrist Sprain

Axial loading on the proximal palm during a fall on an outstretched hand is the leading cause of wrist sprains. This injury is often neglected, leading to chronic wrist pain.

Signs and Symptoms

Assessment reveals point tenderness on the dorsum of the radiocarpal joint. Pain increases with active or passive extension. Because of the shape of the lunate and its position between the large capitate and lower end of the radius, this carpal bone is particularly prone to dislocation during axial loading (FIG. 13.14). The dorsum of the hand is point tender, and a thickened area on the palm can be palpated just distal to the end of the radius if not obscured by swelling. Passive and active motion may not be painful. If the bone moves into the carpal tunnel, compression of the median nerve leads to pain, numbness, and tingling in the first and second fingers.

Management

Immediate treatment involves immobilization, application of cold, elevation, and immediate referral to a physician to rule out a fracture or carpal dislocation.

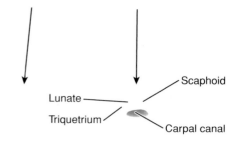

FIGURE 13.14 Lunate dislocation. **A.** The lunate can dislocate during a fall on an outstretched hand when the load from the radius compresses the lunate in a volar direction. **B.** If the bone moves into the carpal tunnel, the median nerve can become compressed, leading to sensory changes in the first and second fingers.

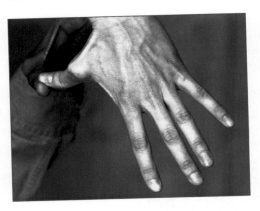

FIGURE 13.15 Clinical appearance of a gamekeeper's thumb.

Thumb and Finger Sprains

Sprains of the thumb and fingers are common. The thumb is exposed to more force than the fingers because of its position on the hand. Integrity of the ulnar collateral ligament at the MCP joint is critical for normal hand function because it stabilizes the joint as the thumb is pushed against the index and middle fingers while performing many pinching, grasping, and gripping motions.

Gamekeeper's Thumb

Gamekeeper's thumb occurs when the MCP joint is near full extension and the thumb is forcefully abducted away from the hand, tearing the ulnar collateral ligament at the MCP joint (FIG. 13.15).

Signs and Symptoms

The palmar aspect of the joint is painful, swollen, and may have visible bruising. Instability is detected by replicating the mechanism of injury or by stressing the thumb in flexion.

Management

Initial treatment includes application of cold, compression, elevation, and referral to a physician for further care.

Finger Sprains and Dislocations

Excessive varus/valgus stress and hyperextension can damage the collateral ligaments of the fingers. Although many individuals will consider the injury to be a simple "jammed finger," this injury often involves an avulsion fracture from a tendon rupture, which requires immediate surgery to repair the damage. Hyperextension of the proximal phalanx can stretch or rupture the volar plate on the palmar side of the joint. As such, it is critical to refer this individual to a physician to rule out a more extensive injury.

Signs and Symptoms

A swollen, painful finger caused by a ball striking the extended finger is the most frequent initial report. An obvious deformity may not be present unless there is a fracture. The most common dislocation in the body occurs at the PIP joint (FIG. 13.16). Pain is present at the joint line and increases when the mechanism of injury is reproduced. Because digital nerves and vessels run along the sides of the fingers and thumb, dislocations here can be potentially serious.

Management

Because of the probability of entrapping the volar plate in an IP joint, which can lead to permanent dysfunction of the finger, no attempt should be made to reduce a finger dislocation by an untrained individual. Immediate treatment for all dislocations involves immobilization in a finger splint, application of cold, and referral to a physician.

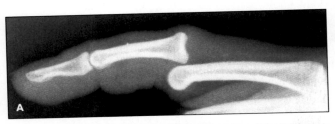

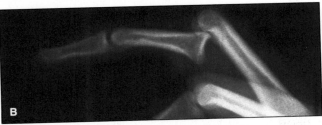

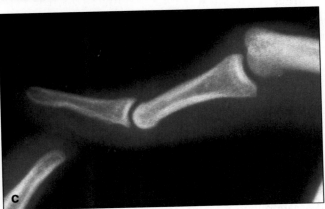

FIGURE 13.16 Dislocation variants of the PIP joint. The most common are (**A**) dorsal, followed by (**B**) volar with a central slip rupture. The least common is (**C**) rotatory subluxation.

STRAINS

Elbow Strains

Muscular strains occur as a result of excessive overload against resistance or overstretching the tendon beyond its normal range. In mild or moderate strains, pain and restricted motion may not be a major factor. In many injuries, muscular strains occur simultaneously with a joint sprain. The joint sprain takes precedence in priority of care, especially with an associated dislocation. As a result, tendon damage may go unrecognized and untreated.

Signs and Symptoms

Injury to the elbow flexors (brachialis, biceps brachii, and brachioradialis) will result in point tenderness on the anterior distal arm. Pain increases with resisted elbow flexion. If the strain is to the triceps, resisted elbow extension produces discomfort. Strains to the common wrist flexor group result in pain on resisted wrist flexion, whereas strains to the wrist extensors produce pain with wrist extension.

Management

If a grade 1 injury is suspected, management involves standard acute care with cold and compression. If the signs and symptoms do not resolve within 2 to 3 days, the coach should require the individual to obtain approval for return to participation from a qualified healthcare professional. If a grade 2 or 3 injury is suspected, cold should be applied and the arm placed in a sling. This injury requires immediate physician referral.

Wrist and Finger Strains

In the hand, muscle strains involving the finger flexors or extensors tend to be more serious. These injuries may involve avulsing the tendon from the bone.

Jersey Finger

A "**jersey finger**" typically occurs when an individual grips an opponent's jersey while the opponent simultaneously twists and turns to get away. This jerking action may force the fingers to rapidly extend, rupturing the flexor digitorum profundus tendon from its attachment on the distal phalanx, and so the name "jersey finger." The ring finger is more commonly involved.

Signs and Symptoms. If avulsed, the tendon can be palpated at the proximal aspect of the involved finger. The individual is unable to flex the DIP joint against resistance.

Management

Treatment involves standard acute care with cold, compression, and elevation. Immediate physician referral is necessary for accurate diagnosis and management.

Mallet Finger

Mallet finger occurs when an object hits the end of the finger while the extensor tendon is taut, such as when catching a ball. The resulting forceful flexion of the distal phalanx avulses the lateral bands of the extensor mechanism from its distal attachment.

Signs and Symptoms

If the common extensor mechanism is avulsed, a characteristic mallet deformity is present (FIG. 13.17), and the individual is unable to fully extend the DIP joint with the forearm pronated.

Management

Treatment is the same as with a jersey finger.

Boutonniere Deformity

A boutonniere deformity is caused by blunt trauma to the dorsal aspect of the PIP joint, or by rapid, forceful flexion

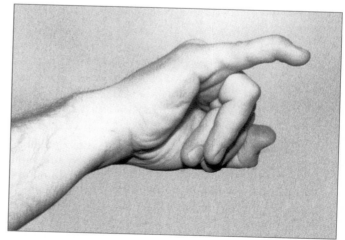

FIGURE 13.17 Mallet finger. The individual was asked to straighten the little finger but was unable to extend the DIP joint, suggesting that the extensor tendon is avulsed from the attachment on the distal phalanx. The tendon may also avulse a small piece of bone, leading to an avulsion fracture.

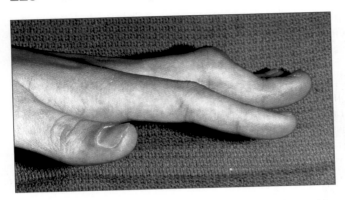

FIGURE 13.18 Boutonniere deformity. In a boutonniere deformity, the proximal joint flexes while the distal joint hyperextends.

of the joint against resistance. The central slip of the extensor tendon ruptures at the middle phalanx, leaving no active extensor mechanism intact over the PIP joint. An injury to the volar plate also can lead to a flexion deformity of the PIP joint that resembles a boutonniere deformity.

Signs and Symptoms

The deformity is not usually present immediately, but develops over 2 to 3 weeks as the lateral slips move in a palmar direction and cause hyperextension at the MCP joint, flexion at the PIP joint, and hyperextension at the DIP joint (FIG. 13.18). Because the head of the proximal phalanx protrudes through the split in the extensor hood, this condition is sometimes referred to as a "buttonhole rupture." The PIP joint is swollen and lacks full extension.

Management

Any injury that limits PIP extension to 30° or less and produces dorsal tenderness over the base of the middle phalanx should be treated as an acute tendon rupture and immediately referred to a physician.

OVERUSE CONDITIONS

The throwing mechanism can lead to significant overuse injuries at the elbow. During the initial acceleration phase, the body is brought rapidly forward, but the elbow and hand lag behind the upper arm. This action results in a tremendous tensile valgus stress placed on the medial aspect of the elbow, particularly the ulnar collateral ligament and adjacent tissues. As acceleration continues, the elbow extensors and wrist flexors contract to add velocity to the throw. This whipping action produces significant valgus stress on the medial elbow and concomitant lateral compressive stress in the radiocapitellar joint (FIG. 13.19).

As the ball is released, the elbow is almost fully extended and is positioned slightly anterior to the trunk. When release takes place, the elbow is flexed approximately 20° to 30°. As these forces decrease, however, the extreme pronation of the forearm places the lateral ligaments under tension.

During deceleration, eccentric contractions of the long head of the biceps brachii, supinator, and extensor muscles decelerate the forearm in pronation. Additional stress occurs on structures around the olecranon as pronation and extension jam the olecranon into the olecranon fossa. Impingement can occur during this jamming.

Medial Epicondylitis

Epicondylitis is a common chronic condition in activities involving pronation and supination, such as tennis, pitching, volleyball, or golf. Often, the individual reveals a pattern of poor technique, fatigue, and overuse. Medial epicondylitis, common in adolescent athletes, is caused by repeated medial tension/lateral compression (valgus) forces placed on the arm during the acceleration phase of the throwing motion. Valgus forces often produce a combined flexor muscle strain, ulnar collateral ligament sprain, and ulnar neuritis. If the medial humeral growth plate is affected, it may be called "**little league elbow.**" However, this term negates that other individuals, such as golfers, gymnasts, tennis players, and wrestlers, are also susceptible to the condition. Simultaneously, lateral compressive forces can damage the lateral condyle of the humerus and radial head. Posterior stresses may lead to triceps strain, olecranon impingement, olecranon fractures, or loose bodies.

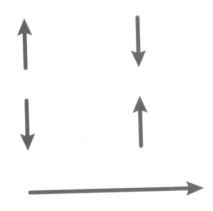

FIGURE 13.19 Traction-compression mechanism. An excessive valgus force can lead to both medial tensile stress and lateral compression stress, causing injury to both sides of the joint.

Signs and Symptoms

Assessment reveals swelling, ecchymosis, and point tenderness directly over the humeroulnar joint, or on the medial epicondyle. Pain is usually severe and aggravated by resisted wrist flexion and pronation and by a valgus stress. If the ulnar nerve is involved, tingling and numbness may radiate into the forearm and hand, particularly the fourth and fifth fingers.

Management

In assessing this condition, it should become apparent to the coach during the history component that the injury is overuse in nature and, as such, the coach should refrain from continuing assessment. Rather, the coach should refer this individual to a physician for accurate diagnosis and treatment options. The coach should not permit the individual to continue activity, as doing so could potentially exacerbate the condition. In addition, the coach could suggest the application of cold to the area to decrease pain and potential spasm.

Lateral Epicondylitis

Lateral epicondylitis is the most common overuse injury in the adult elbow. The condition is typically caused by eccentric loading of the extensor muscles, predominantly the extensor carpi radialis brevis, during the deceleration phase of the throwing motion or tennis stroke. Gripping a racquet too tightly, improper grip size, excessive string tension, excessive racquet weight or stiffness, faulty backhand technique, putting topspin on backhand strokes, or hitting the ball off-center all contribute to this condition.

Signs and Symptoms

Pain is anterior or just distal to the lateral epicondyle and may radiate into the forearm extensors during and after activity. Pain increases with resisted wrist extension or in an action similar to picking up a full cup of coffee.

Management

The management is the same as for medial epicondylitis.

Tendinitis and Stenosing Tenosynovitis

Individuals involved in strenuous and repetitive training often inflame tendons and tendon sheaths in the wrist and hand. In the wrist, the abductor pollicis longus and extensor pollicis brevis are commonly affected. These two tendons share a single synovial tendon sheath that turns sharply, as much as 105°, to enter the thumb when the wrist is in radial deviation. Friction between the tendons, the **stenosing** sheath, and bony process leads to a condition called "**de Quervain's tenosynovitis.**"

Signs and Symptoms

Tendinitis in the wrist flexors or extensors leads to stiffness and an aching pain that is aggravated by activity. It may appear several hours after participation in physical activity. Pain is usually localized over the involved tendons and is aggravated with passive stretching and resisted motion of the affected tendons.

Management

The coach should refer this individual to a physician for accurate diagnosis and treatment options. The coach should not permit the individual to continue activity, as doing so could potentially exacerbate the condition. In addition, the coach could suggest the application of cold to the area to decrease pain and potential spasm.

NERVE ENTRAPMENT SYNDROMES

Nerve entrapment syndromes, or compressive neuropathies, can be subtle and are often overlooked. They occur in activities, such as bowling, cycling, karate, rowing, baseball/softball,

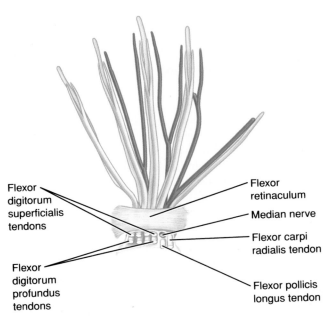

Flexor digitorum superficialis tendons

Flexor digitorum profundus tendons

Flexor retinaculum

Median nerve

Flexor carpi radialis tendon

Flexor pollicis longus tendon

FIGURE 13.20 Carpal tunnel. The flexor tendons of the fingers pass through the carpal tunnel in a single synovial sheath.

field hockey, lacrosse, rugby, weight lifting, and handball, and wheelchair athletics. Mechanisms of injuries most commonly involve repetitive compression, contusion, or traction. A compressive neuropathy may also be caused by anatomical structures, such as anomalous muscles or vessels, fibrous bands, osteofibrous tunnels, or muscle hypertrophy. Pathologic structures, such as ganglia, lipomas, osteophytes, aneurysms, and localized inflammation, can also compress a nerve. The two most common nerve entrapment conditions are **carpal tunnel syndrome** and ulnar entrapment.

Carpal Tunnel Syndrome

The carpal tunnel is formed by the floor of the volar wrist capsule, with the roof formed by the transverse retinacular ligament traveling from the hook of the hamate and pisiform on the lateral side to the volar tubercle of the trapezium and tuberosity of the scaphoid on the medial side. This unyielding tunnel accommodates the median nerve, finger flexors in a common sheath, and flexor pollicis longus in an independent sheath (FIG. 13.20). Any irritation of the synovial sheath covering these tendons can produce swelling or edema that puts pressure on the median nerve.

Carpal tunnel syndrome (CTS) is the most common compression syndrome of the wrist and hand, although it is not commonly seen in the physically active population. Movement of tendons and nerves during prolonged repetitive hand movement may contribute to the development of CTS.[4] In addition, CTS may be caused by direct trauma or anatomical anomalies. It is typically seen in the dominant extremity. Sporting activities that predispose an individual to CTS include activities that involve repetitive or continuous flexion and extension of the wrist, such as cycling, throwing sports, racquet sports, archery, and gymnastics. Etiologies for CTS other than traumatic causes include those of infectious origin (e.g., diphtheria, mumps, influenza, pneumonia, meningitis, malaria, syphilis, typhoid, dysentery, tuberculosis, or gonococcus), or metabolic causes (e.g., hypothyroidism, diabetes, rheumatoid arthritis, gout, vitamin deficiency, heavy metals poisoning, and carbon monoxide poisoning).[5]

Signs and Symptoms

A common sign is pain that awakens the individual in the middle of the night and is often relieved by "shaking out the hands." Pain, numbness, tingling, or a burning sensation may be felt only in the fingertips on the palmar aspect of the thumb, index, and middle finger. Generally, only one extremity is affected. Grip and pinch strength may be limited. A common complaint is difficulty manipulating coins.

Management

The coach should refer this individual to a physician for accurate diagnosis and treatment options. The coach should not permit the individual to continue activity, as doing so could potentially exacerbate the condition. In addition, the coach could suggest the application of cold to the area to decrease pain and potential spasm. Use of a compression wrap should be avoided, because it adds additional compression on the already impinged structures.

Ulnar Nerve Entrapment

In the elbow, the ulnar nerve passes behind the medial epicondyle of the humerus via the ulnar groove, through the cubital tunnel, and underneath the ulnar collateral ligament to enter the forearm (FIG. 13.21). The nerve is vulnerable to compression and tensile stress at this site.

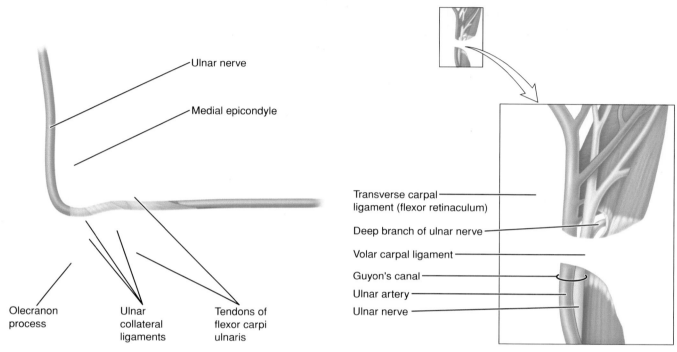

FIGURE 13.21 Ulnar nerve. As the ulnar nerve passes through the cubital tunnel between the ulnar collateral ligament and the olecranon fossa, it passes under the two heads of the flexor carpi ulnaris. This tendon is slack during extension, but becomes taut during flexion, contributing to ulnar nerve compression.

FIGURE 13.22 Impingement of the ulnar nerve. The ulnar nerve can become impinged in the tunnel of Guyon as it runs under the ligament between the hamate and pisiform.

The ulnar nerve can also become entrapped between the hook of the hamate and pisiform. This condition is frequently seen in cycling, racquet sports, and in baseball or softball catchers who experience repetitive trauma to the palm.

Ulnar Tunnel Syndrome

Compression of the ulnar nerve may occur as the nerve enters the ulnar tunnel or as the deep branch curves around the hook of the hamate and traverses the palm (FIG. 13.22). This condition is frequently seen in cycling, racquet sports, and in baseball/softball catchers, hockey goalies, and handball players who experience repetitive compressive trauma to the palmar aspect of the hand. Distal ulnar nerve palsy may also be seen as push-up palsy, following fractures of the hook of the hamate, or as a result of a missed golf shot or baseball swing.

Signs and Symptoms

The lesion may present with motor, sensory, or mixed symptoms. Coincident involvement of the median nerve is common. The individual complains of numbness in the ulnar nerve distribution, particularly in the little finger, and is unable to grasp a piece of paper between the thumb and index finger. Slight weakness in grip strength and atrophy of the **hypothenar** mass may also be present.

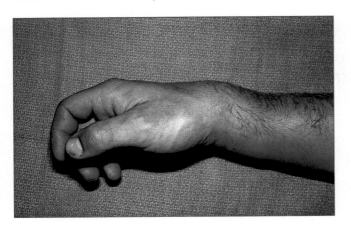

FIGURE 13.23 Clinical view of a Colles' fracture.

Management

The management is the same as for carpal tunnel syndrome.

Cyclist's Palsy

Cyclist's palsy, also linked to ulnar nerve entrapment, occurs when a biker leans on the handlebar for an extended period of time, leading to swelling in the hypothenar area. Symptoms mimic the more serious ulnar nerve entrapment syndrome, but they usually disappear rapidly after completion of the ride. Properly padding the handlebars, wearing padded gloves, varying hand position, and properly fitting the bike to the rider can greatly reduce the incidence of this condition.

FRACTURES

Distal Radial and Ulnar Fractures

Fractures to the distal radius and ulna present a special problem. In adolescents, epiphyseal and metaphyseal fractures are common. These fractures usually heal without residual disability. In older individuals, one or both bones may be fractured, or one bone may be fractured with the other bone dislocated at the elbow or wrist joint. A **Colles' fracture** occurs within 1½ in. of the wrist joint, and results in a "dinner-fork" deformity when the distal segment displaces in a dorsal and radial direction (FIG. 13.23). A reverse of this fracture is **Smith's fracture**, which tends to move toward the palmar aspect (volar). A Monteggia fracture is characterized by a fracture of the proximal one-third of the ulna accompanied by a dislocation of the radial head. In a Galeazzi fracture, the distal radioulnar dislocation is secondary to the marked shortening of the radius caused by the severe ulnar displacement and dorsal angulation of the distal radial fragment. FIG. 13.24 demonstrates the four common fractures of the forearm.

A catastrophic complication from a forearm fracture is a condition called **Volkmann's contracture**. This condition is caused by increased pressure and swelling inside one of the forearm compartments that compromise circulation to the surrounding muscles and nerves. As the pressure builds unabated, **ischemic necrosis** can lead to permanent loss of nerve and muscular function. As a result, the hand is cold, white, and numb. Passive extension of the fingers leads to severe pain. These symptoms indicate a serious problem.

Signs and Symptoms

In adolescents, fractures of the growth plate may present with the distal fragment being dorsally displaced. Other signs and symptoms associated with traumatic fractures include intense pain, swelling, deformity, and a false joint. Swelling and hemorrhage may lead to circulatory impairment, or the median nerve may be damaged as it passes through the forearm.

Management

Fractures should be suspected in all forearm injuries, particularly in adolescents. A suspected fracture should be immobilized and the individual should be referred to a physician immediately.

Scaphoid Fractures

Scaphoid fractures account for more than 70% of all carpal bone injuries in the general population, and are the most common wrist bone fracture in physically active individuals.[6] Peak incidence is between 12 and 15 years of age.[6] In many cases, the individual falls on the wrist, has normal radiographs, and is discharged with a diagnosis of a wrist sprain without further care. However, several months later, the individual continues to experience persistent wrist pain. Radiographs at this time may reveal an established nonunion fracture of the scaphoid. Because of a poor blood supply to the area, **aseptic necrosis**, or death of the tissue, is a common complication with this fracture.

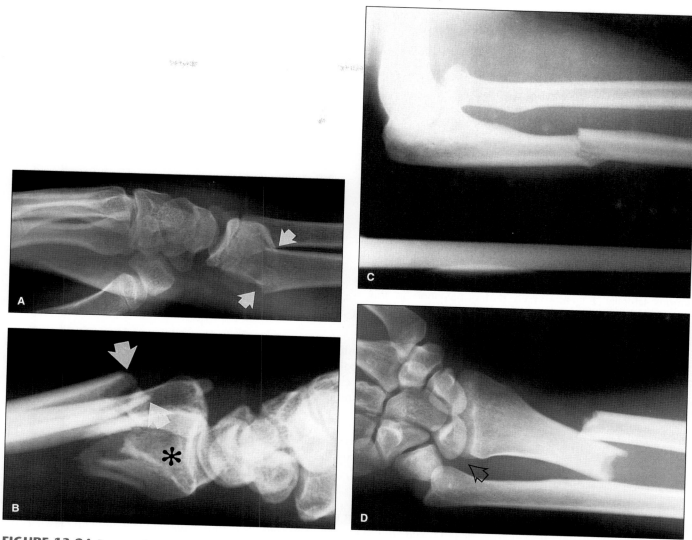

FIGURE 13.24 Forearm fractures. **A.** Colles' fracture: the extra articular distal radial fracture is associated with a fracture of the base of the ulnar styloid. **B.** Smith's fracture: this type of fracture is characterized by a transverse fracture of the distal radius, with volar and proximal displacement of the distal radial fragment. **C.** Monteggia fracture: this type of fracture is characterized by a fracture of the proximal third of the ulna, accompanied by a dislocation of the radial head. **D.** Galeazzi fracture: the distal radioulnar dislocation is secondary to the marked shortening of the radius caused by the severe ulnar displacement and dorsal angulation of the distal radial fragment.

Signs and Symptoms

Assessment reveals a history of falling on an outstretched hand. Pain is present during palpation of the **anatomical snuff box** (Fig. 13.25), which lies directly over the scaphoid, or with inward pressure along the long axis of the first metacarpal bone. Pain increases during wrist extension and radial deviation.

Management

A suspected fracture should be immobilized and the individual should be referred to a physician immediately. Application of cold can help to reduce swelling and inflammation.

Metacarpal Fractures

Uncomplicated fractures of the metacarpals result in severe pain, swelling, and deformity. Unique fractures at the base of the first metacarpal may involve a simple intra-articular fracture (e.g., **Bennett's fracture**). A unique fracture involving the neck of the fourth or fifth metacarpal is called

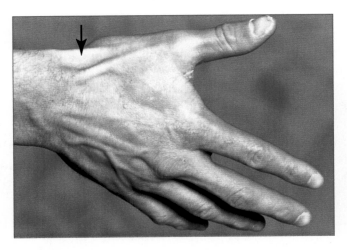

FIGURE 13.25 Anatomical snuff box. The scaphoid forms the floor of the anatomical snuff box. It is bounded by the extensor pollicis brevis medially and the extensor pollicis longus laterally. Increased pain during palpation in this region indicates a possible fracture to the scaphoid bone.

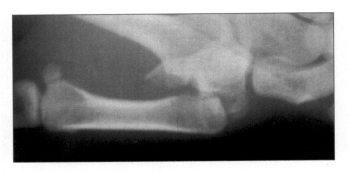

FIGURE 13.26 Bennett's fracture. A Bennett's fracture is usually associated with a dislocation of the MCP joint of the thumb. An avulsion fracture, however, occurs when a segment of the metacarpal is held in place by the deep volar ligament.

a boxer's fracture. It occurs when an individual punches an object with a closed fist, leading to rotation of the head of the metacarpal over the neck. Axial compression on the hand can lead to a fracture-dislocation of the proximal end of the metacarpal. It often goes undetected because edema obscures the extent of injury. Fractures of the shaft of the metacarpal are more easily recognized.

Signs and Symptoms

Increased pain and a palpable deformity are present in the palm of the hand directly over the involved metacarpal. Gentle percussion and compression along the long axis of the bone increase pain at the fracture site.

Management

Fractures should be immobilized in the position of function, with the palm face down and fingers slightly flexed. Cold should be applied to reduce hemorrhage and swelling; an elastic compression bandage should not be applied to a swollen hand, because it may lead to increased distal swelling in the fingers. The individual should be referred immediately to a physician for further assessment.

Bennett's Fracture

A Bennett's fracture is an articular fracture of the proximal end of the first metacarpal and is usually associated with a dislocation. It is typically caused by axial compression, as occurs when a punch is thrown with a closed fist or the individual falls on a closed fist. The pull of the abductor pollicis longus tendon at the base of the metacarpal displaces the shaft proximally. However, a small medial fragment is held in place by the deep volar ligament, leading to a fracture-dislocation (FIG. 13.26).

Signs and Symptoms

Pain and swelling are localized over the proximal end of the first metacarpal, but deformity may or may not be present. Inward pressure exerted along the long axis of the first metacarpal elicits increased pain at the fracture site.

Management

The management is the same as for a metacarpal fracture.

Boxer's Fracture

Fractures involving the distal metaphysis or neck of the fourth or fifth metacarpals are commonly seen in young males involved in punching activities, as such the name boxer's fracture (although the fracture rarely occurs in boxers) (FIG. 13.27). The fracture typically has an apex dorsal angulation and is inherently unstable secondary to the deforming muscle forces and the frequent volar comminution.

Signs and Symptoms

Sudden pain, inability to grip objects, rapid swelling, and possible deformity are present. Palpation reveals tenderness and pain over the fracture site, and possible crepitus and bony deviation. Delayed ecchymosis is common. Pain increases with axial compression of the involved metacarpal and percussion.

Management

The management is the same as for a metacarpal fracture.

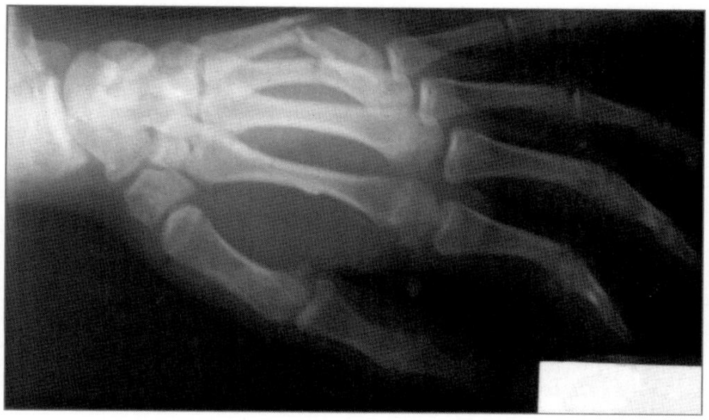

FIGURE 13.27 Boxer's fracture. These fractures usually involve the fourth and fifth metacarpals.

Phalangeal Fractures

Fractures of the phalanges are very common in sport participation. These fractures can be difficult to manage. They may be caused by having the fingers stepped on or impinged between two hard objects such as a football helmet and the ground or by hyperextension that may lead to a fracture-dislocation.

Signs and Symptoms

Increased pain is present with circulative compression around the involved phalanx. Gentle percussion and compression along the long axis of the bone increase pain at the fracture site. Particular attention should be given to a possible fracture of the middle and proximal phalanges. These fractures tend to have marked deformity because of the strong pull of the flexor and extensor tendons. The four fingers move as a unit. Failure to maintain the longitudinal and rotational alignments of the fingers can lead to long-term disability in grasping or manipulating small objects in the palm of the hand. This deformity often results in a finger overlapping another when a fist is made.

Management

The management is the same as for a metacarpal fracture.

THE COACH AND ON-SITE ASSESSMENT OF AN ELBOW, WRIST, OR HAND CONDITION

Injuries to the elbow, wrist, hand, and, in particular, the fingers are sometimes dismissed as minor in the absence of an appropriate assessment. The coach should ensure that injuries to these areas are not overlooked and anticipate that most injuries will require physician referral. Signs and symptoms that necessitate immediate referral to a physician are identified in BOX 13.1.

While the coach should restrict their assessment of injuries to those that are acute in nature, it may be appropriate to ask questions as part of the history component of an assessment that addresses chronic scenarios (APPLICATION STRATEGY 13.2). In doing so, the coach can confirm the presence of an acute or chronic/overuse injury and proceed accordingly. When it becomes apparent that an injury is overuse in nature, the coach should refrain from any continued assessment and, instead, refer the individual to an appropriate healthcare practitioner.

In completing the observation component of the on-site assessment of an acute injury, both arms should be visibly clear, so that a bilateral comparison can be performed. It will be important for the coach to recognize possible fractures and dislocations before moving the elbow, wrist, or hand. If a fracture or dislocation is suspected, the coach should not perform any of the testing components of the assessment. If the individual is in significant pain and/or is unable or unwilling to move the body part, the coach should complete the assessment with the body part in a comfortable position and avoid passively moving the involved or surrounding areas.

APPLICATION STRATEGY 13.2

On-site Assessment of an Acute Elbow, Wrist, or Hand Injury: History, Observation, and Palpation

HISTORY

Chief Complaint
What's wrong?

Mechanism of Injury
What happened?
What were you doing?
Was there a direct blow?
Did you fall? How (outstretched arm; flexed arm; outstretched hand)?
Are you able to demonstrate how it happened?

Acute or Chronic Injury (Onset)
Do you remember when it started hurting?
How long has this been bothering you?

Pain
Location
Where is the pain?
Can you point to a location where it hurts the most?

Type
Can you describe the pain (e.g., sharp, shooting, dull, achy, diffuse)?

Intensity
What is the level of pain on a scale from 1 to 10?

Sounds/Feelings
Did you hear anything when the injury happened (e.g., pop; snap; crack)?
Did you feel any unusual sensations (e.g., tearing; tingling; numbing; cracking) when the injury happened?

Previous History
Have you ever injured your shoulder before? If so, what happened? What was the injury? Were you treated for it?

Other Important/Helpful Information
Have you made any changes in performance technique (e.g., throwing style; swimming strokes)?
Are you able to perform activity-specific skills (e.g., throw, swimming strokes)?
Have you changed your weight training work-outs (e.g., increased weight or number of repetitions; added new exercises)?
Are you able to perform normal motions/ADLs?
Is there anything else you would like to tell me about your condition?

OBSERVATION

General Presentation
Guarding
Moving easily; hesitant to move

Specific to Elbow
The manner in which the individual is holding their arm

Resting position—swelling in the joint may prevent full elbow extension or flexion
Soft tissue symmetry (i.e., muscle atrophy, hypertrophy)

Specific to the Forearm, Wrist, and Hand Posture
Shape and contour of the bony and soft tissue structures
MCP joints and between (peaks and valleys—normal or filled with swelling?)
Angular deformities of the fingers (that may indicate previous fracture or dislocation)
Injury site appearance—deformity; swelling; discoloration

PALPATION

The coach should only perform palpation if there is a clear understanding of what is being palpated and why? A productive assessment appropriate to the standard of care of a coach does not necessitate palpation.

TESTING

Active Range of Motion—Bilateral Comparison
- Elbow flexion and extension
- Forearm supination and pronation
- Wrist flexion and extension
- Ulnar deviation and radial deviation
- Finger flexion and extension at MCP, PIP, and DIP joints
- Abduction and adduction at MCP joints
- Thumb (first CMC joint) flexion and extension
- Thumb abduction and adduction
- Opposition

Passive Range of Motion Should not be Performed by the Coach

Resistive Range of Motion
- The coach should only perform resistive range of motion for the muscles that govern the shoulder if instruction and approval for doing so has been obtained in advance from an appropriate healthcare practitioner.
- Active range of motion is normal and pain-free as a way to assess strength.

ACTIVITY/SPORT-SPECIFIC FUNCTIONAL TESTING

- Performance of active movements typical of the movements executed by the individual during sport or activity participation (including weight training)
- Should assess strength, agility, flexibility, joint stability, endurance, coordination, balance, and activity-specific skill performance

BOX 13.1	Signs and Symptoms that Necessitate Immediate Referral to a Physician

- Possible epiphyseal or apophyseal injuries
- Tingling or numbness in the forearm or hand
- Obvious deformity suggesting a dislocation or fracture
- Excessive joint swelling
- Significantly limited range of motion
- Weakness in a myotome
- Gross joint instability
- Absent or weak pulse
- All adolescent wrist sprains because of possible epiphyseal or apophyseal injuries
- Any unexplained pain

SUMMARY

1. The elbow encompasses three articulations—the humeroulnar, humeroradial, and proximal radioulnar joints.

2. The subcutaneous olecranon bursa is the largest bursa in the elbow region. Bursitis may be acute or chronic. If the skin is warm to the touch, the individual should be referred to a physician.

3. Most ulnar dislocations occur in individuals younger than 20 years, with a peak incidence in early adolescence. The mechanism is usually hyperextension, or a sudden, violent unidirectional valgus force that drives the ulna posterior or posterolateral.

4. Chronic injuries result from inadequate warm-up, excessive training past the point of fatigue, inadequate rehabilitation of previous injuries, or neglect of seemingly minor conditions that progress to major complications.

5. Repetitive throwing motions place a tremendous tensile stress on the medial joint structures (medial collateral ligament, ulnar nerve, and common flexor tendons) and concomitant lateral compressive stress in the radiocapitellar joint.

6. Medial epicondylitis produces severe pain on resisted wrist flexion and pronation, and with a valgus stress.

7. Common extensor tendinitis produces severe pain on resisted wrist extension and supination, and with a varus stress.

8. Most injuries to the wrist are caused by axial loading on the proximal palm during a fall on an outstretched hand.

9. Excessive varus/valgus stress and hyperextension can damage the collateral ligaments of the fingers. Ligament failure usually occurs at its attachment to the proximal phalanx or, less frequently, in the midportion.

10. The most common dislocation in the body occurs at the PIP joint. Because digital nerves and vessels run along the lateral sides of the fingers and thumb, dislocations can be serious if reduced by an untrained individual.

11. Muscular strains occur from excessive overload against resistance or from stretching the tendon beyond its normal range. Ruptures of a muscle tendon may cause the tendon to retract, necessitating surgical reattachment of the tendon in its proper position.

12. CTS is the most common compression syndrome of the wrist and hand. It is characterized by pain and numbness that wakes the individual in the middle of the night, and it is often relieved by shaking the hands.

13. Compression of the ulnar nerve leads to weakness in grip strength, atrophy of the hypothenar mass, and loss of sensation over the little finger.

14. If pain is present during palpation of the anatomic snuff box, suspect a fracture of the scaphoid and refer the athlete immediately to a physician.

15. If a decision is made to refer an individual to a physician for care, the limb should be appropriately immobilized to protect the area and, if tolerable, cold should be applied to reduce swelling and hemorrhage.

APPLICATION QUESTIONS

1. Following practice, a high school lacrosse player is complaining of pain in his right arm after being struck by another player's stick. He reports receiving several blows to the area over the past week. The area, which is over the belly of the deltoid, is sore and very tender to touch. Bilateral strength of the muscles in the area is normal. What condition should the coach suspect? How should the coach manage this situation?

_____

_____

2. While practicing at a private gymnastics facility, a 12-year-old girl misses the vault and falls to the mat on an out-stretched arm. Upon reaching the girl, it is apparent to the coach that she has sustained a posterior dislocation of the elbow. What signs and symptoms would have helped the coach reach that determination? How should the coach manage the situation?

_____

_____

3. During a basketball class, a high school freshman inadvertently falls and lands on a flexed elbow. What questions should the coach ask as part of the history component of an assessment of this injury? How should the coach conduct the observation component of the assessment?

_____

_____

4. Following the second innings of play, a little league baseball pitcher complains of pain on the medial elbow during pitching. The pitcher tells the coach that the pain started a couple weeks ago and has progressively become worse. The pitcher has not yet thrown the maximum number of pitches for the current game. How should the coach mange this situation?

_____

_____

5. During a physical education class, a fourth-grade student falls on an outstretched hand. Assessment of the injury reveals intense pain, swelling, and deformity in the distal wrist. How should the teacher mange this situation?

_____

_____

6. A client in your fitness facility has been participating in spinning classes (i.e., riding a stationary bike) as a means for improving cardiovascular fitness. When the session is finished, the 30-year-old reports that following the past couple of workouts, she has experienced numbness in the region of the little finger and an inability to grasp some objects (i.e., weakness in grip strength). She indicates that the symptoms typically subside in 15 to 20 minutes after the ride. What condition should the fitness specialist suspect? What suggestions could the fitness specialist make with regard to the immediate and on-going management of this condition?

_____

_____

7. During an adult league recreational softball game, a 40-year-old male pitcher sustains a blow to the end of his finger off a line drive hit. Initially, the pitcher reports pain to the area which is visibly swollen. The pitcher is confident that it's just a "jammed finger." How should the condition be managed?

_____

_____

8. In preparation for the outdoor season which begins in 8 weeks, a 45-year-old recreational tennis player would like to strengthen the muscles in her elbow and wrist. She hires a fitness specialist for advice and instruction of accomplishing her goal. What exercise should the fitness specialist recommend? Why?

_____

_____

9. While holding an opponent's jersey tightly, a high school basketball player felt a sharp pain in the distal phalanx of the ring finger. After releasing the jersey, the player was unable to flex the DIP joint of the ring finger. What injury should the coach suspect? What is the management for that condition?

_____

_____

10. A cheerleader is complaining of pain over the right anatomical snuff box. She can't recall a specific mechanism that has occurred in the past several days. She did indicate that her doctor diagnosed a sprain to that wrist about two months ago after she fell and landed on an outstretched hand. She thought her wrist was improving, but states that she has had persistent wrist pain for about 2 weeks. How should the cheerleading coach manage this situation?

_____

_____

REFERENCES

1. Kocker MS, Waters PM, and Micheli LJ. 2000. Upper extremity injuries in the paediatric athlete. Sports Med, 30(2):117–135.
2. Mehlhoff TL, and Bennett JB. Elbow injuries. In The team physician's handbook, edited by MB Mellion, et al. Philadelphia: Hanley & Belfus, 2002.
3. Pugh DM, et al. 2004. Standard surgical protocol to treat elbow dislocations with radial head and coronoid fractures. J Bone Joint Surg, 86-A(6):1122–1130.
4. Ugbolue UC, Hsu W-H, Goitz RJ, and Li Z-M. 2005. Tendon and nerve displacement at the wrist during finger movements. Clin Biomech, 20(1):50–56.
5. Holm G, and Moody LE. 2003. Carpal tunnel syndrome: Current theory, treatment, and the use of B6. Clin Pract, 15(1):18–22.
6. McNally C, and Gillespie M. 2004. Scaphoid fractures. Emerg Nurse, 12(1):21–25.

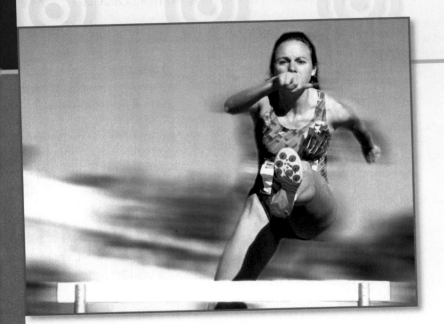

PELVIS, HIP, AND THIGH CONDITIONS

KEY TERMS

- hip pointer
- innominate
- Legg-Calvé-Perthes disease
- lumbar plexus
- myositis ossificans
- osteochondrosis
- sacral plexus
- snapping hip syndrome

LEARNING OUTCOMES

1. Describe the major articulations that comprise the pelvis and hip.

2. Identify the major motions available at the hip.

3. Explain general principles used to prevent injuries to the pelvis, hip, and thigh.

4. Describe common injuries and conditions sustained by physically active individuals to the pelvis, hip, and thigh, including their signs, symptoms, and immediate management.

5. Describe an on-site assessment of an acute pelvis, hip, or thigh injury appropriate for use by a coach.

Although the pelvis, hip, and thigh have a sturdy anatomical composition, this region can be subjected to large, potentially injurious forces when individuals engage in sports or exercise. For example, the soft tissues of the anterior thigh often sustain compressive forces, particularly during contact sports. Although the resulting contusions are not usually serious, mismanagement of these injuries can lead to more serious problems. Daily activities, such as sitting, walking, and climbing stairs, rarely involve stretching of the hamstrings. A lack of hamstring flexibility combined with a strength imbalance between the hamstrings and the quadriceps increases the risk for sustaining a hamstring strain. Because of their strong bony stability, the hip and pelvis are seldom injured. However, because the hip sustains repetitive forces of four to seven times body weight during walking and running, the joint is subject to stress-related injuries.

This chapter begins with a general anatomy review of the pelvis, hip, and thigh. Next, preventative measures are discussed, followed by an overview of common injuries to the region. Information pertaining to mechanism of injury, signs and symptoms, and management by the coach will be provided. Finally, a basic assessment of the region is presented.

ANATOMY REVIEW OF THE PELVIS, HIP, AND THIGH

The pelvis, hip, and thigh have an extremely stable bony structure that is further reinforced by a number of large, strong ligaments and muscles. This region is well suited anatomically for withstanding the large forces to which it is subjected during daily activities.

The Pelvis

The pelvis, or pelvic girdle, consists of a protective bony ring formed by four fused bones, namely the two **innominate** bones, sacrum, and coccyx (FIG. 14.1). The innominate bones articulate with each other anteriorly at the pubic symphysis and with the sacrum posteriorly at the sacroiliac (SI) joints. Each innominate bone consists of three fused bones, namely the ilium, ischium, and pubis. Among these, the ilium forms the major portion of the innominate bone, including the prominent iliac crests. The anterior superior iliac spine (ASIS) is a readily palpable landmark on the iliac crest. The posterior superior iliac spine (PSIS) is typically marked by an indentation in the soft tissues just lateral to the sacrum. The pelvis protects the enclosed inner organs, transmits loads between the trunk and lower extremity, and provides a site for a number of major muscle attachments.

Sacroiliac Joints

The SI joints form the critical link between the two pelvic bones. Working with the pubic symphysis, they help to transfer the weight of the torso and skull to the lower limbs, provide elasticity to the pelvic ring, and conversely, act as a buffer to decrease impact forces from the foot as they are transmitted to the spine and upper body.

Sacrococcygeal Joint

The sacrococcygeal joint is usually a fused line (i.e., symphysis) united by a fibrocartilaginous disc. Occasionally, the joint is freely movable and synovial, but with advanced age, the joint may fuse and be obliterated.

Pubic Symphysis

The pubic symphysis is a cartilaginous joint with a disc of fibrocartilage, called the interpubic disc, located between the two joint surfaces. A small degree of spreading, compression, and rotation occurs between the two halves of the pelvic girdle at this joint.

The Femur

The femur, a major weight-bearing bone, is the longest, largest, and strongest bone in the body (see FIG. 14.1). Its weakest component is the femoral neck, which is smaller in diameter

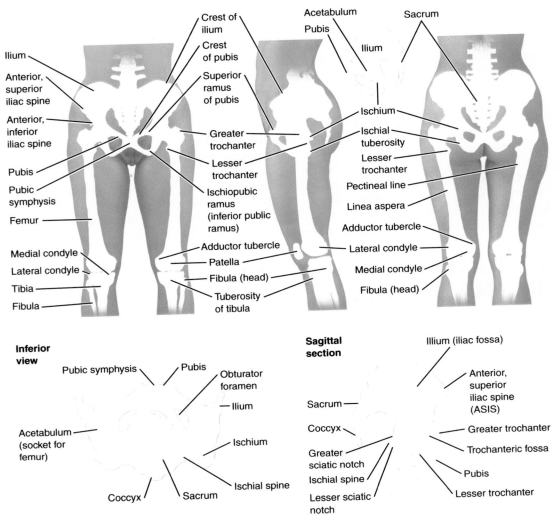

FIGURE 14.1 Skeletal features of the pelvis, hip, and thigh.

than the rest of the bone, and is weak internally because it is primarily composed of cancellous bone. The femur angles medially downward from the hip during the support phase of walking and running, enabling single leg support beneath the body's center of gravity. Because women have a wider pelvis, this angulation tends to be more pronounced in women.

The Hip Joint

The hip is the articulation between the concave acetabulum of the pelvis and the head of the femur. It functions as a classic ball-and-socket joint. Because the socket is deep, it provides considerable bony stability to the joint. Both articulating surfaces are covered with friction-reducing joint cartilage. The cartilage on the acetabulum is thickened around the periphery where it merges with the U-shaped fibrocartilaginous acetabular labrum, which further contributes to stability of the joint.

The joint capsule of the hip, the coxofemoral joint, is large and loose. It completely surrounds the joint, attaching to the labrum of the acetabular socket. The labrum forms a seal around the joint, with increased fluid pressure within the labrum contributing to lubrication of the joint.[1]

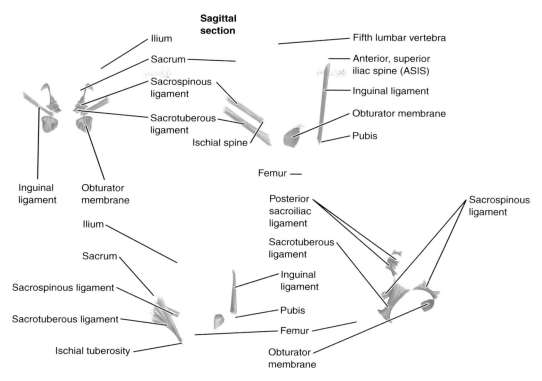

FIGURE 14.2 Ligaments of the pelvis and hip.

Several large, strong ligaments support the hip (FIG. 14.2). The anterior aspect of the hip includes the extremely strong Y-shaped iliofemoral ligament, sometimes referred to as the Y ligament of Bigelow, limits hip hyperextension and plays a major role in maintaining upright posture at the hip. The pubofemoral ligament limits hip extension and abduction. The ischiofemoral ligament, the weakest of the three, reinforces the hip posteriorly and along with the other two ligaments, acts to twist the head of the femur into the acetabulum upon hip extension, as occurs when a person rises from a seated position.

Femoral Triangle

The femoral triangle is formed by the inguinal ligament superiorly, the sartorius laterally, and the adductor longus medially (FIG. 14.3). This region is significant in that the femoral nerve, artery, and vein are located within the area. The femoral pulse can be palpated as it crosses the crease between the thigh and abdomen. In addition, if there is an infection or active inflammation in the lower extremity, enlarged lymph nodes may be palpated in this region.

Bursae

Four primary bursae are present in the hip and pelvic region (FIG. 14.4). The iliopsoas bursa is positioned

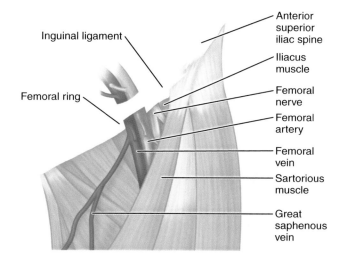

FIGURE 14.3 Femoral triangle. The triangle is bounded by the inguinal ligament superiorly, the adductor longus medially, and the sartorius laterally. The femoral artery, vein, and nerve pass through this area to enter the thigh.

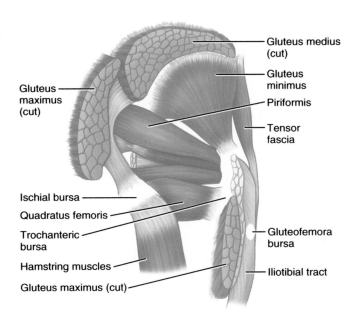

Gluteus medius
(cut)

Gluteus
minimus

Piriformis

Tensor
fascia

Gluteus
maximus
(cut)

Ischial bursa

Quadratus femoris

Trochanteric
bursa

Hamstring muscles

Gluteus maximus (cut)

Gluteofemora
bursa

Iliotibial tract

FIGURE 14.4 Bursa of the hip. Bursitis at the hip may involve the trochanteric bursa, iliopsoas bursa, or ischial bursa.

between the iliopsoas and articular capsule, serving to reduce the friction between these structures. The deep trochanteric bursa provides a cushion between the greater trochanter of the femur and the gluteus maximus at its attachment to the iliotibial tract. The gluteofemoral bursa separates the gluteus maximus from the origin of the vastus lateralis. Finally, the ischial bursa serves as a weight-bearing structure when an individual is seated, cushioning the ischial tuberosity at the site where it passes over the gluteus maximus.

NERVES AND BLOOD VESSELS OF THE PELVIS, HIP, AND THIGH

The major nerve supply to the pelvis, hip, and thigh arises from the lumbar and sacral plexi. The **lumbar plexus** is formed from the first four lumbar spinal nerves (see FIG. 14.5). It innervates portions of the abdominal wall and psoas major, with branches into the thigh region. The largest branch is the femoral nerve (L2—to L4), which supplies muscles and skin of the anterior thigh. Another branch, the obturator nerve (L2—to L4), provides innervation to the hip adductor muscles.

The **sacral plexus** is positioned just anterior to the lumbar plexus, and has some intermingling of fibers with the lumbar plexus. The lower spinal nerves, including L4 through S4, spawn the sacral plexus (FIG. 14.5). Twelve nerve branches arise from the sacral plexus. The major nerve is the sciatic nerve (L4, L5, S1—to S3), which is the largest and longest single nerve in the

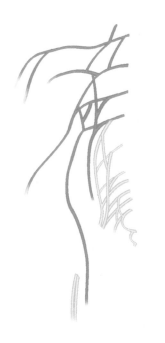

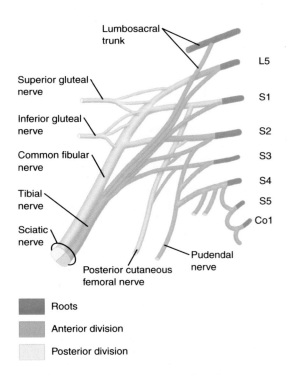

Lumbosacral
trunk

L5

Superior gluteal
nerve

S1

Inferior gluteal
nerve

S2

Common fibular
nerve

S3

S4

Tibial
nerve

S5

Co1

Sciatic
nerve

Pudendal
nerve

Posterior cutaneous
femoral nerve

Roots

Anterior division

Posterior division

FIGURE 14.5 Arterial supply to the hip and thigh region. **A.** Anterior view. **B.** Posterior view.

body. The sciatic nerve passes through the greater sciatic notch of the pelvis, courses through the gluteus maximus muscle, and then innervates the hamstrings and adductor magnus. The tibial and common peroneal nerves branch from the sciatic nerve in the posterior thigh region.

The external iliac arteries become the femoral arteries at the level of the thighs (FIG. 14.6). The femoral artery gives off several branches in the thigh region, including the deep femoral artery, which serves the posterior and lateral thigh muscles, and the lateral and medial femoral circumflex arteries, which supply the region of the femoral head.

KINEMATICS AND MAJOR MUSCLE ACTIONS OF THE HIP

A large number of muscles cross the hip (FIGS. 14.7, 14.8, and 14.9). Identifying the actions of these muscles is complicated by the fact that several muscles are two-joint muscles.

Because the hip is a ball-and-socket joint, the femur can move in all planes of motion (FIG. 14.10). However, the massive muscles crossing the hip tend to limit range of motion (ROM), particularly in the posterior direction.

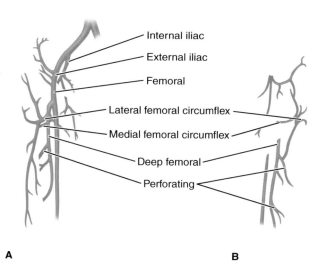

A   **B**

FIGURE 14.6 Sacral plexus. The sacral plexus is formed by the segmental nerves L4:S5. This plexus innervates the lower leg, ankle, and foot via the tibial and common peroneal nerves.

Flexion

The major hip flexors are the iliacus and psoas major, referred to jointly as the iliopsoas because of their common attachment at the femur. Four other muscles cross the anterior aspect of the hip to contribute to hip flexion. These include the pectineus, rectus femoris, sartorius, and tensor fascia latae. Because the rectus femoris is a two-joint muscle active during both hip flexion and knee extension, it functions more effectively as a hip flexor when the knee is in flexion, as occurs when a person kicks a ball. The sartorius is also a two-joint muscle. Crossing from the ASIS to the medial surface of the proximal tibia just below the tuberosity, the sartorius is the longest muscle in the body.

Extension

The hip extensors are the gluteus maximus and the three hamstrings: the biceps femoris, semitendinosus, and semimembranosus. The gluteus maximus is usually active only when the hip is in flexion, as occurs during stair climbing or cycling, or when extension at the hip is resisted. The nickname "hamstrings" derives from the prominent tendons of the three muscles, which are readily palpable on the posterior aspect of the knee. The hamstrings cross both the hip and knee, contributing to hip extension and knee flexion.

Abduction

The gluteus medius is the major abductor at the hip, with assistance from the gluteus minimus. The hip abductors are active in stabilizing the pelvis during single-leg support of the body, and during the support phase of walking and running. For example, when body weight is supported by the right foot during walking, the right hip abductors contract isometrically and eccentrically to prevent the left side of the pelvis from being pulled downward by the weight of the swinging left leg. This allows the left leg to move freely through the swing phase without scuffing the toes. If the hip abductors are too weak to perform this function, then lateral pelvic tilt occurs with every step.

Adduction

The hip adductors include the adductor longus, adductor brevis, and adductor magnus. These muscles are active during the swing phase of gait, bringing the foot beneath the body's center of

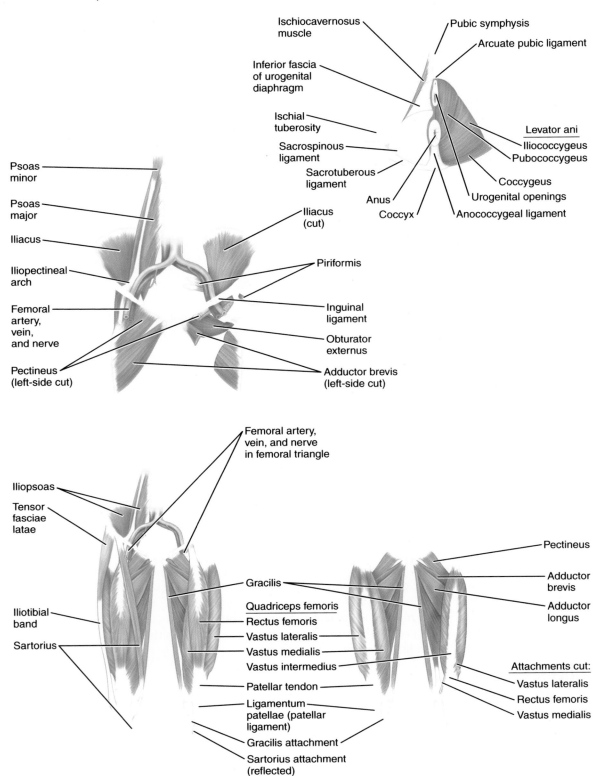

FIGURE 14.7 Muscles of the pelvis, hip, and thigh. Anterior view.

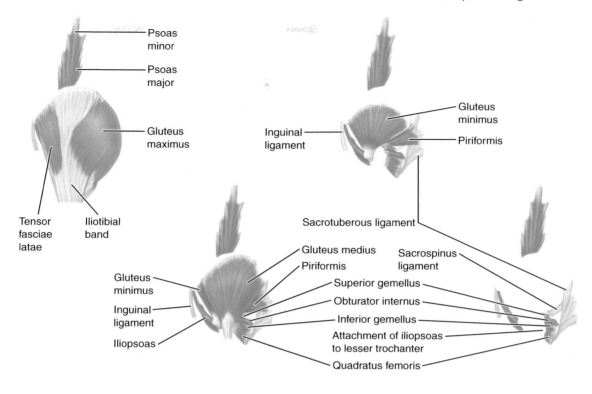

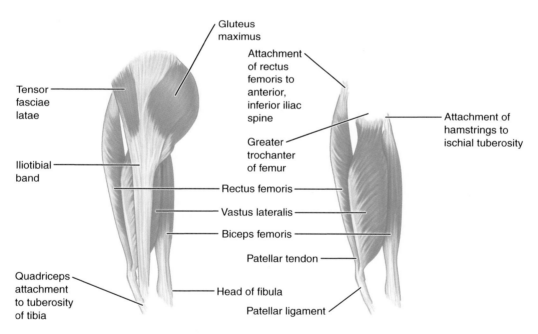

FIGURE 14.8 Muscles of the pelvis, hip, and thigh. Lateral view.

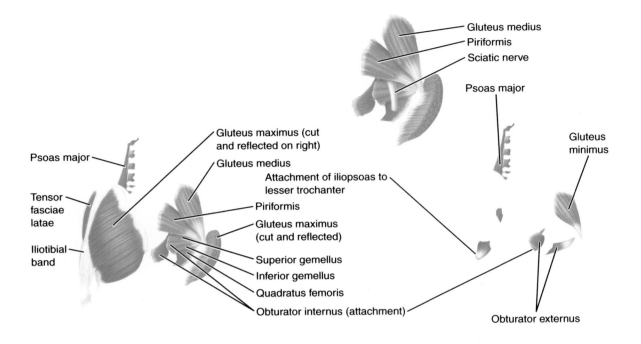

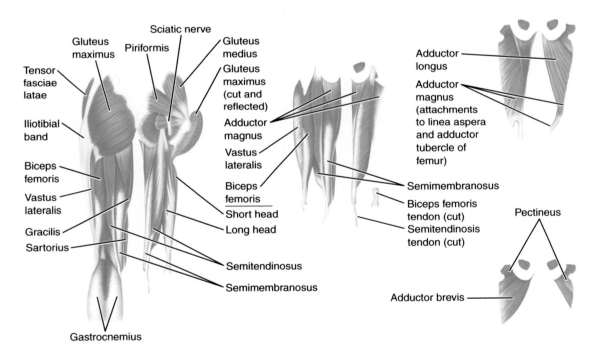

FIGURE 14.9 Muscles of the pelvis, hip, and thigh. Posterior view.

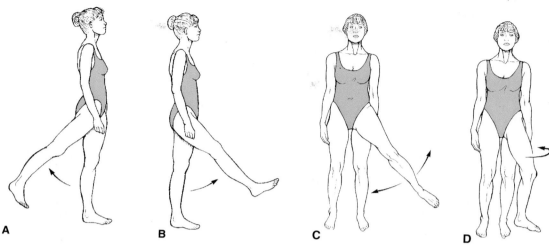

FIGURE 14.10 Motions at the hip.

gravity for placement during the support phase. The relatively weak gracilis assists with hip adduction. The hip adductors also contribute to flexion and internal rotation at the hip, especially when the femur is externally rotated.

Medial and Lateral Rotation of the Femur

Although several muscles contribute to lateral rotation of the femur, there are six that function solely as lateral rotators. These are the piriformis, gemellus superior, gemellus inferior, obturator internus, obturator externus, and quadratus femoris. The femur of the swinging leg rotates laterally to accommodate the lateral rotation of the pelvis during the stride.

The major medial rotator of the femur is the gluteus minimus, with assistance from the tensor fascia latae, semitendinosus, semimembranosus, gluteus medius, and the four adductor muscles. The medial rotators are relatively weak; the estimated strength is approximately one-third that of the lateral rotators.

PREVENTION OF PELVIS, HIP, AND THIGH CONDITIONS

The hip joint is well protected within the pelvic girdle and is seldom injured. Even still, several factors, such as wearing protective equipment, wearing shoes with adequate cushion and support, and participating in an extensive physical conditioning program, can reduce the incidence of acute and chronic injuries to the region.

Physical Conditioning

Because several of the muscles in the pelvis, hip, and thigh are two joint muscles, physical conditioning should include ROM and strengthening exercises for both the hip and knee. APPLICATION STRATEGY 14.1 demonstrates specific exercises for the hip flexors, extensors, adductors, abductors, and medial and lateral rotators. Exercises for the muscles that govern the knee are presented in Chapter 15.

Protective Equipment

Several collision and contact sports require special pads composed of hard polyethylene covered with layers of specialized foam rubber to protect vulnerable areas, such as the iliac crests, sacrum and coccyx, and genital region. A girdle with special pockets can hold the pads in place. The male genital region is best protected by a protective cup placed in an athletic supporter. Special commercial thigh pads may also be used to prevent contusions to the anterior thigh, and

APPLICATION STRATEGY 14.1

Exercises to Prevent Injury at the Thigh, Hip, and Pelvis

The following exercises can be performed for motions at the hip. Exercises for the hamstrings, quadriceps, and iliotibial band, which also cross the knee joint, can be seen in Chapter 15.

A. Hip flexor stretch (lunge). Place the leg to be stretched in front. Bend the contralateral knee as the hips are moved forward. Keep the back straight. Alternative method: Place the foot on a chair or table and lean forward until a stretch is felt.

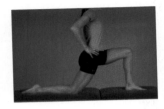

B. Lateral rotator stretch, seated position. Cross one leg over the thigh and place the elbow on the outside of the knee. Gently stretch the buttock muscles by pushing the bent knee across the body while keeping the pelvis on the floor.

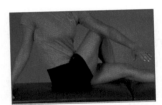

C. Adductor stretch, standing position. Place the leg to be stretched out to the side. Slowly bend the contralateral knee. Keep the hips in a neutral or extended position.

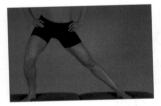

D. Elastic tubing exercises. Secure elastic tubing to a table. Perform hip flexion, extension, abduction, adduction, and medial and lateral rotation in a single plane or in multidirectional patterns.

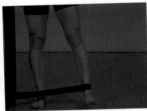

E. Full squats. A weight belt should be worn during this exercise. Place the feet at shoulder width or wider. Keep the back straight by keeping the chest out and the head up at all times. Flex the knees and hips to no greater than 90°. Begin the upward motion by extending the hips first.

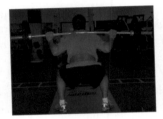

F. Hip extension. With the trunk stabilized and the back flat, extend the hip while keeping the knee flexed. Alternate legs.

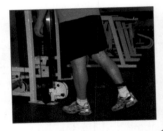

neoprene sleeves can provide uniform compression, therapeutic warmth, and support for a quadriceps or hamstrings strain.

Shoe Selection

Sport and physical activities take place on a variety of terrains and floor surfaces. Shoes should adequately cushion impact forces as well as support and guide the foot during the stance and final push-off phases of running, regardless of the terrain or surface. Inadequate cushioning in the heel region can transmit forces up the leg, leading to inflammation of the hip joint, or stress fractures of the femoral neck or pubis. Therefore, it is important to purchase shoes that provide an adequate heel cushion and a thermoplastic heel counter, which can maintain its shape and firmness even in adverse weather conditions. The soles should be designed for the specific type of playing surface to avoid slipping or sliding.

CONTUSIONS

Direct impact to soft tissue, such as a kick to the thigh or a fall onto a hard surface, causes a compressive force to crush soft tissue. The condition may be mild and resolve itself in a matter of days, or the bleeding and swelling may be more extensive, resulting in a large, deep hematoma that takes months to resolve. Contusions may occur anywhere in the hip region, but are typically seen on the crest of the ilium or in the quadriceps muscle group.

Hip Pointer

A **hip pointer** refers to a contusion of the iliac crest. Most injuries are sustained when a direct blow impacts the iliac crest. It can also be caused by a fall onto the hip. The trauma can include the muscles that attach to the iliac crest (e.g., abdominal muscles; hip flexors).

Signs and Symptoms

Because so many trunk and abdominal muscles attach to the iliac crest, any movement of the trunk is painful, including coughing, laughing, and even breathing. Immediate pain, discoloration, spasm, and loss of function prevent the individual from rotating the trunk or laterally flexing the trunk toward the injured side. Extreme tenderness is present over the iliac crest, and abdominal muscle spasm may be present. Within 24 to 48 hours, the swelling is more diffuse, and ecchymosis is visibly evident. In severe injury, the individual may be unable to walk or bear weight, even with crutches, because of the intense pain caused by muscular tension at the injury site.

Management

The immediate management involves the application of cold and compression to the area. The use of crutches is warranted if walking is painful or with a limp. If intense pain is palpated directly over the iliac crest, the individual should be referred to a physician to rule out a fracture of the iliac crest, as the same mechanism of injury may cause both injuries. This injury often requires total rest during the first 2 to 3 days following injury. When return to play is permitted, the area should be protected with padding to prevent reinjury.

Quadriceps Contusion

The most common site for a quadriceps contusion is the anterolateral thigh. Contusions within the muscle itself are often associated with greater tearing, hemorrhage, and pain, and a greater tendency toward abnormal pathology. Severity of the injury is almost always underestimated and undertreated.

Signs and Symptoms

Pain and swelling may be extensive immediately after impact. In a mild (Grade I) contusion, the individual has mild pain and swelling, and is able to walk without a limp. Passive flexion beyond 90° may be painful, but resisted knee extension may cause less discomfort. In a moderate (Grade II) contusion, the individual can flex the knee between 45° and 90°, and walks with a noticeable limp. If severe (Grade III), the individual is unable to bear weight or fully flex the knee.

Management

Treatment involves ice application and a compressive wrap for the first 24 to 48 hours applied with the knee in maximal flexion (FIG. 14.11). This position preserves the needed flexion and limits intramuscular bleeding and spasm. If unable to perform a pain-free gait, the individual should be placed on crutches. Continued swelling despite proper acute care protocol indicates continued hemorrhage. In these cases, immediate referral to a physician is necessary to assess the level of bleeding.

Myositis Ossificans

Myositis ossificans is an abnormal ossification involving bone deposition within muscle tissue. It may stem from a single traumatic blow, or repeated blows, to the quadriceps. Several risk factors

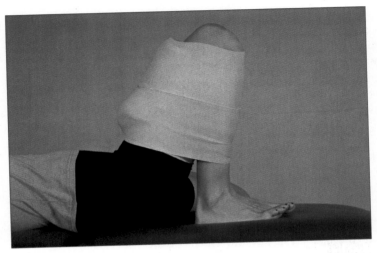

FIGURE 14.11 Management of a quadriceps contusion. Ice should be applied, with the knee in maximal flexion to place the muscles on stretch.

following a quadriceps contusion can predispose an individual to this condition (see BOX 14.1). Common sites are the anterior and lateral thigh. Although the precise mechanism that triggers the bone formation has yet to be established, it is thought that during resolution of the hematoma, within a week after injury, the existing fibroblasts involved in the repair process begin to differentiate into osteoblasts. The evidence of calcification on a radiograph becomes visible after 2 to 4 weeks. As the calcification continues to progress, a palpable, firm mass can be felt in the deep tissues. After 6 to 7 weeks, the mass generally stops growing and resorption occurs. However, total resorption may not fully occur, leaving a visible cortical-type bony lesion (FIG. 14.12).

Signs and Symptoms

Examination reveals a warm, firm, swollen thigh nearly 2 to 4 cm larger than the unaffected side. A palpable, painful mass may limit passive knee flexion to 20° to 30°. Active quadriceps contractions and straight-leg raises may be impossible.

Management

This individual should be referred to a physician. Treatment includes ice, compression, elevation, crutches, and protected rest.

BURSITIS

Bursitis is common in runners and joggers. It typically affects the greater trochanteric bursa, iliopsoas bursa (iliopectineal), and ischial bursa. The common mechanism is inflammation secondary to excessive friction or shear forces caused by overuse.

Greater Trochanteric Bursitis

The greater trochanteric bursa lies between the greater trochanter and the gluteus maximus and tensor fascia latae (iliotibial tract). Inflammation of this bursa is seen more often in females because of the wider pelvis and larger Q-angle. It is also seen in runners who cross their feet over the midline as they run, as that action functionally increases the Q-angle. Because streets are crowned to allow for run-off, individuals who typically run on streets are at increased susceptibility for irritating the greater trochanteric bursa. The down leg (i.e., the leg closest to the gutter) is usually affected.

BOX 14.1	**Risk Factors for Developing Myositis Ossificans**

- **Innate predisposition to ectopic bone formation**
- **Continuing to play after injury**
- **Passive, forceful stretching**
- **Too rapid a progression in rehabilitation program**
- **Premature return to play**
- **Reinjury of the same area**

Signs and Symptoms

The individual reports a burning or aching pain over or just posterior to the tip of the greater trochanter that intensifies with walking or exercise. The condition is aggravated by contraction of the hip abductors against resistance, or during hip flexion and extension on weight-bearing.

Iliopsoas Bursitis

The iliopsoas bursa, the largest bursa in the body, can be irritated when the iliopsoas muscle repeatedly compresses the bursa against either the joint capsule of the hip or the lesser trochanter of the femur. Osteoarthritis of the hip may also lead to the condition.

Signs and Symptoms

Pain is felt more medial and anterior to the joint, and cannot be easily palpated. Passive rotary motions at the hip, and resisted hip flexion, abduction, and external rotation, may produce increased pain.

Ischial Bursitis

Direct bruising from a fall can lead to compression of the ischial bursa. However, there is often a history of prolonged sitting (resulting in the nickname bench warmer's bursitis), especially with the legs crossed or on a hard surface. Although it is relatively uncommon, it must be differentiated from a hamstring tear at the tendinous attachment or an epiphyseal fracture.

Signs and Symptoms

Pain is aggravated by prolonged sitting, uphill running, and even carrying a wallet in the back pocket. Pain increases with passive and resisted hip extension.

Management of Bursitis

The individual should be referred to a qualified healthcare practitioner for a definitive diagnosis and ongoing treatment options. The coach should not permit the individual to continue activity, as doing so could potentially exacerbate the condition. In addition, the coach could suggest the application of cold to the area to decrease pain and inflammation.

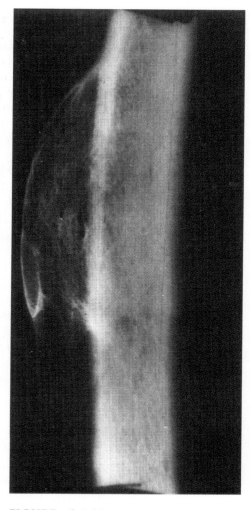

FIGURE 14.12 Myositis ossificans. In myositis ossificans, full resorption of the calcification may not occur, leaving a visible, cortical type bony lesion.

SNAPPING HIP SYNDROME

Chronic bursitis can lead to **snapping hip syndrome**, a condition very prevalent in dancers, runners, and cheerleaders, which may develop secondary to a variety of both intra-articular and extra-articular causes.

Signs and Symptoms

Snapping hip syndrome is characterized by a snapping sensation, rather than pain, either heard or felt during certain motions at the hip. It usually occurs when an individual laterally rotates and flexes the hip joint while balancing on one leg. If the iliopsoas bursa is affected, the individual may complain of snapping, chronic pain, or both in the femoral triangle of the medial groin.

Management

The management for this condition is the same as bursitis.

SPRAINS AND DISLOCATIONS

Hip joint sprains are rare because of the multitude of movements allowed at the ball-and-socket joint and the level of protection provided by layers of muscles that add to its stability. Injury can occur in violent twisting actions or in catastrophic trauma when the knee strikes a stationary object, such as in an automobile accident when the knee is driven into the dashboard. Traumatic hip dislocations in children are rare, but are more common than femoral neck fractures. This may largely result from the pliable cartilage composition of the acetabulum during the early- to mid-teen years.

Signs and Symptoms

Symptoms of a mild or moderate hip sprain involve pain on hip rotation. Severe hip sprains and dislocations result in immediate, intense pain and an inability to walk or even move the hip. The hip remains in a characteristic flexed and internally rotated position, which indicates a posterior, superior dislocation (FIG. 14.13).

Management

The immediate management for a mild or moderate sprain involves the application of cold to the area, the use of crutches if walking is painful or with a limp, and referral to a qualified healthcare practitioner for a definitive diagnosis and ongoing treatment options. A hip dislocation is considered a medical emergency. As such, it requires activation of the emergency plan, including activation of EMS. The coach should not move the individual because of a possible fracture to the acetabulum or head of the femur. In addition, while waiting for EMS to arrive, the coach should monitor the individual's vital signs and anticipate the need to treat the individual for shock.

STRAINS

Muscular strains of the hip and thigh muscles are frequently seen not only in sport and physical activity but also in many occupations involving repetitive motions. Strains may range from mild to severe, with the severity of symptoms paralleling the amount of disruption to the fibers.

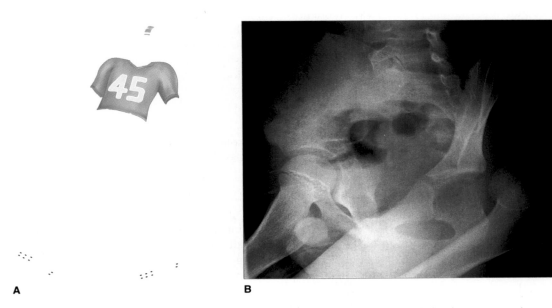

A   **B**

FIGURE 14.13 Hip dislocation. Most hip dislocations drive the head of the femur posterior and superior, leaving the leg in a characteristically flexed and internally rotated position. **A**. External presentation. **B**. X-ray view.

Quadriceps Strain

A strain of the quadriceps is less common than hamstring strains. An explosive muscular contraction of the rectus femoris can lead to an avulsion fracture at the proximal attachment on the anterior inferior iliac spine (AIIS), but tears more commonly occur in the midsubstance of the muscle belly. Because the rectus femoris is the most superficial muscle of the quadriceps, any disruption in its continuity is easily visible.

Signs and Symptoms

In a Grade I injury, the individual complains of tightness in the anterior thigh, but gait is normal. Passive knee flexion beyond 90° may be painful. In a Grade II injury, the individual reports a snapping or tearing sensation during an explosive jumping, kicking, or running motion, followed by immediate pain and loss of function. The knee may be held in extension as a means for protecting the injured area. Passive knee flexion is painful. There is pain and weakness with knee extension. Grade III strains are extremely painful, and ambulation is not possible. An obvious defect in the muscle may be visible. Resisted knee extension is not possible, and ROM is severely limited.

Hamstrings Strains

During the initial swing phase of gait, the hamstrings act to flex the knee. In late swing, the hamstrings contract eccentrically to decelerate knee extension and re-extend the hip in preparation for the stance phase. The hamstrings are the most frequently strained muscles in the body and are typically caused by a rapid contraction of the muscle during a ballistic action or a violent stretch. Several factors can increase the risk of sustaining a hamstring strain (see Box 14.2).

Signs and Symptoms

In mild strains, the individual complains of tightness and tension in the muscle. Passive stretching of the hamstrings may be painful. In second- and third-degree strains, the individual may report a tearing sensation or feeling a "pop," leading to immediate pain and weakness in knee flexion. In more severe cases, a sharp pain is present in the posterior thigh that may occur during midstride. The individual limps and is unable to do heel-strike or fully extend the knee. Pain and muscle weakness are elicited during active knee flexion.

A hamstrings strain has a reputation of being both chronic and recurring. Rehabilitation should focus on regaining flexibility and strengthening the muscles. It is important to maintain an appropriate strength balance between the quadriceps and hamstrings.

Adductor (Groin) Strain

Adductor strains are common in activities that require quick changes of direction, and explosive propulsion and acceleration. A strength imbalance between the hip abductors and adductors may be a predisposing factor in many of these injuries. The more severe strains are typically at the muscles' proximal attachment on the hip, particularly the adductor longus. Milder strains tend to occur more distally at the musculotendinous junction.

BOX 14.2   **Risk Factors for Hamstring Strains**

- **Poor flexibility**
- **Poor posture**
- **Muscle imbalance**
- **Improper warm-up**
- **Muscle fatigue**

- **Lack of neuromuscular control**
- **Previous injury**
- **Overuse**
- **Improper technique**

Signs and Symptoms

The individual often experiences an initial "twinge" or "pull" of the groin muscles, and is unable to walk because of the intense, sharp pain. As the condition worsens, increased pain, stiffness, and weakness in hip adduction and flexion become apparent. Running straight ahead or backward may be tolerable, but any side-to-side movement leads to more discomfort and pain. Increased pain is present during passive stretching with the hip extended, abducted, and externally rotated, and with resisted hip adduction.

Management of Strains

If a Grade I injury is suspected, management involves standard acute care with cold and compression. If the signs and symptoms do not resolve within 2 to 3 days, the coach should require the individual to obtain approval for return to participation from a qualified healthcare professional.

If a Grade II or III injury is suspected, standard acute management, including the use of crutches, should be used. The individual should be referred to a qualified healthcare practitioner for a definitive diagnosis and ongoing treatment options.

VASCULAR AND NEURAL DISORDERS

Vascular disorders should be suspected in any lower extremity injury caused by a high-velocity, low-mass projectile, and in an injury where no physical findings support the continued discomfort. If an acute circulatory problem exists, the lower leg and foot may appear pale or cyanotic, be cool to the touch, or have diminished or totally absent pulse. In these cases, immobilization of the limb and transportation to the nearest medical center is warranted. Other vascular problems are more insidious, but can be just as serious.

Legg-Calvé-Perthes Disease

Legg-Calvé-Perthes disease, or avascular necrosis of the capital femoral epiphysis, is a noninflammatory, self-limiting disorder of the hip seen in young children, especially males, between the ages of 3 and 8.[2] It is considered to be an **osteochondrosis** condition of the femoral head, caused by diminished blood supply to the capital region of the femur. This leads to a progressive necrosis of the bone and marrow of the epiphysis of the femoral head (FIG. 14.14).

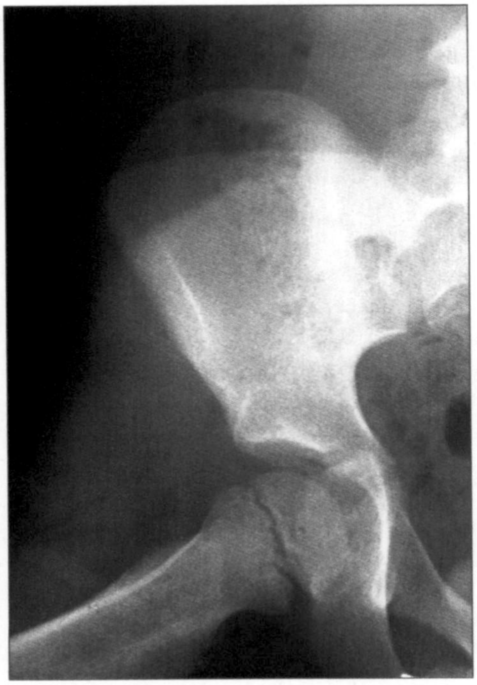

Signs and Symptoms

The most common complaint is a gradual onset of a limp and mild hip or knee pain of several months' duration. The pain is most often referred to the groin region, but up to 15% of patients report knee pain as the primary symptom.[2] Pain is generally activity related, which often contributes to delayed recognition. Examination reveals a decreased ROM in hip abduction, extension, and external rotation caused by muscle spasm in the hip flexors and adductors.

Management

This condition should be suspected in young children when pain in the groin, anterior thigh, or knee region cannot be explained. If pain persists for more than 1 week after initial acute care, or if the individual continues to limp after activity, the individual should be referred to a physician for a definitive diagnosis and ongoing treatment options. The coach should not permit the individual to continue activity, as doing so could potentially exacerbate the condition.

FIGURE 14.14 Osteochondrosis of the left femoral head (Legg-Calve-Perthes disease). This picture demonstrates the destruction of articular cartilage.

FRACTURES

Major fractures of the pelvic girdle, hip, and femur often result from severe direct trauma. In some sports (e.g., football and ice hockey), the pelvic region is usually adequately protected by padding to prevent such injuries. However, susceptibility to some fractures is not influenced by the use of protective padding.

Avulsion Fractures

Individuals who perform rapid, sudden acceleration and deceleration moves are at risk for the following avulsion fractures:

- The ASIS with sartorius displacement
- The AIIS with rectus femoris displacement
- The ischial tuberosity with hamstrings displacement
- The lesser trochanter with iliopsoas displacement.

Many of these apophyseal sites do not unite with the bone until ages 18 to 25, and as such, continue to be prone to fracture.

Signs and Symptoms

The individual complains of sudden, acute, localized pain that may radiate down the muscle. Examination reveals severe pain, swelling, and discoloration directly over the tendinous attachment on the bony landmark. In a completely displaced avulsion fracture, a gap may be palpated between the tendon's attachment and the bone. Pain increases with passive stretching of the involved muscle and active/resisted ROM.

Management

The individual should be referred immediately to a physician. Because of pain associated with walking, provisions need to be made to transport the individual (e.g. fit with crutches; activate the emergency plan). This condition will necessitate radiograph examination.

Slipped Capital Femoral Epiphysis

The capital femoral epiphysis is the growth plate at the femoral head. A fracture to this area, sometimes referred to as adolescent coxa vara, is seen in adolescent boys ages 12 to 15. In particular, the condition is commonly seen in obese adolescents with underdeveloped sexual characteristics and, occasionally, in rapidly growing slender boys. In a slipped capital femoral epiphysis, the femoral head slips at the epiphyseal plate and displaces inferiorly and posteriorly relative to the femoral neck (FIG. 14.15). As the proximal femoral growth plate deteriorates, the individual begins to develop a painful limp with groin pain. Pain may also be referred to the anterior thigh or knee region.

Signs and Symptoms

Early signs and symptoms may go undetected. Frequently, the only complaint is diffuse knee pain. In later stages, the individual feels more comfortable holding the leg in slight flexion. The individual is unable to touch the abdomen with the thigh because the hip externally rotates with flexion, and the individual is unable to rotate the femur internally or stand on one leg.

Management

The individual should be referred to a physician for a definitive diagnosis and ongoing treatment options. The coach should not permit the individual to continue activity, as doing so could potentially exacerbate the condition. In addition, the coach could suggest the use of crutches for ambulation.

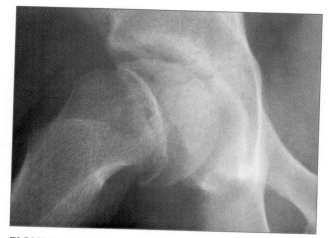

FIGURE 14.15 Slipped capital femoral epiphysis. An epiphyseal fracture, seen in adolescents from 12 to 15 years of age, occurs through the growth plate at the femoral head. An individual who sustains this fracture will not be able to rotate the femur internally.

BOX 14.3	**Risk Factors for Stress Fractures**

- **Sudden increase in training (mileage, intensity, or frequency)**
- **Change in running surface or terrain**
- **Improper footwear**
- **Biomechanical abnormalities**
- **Nutritional and hormonal factors (anorexia, amenorrhea, osteopenia)**

Stress Fractures

Stress fractures to the pubis, femoral neck, and proximal third of the femur are seen in individuals who engage in extensive jogging or aerobic dance activities, to the point of muscle fatigue. Several factors can increase the risk of sustaining a stress fracture of the femur (see BOX 14.3).

Signs and Symptoms

Signs and symptoms usually involve a diffuse or localized aching pain in the anterior groin or thigh region during weight-bearing activity that is relieved with rest. Night pain is a frequent complaint. An antalgic gait may be present. Increased pain on the extremes of hip rotation, an abduction lurch, and an inability to stand on the involved leg may indicate a femoral neck stress fracture.

Management

The individual should be referred to a physician for a definitive diagnosis and ongoing treatment options. The coach should not permit the individual to continue activity, as doing so could potentially exacerbate the condition.

Displaced and Nondisplaced Pelvic Fractures

Major fractures of the pelvis seldom occur in sport participation except in activities such as equestrian sports, ice hockey, rugby, skiing, and football. There are three distinct mechanisms involved in traumatic pelvic fractures:

- Avulsion or traction injury of the bony origin or attachment of muscle
- Direct compression, with disruption of the pelvic osseous ring
- Direct blow to the pelvis

Because the pelvis is a closed ring, an injury to one location in the pelvis can cause a countercoup fracture or sprain on the other side of the pelvic ring. For example, if the superior and inferior pubic rami are fractured on the right side, there is often SI disruption on the left side.

Signs and Symptoms

This crushing injury produces severe pain, total loss of function, and in many cases, severe loss of blood leading to hypovolemic shock. The extent of blood loss is unknown because hemorrhage within the pelvic cavity is not visible. In addition, possible internal injuries to the genitourinary system, such as rupture of the bladder or laceration of the urethra, may also occur.

Management

If a fracture is suspected, the emergency plan should be activated, including summoning EMS. While waiting for EMS to arrive, the coach should assess vital signs and treat for shock as necessary.

Sacral and Coccygeal Fractures

Fractures of the sacrum and coccyx rarely occur in sports. They are typically caused by a direct blow onto the sacrococcygeal area subsequent to a fall on the buttock region.

5. An elementary school physical education teacher began to notice that a second-grade student (an 8-year-old) was limping after class every day for the last week. When asked about a possible injury, the boy told the teacher that his groin and knee have hurt ever since the start of the year, nearly 10 weeks ago. When the teacher questioned the parents about the pain, they reported that the pain comes and goes and have not thought that it was serious enough to see a physician. Should the physical education teacher permit the student to continue to participate in activity? Why?

_____

_____

6. During a high school physical education class, a student is down on the field after receiving a severe blow to the anterior right thigh. When the teacher reaches the student, she notices that the thigh is externally rotated and severely angulated and the involved limb appears shorter. The student is in severe pain. What injury should be expected? How should the physical education teacher mange this situation?

_____

_____

7. A 45-year-old apparently healthy male comes to your exercise facility indicating that he has just finished undergoing physical therapy for a hip injury. His physical therapist strongly advised that he continue to work on increasing the flexibility and strength of the muscles governing the hip joint. Demonstrate exercises used to increase flexibility and strength of the hip musculature.

_____

_____

8. During the start of the 100 m hurdles, a hurdler pulls up and grabs his distal posterior thigh. The assessment by the coach reveals a moderate to severe hamstring strain. How should the coach manage this injury?

_____

_____

REFERENCES

1. Ferguson SJ, Bryant JT, Ganz R, and Ito K. 2003. An in vitro investigation of the acetabular labral seal in hip joint mechanics. J Biomech, 36(2):171–178.

2. Esposito PW. Pelvis, hip and thigh injuries. In The team physician's handbook, edited by MB Mellion, et al. Philadelphia, PA: Hanley & Belfus, 2002.

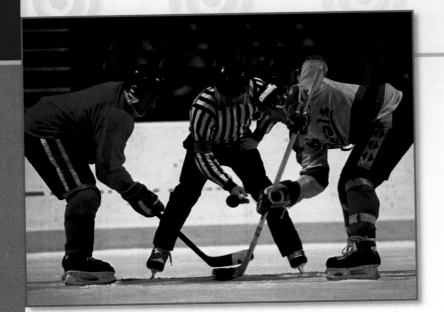

KNEE CONDITIONS

KEY TERMS

chondral

chondromalacia

extensor mechanism

hemarthrosis

menisci

neoplasms

Osgood-Schlatter's disease

osteochondral

Q-angle

screw-home mechanism

valgus

varus

LEARNING OUTCOMES

1. Describe the major articulations that comprise the knee.

2. Identify the motions available at the knee.

3. Explain general principles used to prevent knee injuries.

4. Describe common injuries and conditions sustained by physically active individuals to the knee, including their sign, symptoms, and immediate management.

5. Describe an on-site assessment of an acute knee injury appropriate for use by a coach.

The knee is a complex joint that is frequently injured in participation in physical activity. During walking and running, the knee moves through a considerable range of motion (ROM) while bearing loads equivalent to three to four times body weight. Because the knee is positioned between the two longest bones in the body (i.e., femur and tibia), there is the potential for creating large, injurious torques at the joint. These factors, coupled with minimal bony stability, make the knee susceptible to injury. The knee is the predominant site of injury among runners, and is one of the most frequently injured joints in sport participants.[1]

This chapter begins with a review of the anatomy of the knee complex. General principles to prevent injuries are followed by discussion of common injuries to the knee complex. Information pertaining to mechanism of injury, signs and symptoms, and management by the coach will be provided. Finally, a basic assessment of the region is presented.

ANATOMY REVIEW OF THE KNEE

The knee is a large synovial joint including three articulations within the joint capsule. The weight-bearing joints are the two condylar articulations of the tibiofemoral joint. The third articulation is the patellofemoral joint. The soft tissue connections of the proximal tibiofibular joint also exert a minor influence on knee motion.

Tibiofemoral Joint

The distal femur and proximal tibia articulate to form two side-by-side condyloid joints collectively known as the tibiofemoral joint (FIG. 15.1). These joints function together primarily as a modified hinge joint. Because of the restricting ligaments, some lateral and rotational motions are allowed at the knee. The medial and lateral condyles of the femur differ somewhat in size, shape, and orientation. As a result, the tibia rotates laterally on the femur during the last few degrees of extension to produce "locking" of the knee. This phenomenon, known as the **"screw-home"** mechanism, brings the knee into the close packed position of full extension.

Menisci

The **menisci**, also known as semilunar cartilages because of their half-moon shapes, are discs of fibrocartilage firmly attached to the superior plateaus of the tibia by the coronary ligaments

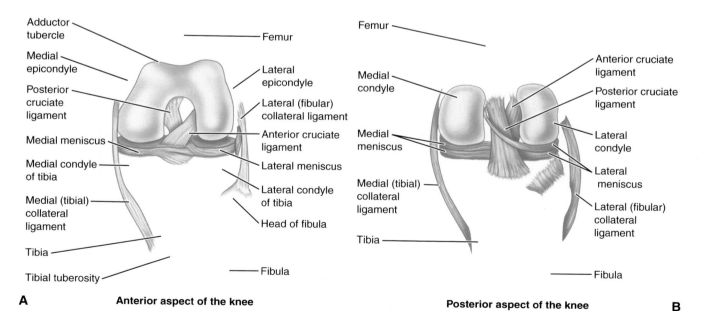

A   **Anterior aspect of the knee**

Posterior aspect of the knee   **B**

FIGURE 15.1 Structures of the knee. **A.** Anterior view. The joint is flexed, and the patella is removed. **B.** Posterior view. The knee is in extension.

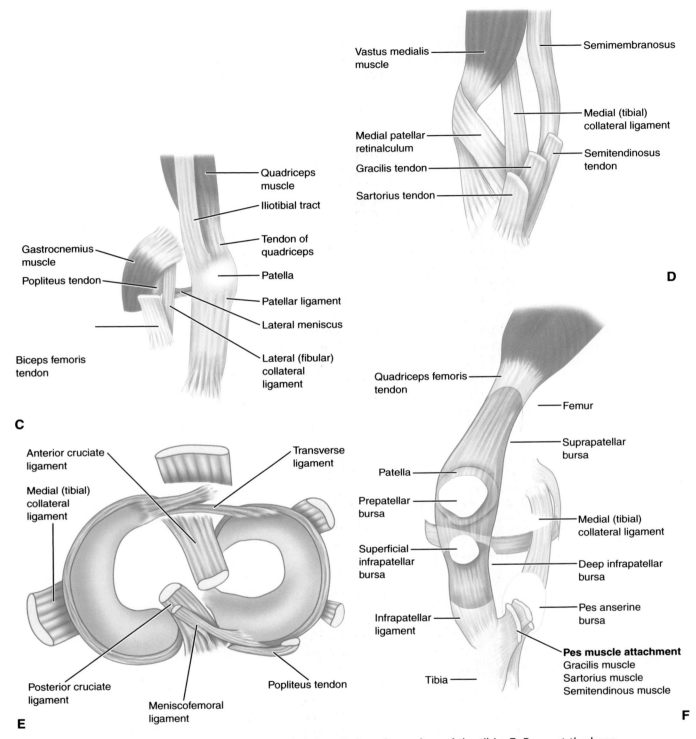

FIGURE 15.1 *(Continued)* **C**. Lateral view. **D**. Medial view. **E**. Superior surface of the tibia. **F**. Bursa at the knee.

and joint capsule. They provide several functional advantages, including absorption and dissipation of force and significantly improved congruency of the joint surfaces to even stress distribution across the joint. Additionally, because 74% of the total weight of the menisci is water, when the knee undergoes compression during weight bearing, much of the fluid is squeezed out into the joint space, providing lubrication to promote gliding of the joint structures.[2]

The menisci also increase knee stability by serving as soft tissue restraints that resist anterior tibial displacement. In addition, the medial meniscus has an attachment to the medial collateral ligament (MCL) and fibers from the semimembranosus muscle. It is injured much more frequently than the lateral meniscus. This is partly because the medial meniscus is more securely attached to the tibia, and therefore less mobile. In comparison, the lateral meniscus is a smaller and more freely moveable structure.

Bursae

The joint capsule at the knee is large and lax, encompassing both the tibiofemoral and patellofemoral joints. Anteriorly, it extends above the patella to attach along the edges of the superior patellar surface. The deep bursa formed by this capsule above the patella, the suprapatellar bursa, is the largest bursa in the body. It lies between the femur and quadriceps femoris tendon and it reduces friction between the two structures. Posteriorly, the subpopliteal bursa lies between the lateral condyle of the femur and popliteal muscle, and the semimembranosus bursa lies between the medial head of the gastrocnemius and semimembranosus tendons.

Three other key bursae associated with the knee, but not contained in the joint capsule, are the prepatellar, superficial infrapatellar, and deep infrapatellar bursae. The prepatellar bursa is located between the skin and anterior surface of the patella, allowing free movement of the skin over the patella during flexion and extension. The superficial infrapatellar bursa is located between the skin and patellar tendon. The deep infrapatellar bursa is located between the tibial tubercle and the infrapatellar tendon and is separated from the joint cavity by the infrapatellar fat pad. This bursa reduces friction between the ligament and the bony tubercle.

Ligaments of the Knee

Because the shallow articular surfaces of the tibiofemoral joint contribute minimally to knee stability, the stabilizing role of the ligaments crossing the knee is of great significance. Two major ligaments of the knee are the anterior and posterior cruciate ligaments (PCLs) (see FIG. 15.1). The name cruciate is derived from the fact that the two ligaments cross each other, with anterior and posterior referring to their respective tibial attachments.

The anterior cruciate ligament (ACL) stretches from the anterior aspect of the intercondyloid fossa of the tibia just medial and posterior to the anterior tibial spine in a superior, posterior direction to the posterior medial surface of the lateral condyle of the femur. The ACL is a critical stabilizer that prevents

- Anterior translation (movement) of the tibia on a fixed femur
- Posterior translation of the femur on a fixed tibia
- Internal and external rotation of the tibia on the femur
- Hyperextension of the knee

The shorter and stronger PCL runs from the posterior aspect of the tibial intercondyloid fossa in a superior, anterior direction to the lateral anterior medial condyle of the femur. The PCL is considered to be the primary stabilizer of the knee and resists posterior displacement of the tibia on a fixed femur.

The medial and lateral collateral ligaments (LCLs) are also referred to as the tibial and fibular collateral ligaments, respectively, after their distal attachments. Formed by two layers, the deep fibers of the MCL merge with the joint capsule and medial meniscus to connect the medial epicondyle of the femur to the medial tibia. The superficial layer originates from a broad band just below the adductor tubercle and is separated from the deep layer by a bursa. The two layers insert just below the pes anserinus, the common attachment of the semitendinosus, sartorius, and gracilis, thereby positioning the ligament to resist medially directed shear (i.e., **valgus**) and rotational forces acting on the knee.

The LCL connects the lateral epicondyle of the femur to the head of the fibula, contributing to lateral stability of the knee. The ligament is separated from the lateral meniscus by a small fat pad. The LCL is the primary restraint against **varus** forces when the knee is between full extension and 30° of flexion, and provides secondary restraint against external rotation of the tibia on the femur.

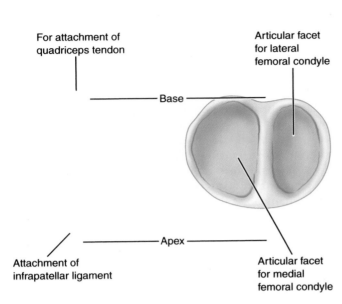

For attachment of
quadriceps tendon

Articular facet
for lateral
femoral condyle

Base

Attachment of
infrapatellar ligament

Apex

Articular facet
for medial
femoral condyle

FIGURE 15.2 Patella. **A**. Anterior view. **B**. Posterior view.

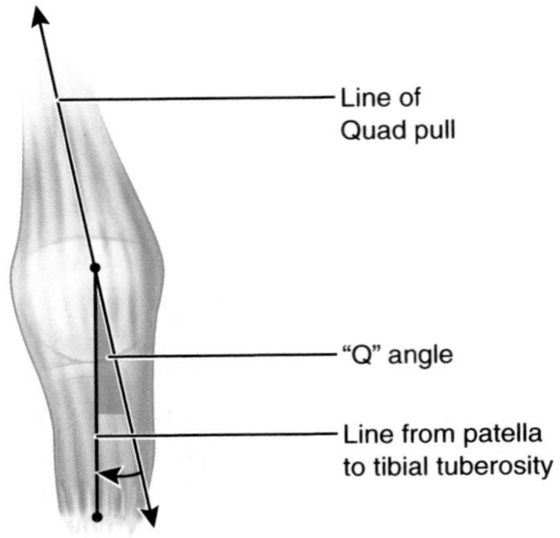

Line of
Quad pull

"Q" angle

Line from patella
to tibial tuberosity

FIGURE 15.3 Q-angle. The Q-angle is formed between the line of quadriceps pull and the imaginary line connecting the center of the patella to the center of the tibial tubercle.

Patellofemoral Joint

The patella (kneecap) is a triangular bone that rests between the femoral condyles to form the patellofemoral joint (FIG. 15.2). The posterior surface of the patella is composed of three distinct facets, although the number, size, and shape of these facets vary from person to person.[3] Because of its location, the patella provides some protection for the anterior aspect of the knee. In addition, the patella serves to increase the angle of pull of the patellar tendon on the tibia and, in doing so, improves the mechanical advantage of the quadriceps muscles to produce knee extension.

Q-ANGLE

The **Q-angle** is defined as the angle between the line of resultant force produced by the quadriceps muscles and the line of the patellar tendon (FIG. 15.3). One line is drawn from the middle of the patella to the anterior superior iliac spine of the ilium, and a second line is drawn from the tibial tubercle through the center of the patella. The normal Q-angle ranges from approximately 13° in males to approximately 18° in females, when the knee is fully extended. A Q-angle less than 13° or greater than 18° is considered abnormal, and can predispose individuals to patellar injuries or degeneration. Cadaver studies show that increasing the Q-angle increases lateral patellofemoral contact pressures and could promote lateral patellar dislocation, whereas decreasing the Q-angle could increase the medial tibiofemoral contact pressure.[4] Factors that contribute to an increased angle in women include a wider pelvis, increased femoral anteversion, increased knee valgus, external tibial torsion, increased ligamentous laxity, and hyperpronation of the foot.[5]

NERVES AND BLOOD VESSELS OF THE KNEE

The tibial nerve (L4, L5, S1—to S3) is the largest and most medial continuation of the sciatic nerve. It innervates all of the muscles in the hamstring group except the short head of the biceps femoris, and also supplies all muscles in the calf of the leg (FIG. 15.4).

The common peroneal nerve (L4, L5, S1, S2) is the lateral branch of the sciatic nerve (see FIG. 15.4). It innervates the short head of the biceps femoris in the thigh. Proceeding inferiorly, it passes through the popliteal fossa to wind laterally along the subcutaneous surface to just

Muscular distribution

Muscular distribution

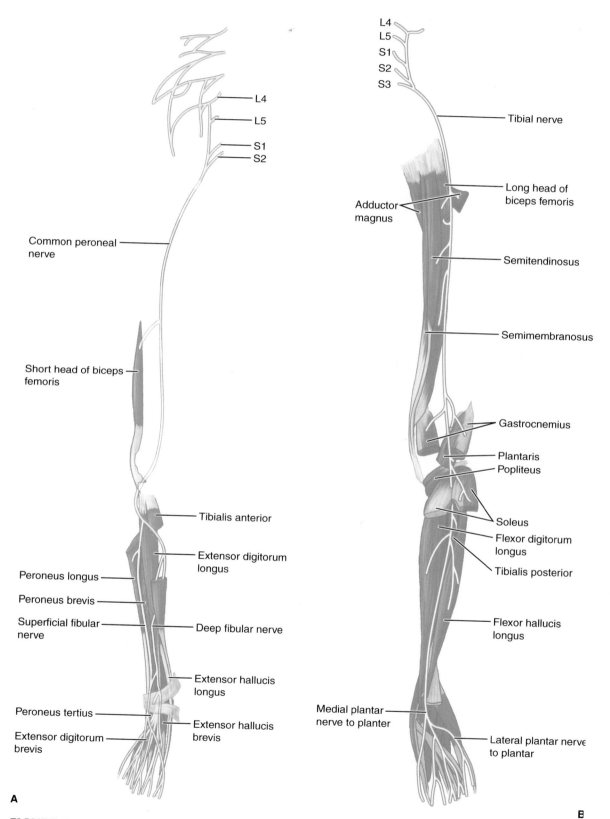

L4
L5
S1
S2

Common peroneal nerve

Short head of biceps femoris

Tibialis anterior

Extensor digitorum longus

Peroneus longus

Peroneus brevis

Superficial fibular nerve

Deep fibular nerve

Extensor hallucis longus

Peroneus tertius

Extensor hallucis brevis

Extensor digitorum brevis

A

L4
L5
S1
S2
S3

Tibial nerve

Long head of biceps femoris

Adductor magnus

Semitendinosus

Semimembranosus

Gastrocnemius

Plantaris
Popliteus

Soleus

Flexor digitorum longus

Tibialis posterior

Flexor hallucis longus

Medial plantar nerve to planter

Lateral plantar nerve to plantar

B

FIGURE 15.4 Innervation of the knee. **A**. Anterior view. **B**. Posterior view.

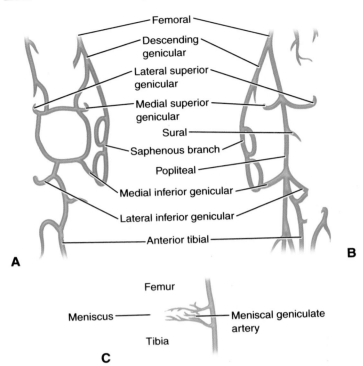

below the proximal head of the fibula, where it can be easily damaged. As it passes between the fibula and the peroneus longus muscle, it subdivides into the superficial and deep peroneal nerves.

The femoral nerve (L2—to L4) courses down the anterior aspect of the thigh adjacent to the femoral artery to supply the quadriceps group. The L2 and L3 branches of the femoral nerve also innervate the sartorius.

Just proximal to the knee, the main branch of the femoral artery becomes the popliteal artery. The popliteal artery courses through the popliteal fossa and then branches, forming the medial and lateral superior genicular, the middle genicular, and the medial and lateral inferior genicular arteries that supply the knee (FIG. 15.5). The superior and inferior genicular arteries intertwine with each other about the knee.

FIGURE 15.5 Collateral circulation around the knee. **A.** Anterior view. **B.** Posterior view. **C.** Circulation to meniscus.

KINEMATICS AND MAJOR MUSCLE ACTIONS OF THE KNEE

The knee functions primarily as a hinge joint. However, the different shapes of the femoral condyles serve to complicate joint function.

Flexion and Extension

The primary motions permitted at the tibiofemoral joint are flexion and extension (FIG. 15.6). Knee flexion is performed primarily by the hamstrings and assisted by the popliteus, gastrocnemius, gracilis, and sartorius. In addition, the flexor musculature has a secondary responsibility of rotating the tibia. The flexors attaching on the tibia's medial side (i.e., semitendinosus, semimembranosus, gracilis, and sartorius) internally rotate the tibia, while those attaching on the lateral side (i.e., biceps femoris) externally rotate the tibia. Knee extension is carried out by the quadriceps femoris muscle group. Although the name implies four

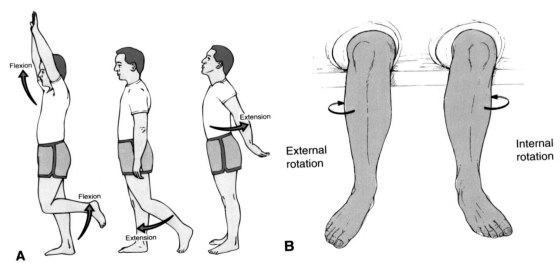

FIGURE 15.6 Motions at the knee. **A.** Flexion and extension. **B.** Supination of the subtalar joint in the foot results in external rotation of the tibia. Pronation is linked with internal rotation of the tibia.

muscles, most clinicians describe five, namely the vastus lateralis, vastus intermedius, vastus medialis (VM), vastus medialis oblique (VMO), and rectus femoris. Each muscle has a common attachment on the tibial tubercle via the patella and infrapatellar ligament.

In the terminal 20° of knee extension, the tibia externally rotates approximately 15° in what is called the "screw-home" mechanism. In full extension, the joint's close packed position, maximal bony contact occurs between the femur and tibia, resulting in the joint being anatomically "locked." This rotation occurs because the articulating surface of the medial condyle of the femur is longer than that of the lateral condyle in this locked position, rendering motion almost completely impossible. Initiation of flexion from a position of full extension requires that the knee must first be "unlocked." The role of locksmith in the closed kinetic chain is provided by the popliteus, which acts to externally rotate the femur with respect to the tibia, and, in doing so, freeing the joint for motion.

Rotation and Passive Abduction and Adduction

Rotational capability of the tibia with respect to the femur is maximal at approximately 90° of knee flexion. A few degrees of passive abduction and adduction are permitted when the joint is positioned in the vicinity of 30° of flexion.

Patellofemoral Joint Motion

During knee flexion and extension movements, the patella glides in the trochlear groove, primarily in a vertical direction. Tracking of the patella against the femur is dependent on the direction of the net force produced by the attached quadriceps. The vastus lateralis tends to pull the patella laterally in the direction of the muscle's action line, parallel to the femoral shaft. The IT band and lateral extensor retinaculum also exert a lateral force on the patella. Although there is considerable debate as to the role of the VMO, it seems to oppose the lateral pull of the vastus lateralis, and, in doing so, keeps the patella centered in the patellofemoral groove. If the magnitude of the force produced by the vastus lateralis exceeds that produced by the VMO, the patella is pulled laterally out of its groove during tracking. Mistracking of the patella during knee flexion/extension can be extremely painful and lead to several chronic patellofemoral conditions.

PREVENTION OF KNEE CONDITIONS

Because many of the muscles that move the knee also move the hip, prevention of knee injuries must focus on a physical conditioning program. Although much debate continues as to the effectiveness of prophylactic knee braces, recent rule changes and improved shoe design have contributed significantly to a reduction of injuries at the knee.

Physical Conditioning

The development of a well-rounded physical conditioning program is the key to injury prevention. Exercises should include flexibility and muscular strength, endurance, and power, as well as speed, agility, balance, and cardiovascular fitness. Stretching exercises should focus on the quadriceps, hamstrings, gastrocnemius, IT band, and adductors. Because many of these muscles contribute to knee stability, strengthening programs should also focus on these muscle groups. Specific exercises to prevent injury to the musculature that moves the knee are provided in APPLICATION STRATEGY 15.1. Additional exercises for muscles that cross the hip region are demonstrated in APPLICATION STRATEGY 14.1.

Rule Changes

Rule changes in contact sports, particularly football, have significantly reduced injuries to the knee region. Modifications in acceptable techniques that prohibit blocking at or below the knee and blocking from behind have reduced traumatic injuries. Proper training methods on correct technique should continue throughout the season to ensure compliance with specific rules designed to prevent injury.

APPLICATION STRATEGY 15.1

Exercises to Prevent Injury at the Knee

A. Hamstrings stretch, seated position. Place the leg to be stretched straight out with the opposite foot tucked toward the groin. Reach toward the toes until a stretch is felt.

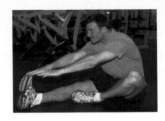

2. Squats (Never below 85° to 90°)

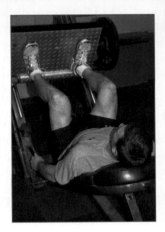

B. Quadriceps stretch, prone position. Push the heel toward the buttocks, and then raise the knee off the floor until tension is felt.

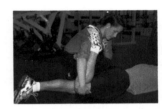

C. Iliotibial band stretch, supine position. With the trunk stabilized, adduct the leg to be stretched over the other leg and allow gravity to passively stretch the iliotibial band.

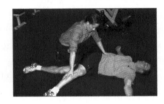

3. Leg press

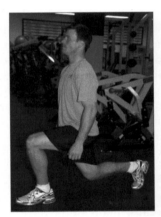

D. Iliotibial band stretch, standing position. Cross the limb to be stretched behind the other, extending and adducting the hip as far as possible.

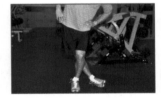

4. Lunges

E. Closed chain exercises:
1. Step-ups, step-downs, and lateral step-ups

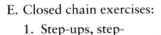

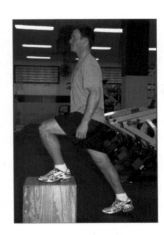

continued on page 271

APPLICATION STRATEGY 15.1 *continued*

Exercises to Prevent Injury at the Knee

F. Open-chain exercises:
   1. Knee extension
       (quadriceps)

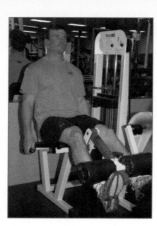

2. Knee flexion
    (hamstrings)

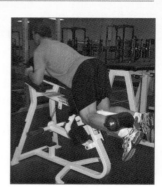

Shoe Design

Shoe design can also prevent injury. In field sports, shoes may have a flat-sole, long-cleat, short-cleat, or multicleated design. The cleats should be properly positioned under the major weight-bearing joints of the foot and should not be felt through the sole of the shoe. Shoes with longer irregular cleats placed at the peripheral margin of the sole with a number of smaller pointed cleats in the middle produce higher torsional resistance and are associated with a significantly higher ACL injury rate when compared with shoe models with flat cleats and screw-in cleats, or with pivot disc models.[6] In football, a cleated shoe with a higher number of shorter, broader cleats can prevent the foot from becoming fixed to the ground, yet still allow for good traction on running and cutting maneuvers.

CONTUSIONS

Contusions resulting from compressive forces (i.e., a kick or falling on the knee) are common at the knee. General signs and symptoms include localized tenderness, pain, swelling, and ecchymosis. Other injuries may be obscured if swelling is extensive. For example, being kicked on the medial aspect of the tibia may appear as a contusion, when in fact the impact may have caused an avulsion fracture of the MCL or an epiphyseal injury in an adolescent. Extreme point tenderness and positive findings on any of the special tests should indicate a more serious injury, and referral to a physician is indicated.

Fat Pad Contusion

The infrapatellar fat pad may become entrapped between the femur and tibia, or inflamed during arthroscopy, leading to a tender, puffy, fat pad contusion.

Signs and Symptoms

Signs and symptoms include locking, catching, giving way, palpable pain on either side of the patellar tendon, and extreme pain on forced extension.

Management

The immediate management includes standard acute care with cold and compression. Participation in sport and physical activity is usually not limited but the area should be protected to prevent further insult. If the signs and symptoms do not resolve within 2 to 3 days, the coach should require the individual to obtain approval for return to participation from a qualified healthcare professional.

Peroneal Nerve Contusion

The common peroneal nerve leaves the popliteal space and winds around the fibular neck to supply motor and sensory function to the anterior and lateral compartments of the lower leg (see FIG. 15.4). A kick or blow to the posterolateral aspect of the knee can contuse this nerve, leading to temporary or permanent paralysis. The nerve may also be injured by prolonged compression from a knee brace or elastic wrap, prolonged squatting (e.g., baseball or softball catcher), or by traction because of a varus stress or hyperextension at the knee.

Signs and Symptoms

In a mild acute injury, an immediate "shocking" feeling of pain may radiate down the lateral aspect of the leg and foot. If the actual nerve is not damaged, tingling and numbness may persist for several minutes. In severe cases where the nerve is crushed, initial pain is not immediately followed by tingling or numbness. Rather, as swelling increases within the nerve sheath, muscle weakness in dorsiflexion or eversion, and loss of sensation on the dorsum of the foot, particularly between the great and second toes, may progressively occur days or weeks later.

Management

Treatment involves standard acute care for contusions. However, caution should be exercised in applying a compression wrap, as the position of the wrap could further compress the nerve. If the condition does not rapidly improve or the individual experiences sensory or motor deficits, immediate referral to a physician is warranted.

BURSITIS

Bursitis can be caused by direct trauma, overuse, infections, metabolic abnormalities, rheumatic afflictions, and **neoplasms** (tumors).

Prepatellar Bursitis

Because of its location, the prepatellar bursa is the most commonly injured bursa in the knee as a result of direct blows and shearing forces.

Signs and Symptoms

Swelling can occur immediately or over a 24-hour period, obscuring the visible outline of the patella. Direct pressure over the bursa and passive flexion of the knee lead to considerable pain. Chronic prepatellar bursitis is more common than an acute episode, and is usually the result of repeated episodes of microtrauma. The condition may remain asymptomatic, except for mild discomfort when firm pressure is applied directly over the bursa.

Deep Infrapatellar Bursitis

Inflammation of the deep infrapatellar bursa is usually caused by overuse and subsequent friction between the patellar tendon and structures behind it (i.e., fat pad and tibia). Because this bursa lies posterior to the patellar tendon, inflammation of the bursa is often confused with **Osgood-Schlatter's disease** (OSD) in adolescents and patellar tendinitis in older individuals.

Signs and Symptoms

This condition is associated with swelling and pain in the distal patellar tendon region. In addition, knee flexion produces pain deep to the patellar tendon.

Pes Anserine Bursitis

Inflammation of the pes anserine bursa typically develops from friction, but may also occur in direct trauma. It is often seen in runners, cyclists, and swimmers who are subjected to excessive valgus stress at the knee or in individuals who have tight hamstrings.

Signs and Symptoms

Initial symptoms include point tenderness beneath the pes tendons (usually 2 cm below the joint line), localized swelling, and crepitation. When inflamed, contraction of the hamstring muscles, rotational movements of the tibia, and direct pressure over the bursa produce pain. Inflammation of this bursa is more commonly seen in middle-aged or older overweight women, many with osteoarthritis of the knee.[7] In order to avoid recurrence, the individual should begin an extensive flexibility program for the hamstrings and gastrocnemius-soleus complex.

Management of Bursitis

Treatment consists of application of cold, a compressive wrap, NSAIDs, avoiding activities that irritate the condition, or total rest until acute symptoms subside. A protective foam, or dough-nut pad, may protect the area from further insult. There is a risk of infection if the skin is broken during the initial injury, in which case, the individual should be referred to a physician immediately. The physician may culture any aspirated fluid to detect bacteria and subsequently prescribe medication.

LIGAMENTOUS CONDITIONS

Knee joint stability depends on a static, passive system of support from its ligaments and capsular structures. The American Academy of Orthopaedic Surgeons (AAOS) classifies ligamentous injuries at the knee according to the functional disruption of a specific ligament, or amount of laxity and the direction of laxity.

Ligamentous damage can result in unidirectional or multidirectional instability. A straight plane (unidirectional) instability implies instability in one of the cardinal planes. Injury to the ACL or PCL results in instability in the sagittal plane, allowing for equal anterior or posterior translation (shifting) of the medial and lateral tibial plateaus on the femur. Injury to the MCL and LCL leads to valgus or varus instability in the frontal plane. While several structures may be damaged, the resulting instability involves a single plane. Whereas unidirectional instability involves damage that results in instability to a single plane, multidirectional instability involves instability in more than one plane. While both unidirectional and multidirectional injuries can be significant injuries, the explanation that follows will focus on unidirectional instabilities.

Straight Medial Instability

In straight medial instability, or **valgus** instability, lateral forces cause tension on the medial aspect of the knee, potentially damaging the MCL and posteromedial capsular ligaments, as well as the PCL (FIG. 15.7A).

Signs and Symptoms

A Grade I sprain is characterized by mild pain on the medial joint line, little to no joint effusion, and full ROM that may include some discomfort. In a Grade II or III injury, the individual may be unable to fully extend the leg, and often walks on the ball of the foot, unable to keep the heel flat on the ground.

Straight Lateral Instability

Straight lateral instability, or **varus** instability, results from medial forces that produce tension on the lateral compartment, damaging the LCL, lateral capsular ligaments, PCL, and joint structures (Fig. 15.7B). This isolated injury is rare because the biceps femoris, IT band, and popliteus provide a strong stabilizing effect. A potential mechanism for this injury can be seen in the sport of wrestling when an opponent is often between the individual's legs and is able to deliver an excessive varus force that can lead to injury.

Signs and Symptoms

Damage to the LCL follows general signs and symptoms associated with an MCL sprain. Occasionally, the individual may hear or feel a pop, accompanied by sharp lateral pain. Swelling is minimal because the ligament is not attached to the joint capsule. Instability is subtle because other structures are intact. If pain is detected on the head of the fibula, an avulsion fracture should be suspected.

Straight Anterior Instability

In a straight anterior instability, the tibia is displaced anteriorly damaging the ACL. Damage to the ACL commonly occurs during a cutting or turning maneuver, landing, or sudden deceleration (Fig. 15.7C). Isolated anterior instability is rare. Instead, an anteromedial or anterolateral laxity usually occurs.

The rate of ACL injuries is higher in women, particularly for those in jumping and pivoting sports. Several theories have been put forth to explain this phenomenon (Box 15.1). Recent research has begun to look at muscle strength imbalance between the hamstrings and quadriceps in both men and women. During a landing/deceleration maneuver, flexion moments are occurring at the hip and knee. Simultaneous eccentric contractions of the quadriceps to stabilize the knee and hamstrings to stabilize the hip decelerate the horizontal velocity of the body. The hamstrings also act to neutralize the tendency of the quadriceps to cause anterior tibial translation. If the muscles are unable to meet the demand of stabilization, inert internal tissues, such as ligaments, cartilage, and bone, are at risk for injury. Therefore, a deficit in eccentric hamstrings strength relative to eccentric quadriceps strength could predispose an individual to an ACL injury. Prophylactic bracing has not been shown to prevent ACL injuries.[8]

Signs and Symptoms

Pain can range from minimal and transient to severe and lasting. It may be described as being deep in the knee, but is more often felt anterior on either side of the patellar tendon or laterally on the joint line. In about 80% of ACL injuries, individuals experience a popping, snapping, or tearing sensation, and a similar percentage note a rapid onset (i.e., usually within 3 hours) of swelling (**hemarthrosis**). Weight bearing leads to a feeling of the knee giving way or "just not feeling right."

Straight Posterior Instability

In straight posterior instability, the tibia is displaced posteriorly, damaging the PCL. Hyperextension is the most common mechanism. However, the PCL can also be damaged during a fall on a flexed knee with the foot plantar flexed, resulting in a blow to the tibial tubercle which drives the tibia posteriorly (Fig. 15.7D).

Signs and Symptoms

In milder cases, intense pain and a sense of stretching are felt in the posterior aspect of the knee. In a total rupture, a characteristic pop or snap is felt and heard, and may be followed by autonomic symptoms of dizziness, sweating, faintness, or slight nausea.[8] Large effusion and hemarthrosis usually occur within the first 2 hours after the acute injury. Knee extension is limited because of the effusion and stretching of the posterior capsule and gastrocnemius.

Management of Ligamentous Conditions

The immediate management for a suspected ligament injury involves standard acute care with cold and compression. If the individual is unable to walk normally, crutches should be

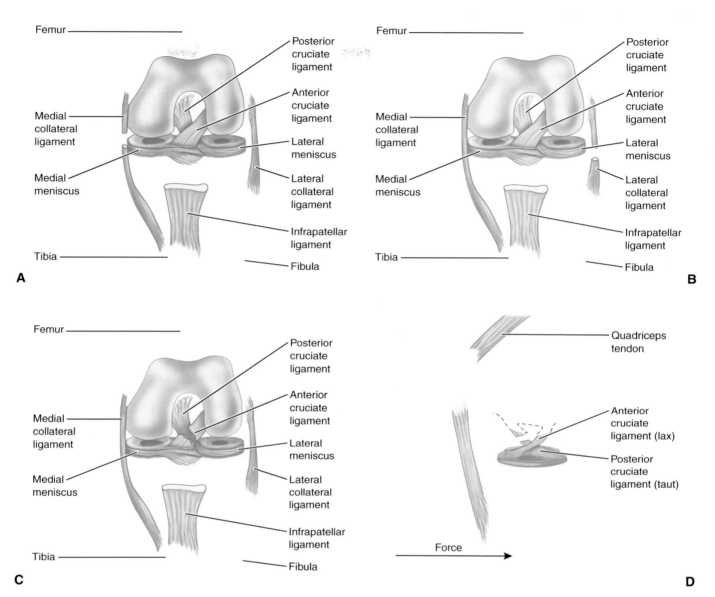

FIGURE 15.7 Knee instability. **A.** When a valgus force is applied to the knee, the medial collateral ligament and medial capsular ligaments are damaged, leading to valgus laxity. **B.** An isolated varus force damages the lateral collateral ligament, leading to varus laxity. **C.** When changing directions during deceleration, the anterior cruciate ligament can be damaged. **D.** During hyperextension of the knee or when the knee is flexed and the tibia is driven posterior, the posterior cruciate ligament can be damaged.

BOX 15.1	Possible Factors Influencing Increased Rate of Anterior Cruciate Ligament Injuries in Women

- **Intrinsic Factors**
  - Ligament size and laxity
  - Intercondylar notch dimensions
  - Limb alignment (wider pelvis, femoral anteversion, genu valgum, and external tibial torsion)
  - Estrogen and estrogen receptors
  - Cruciate-dependent knee
- **Extrinsic factors**
  - Level of skill and experience
  - Shoe-floor friction

- Ankle prophylactic braces
- Stylistic differences in sport play
- Plant and cut
- Straight leg landing
- One-step stop landing with the knee hyperextended
- Pivoting with sudden deceleration
- Muscle strength imbalance (eccentric hamstrings strength relative to eccentric quadriceps strength), endurance, and muscle recruitment

used. The individual should be referred to a qualified healthcare practitioner for a definitive diagnosis and ongoing treatment options. It is important to note that the initial symptoms associated with a ligament injury could resolve within a week, including the ability to walk with a normal gait. However, the change in symptoms is not an accurate indicator of the severity of the injury. While ligament injuries do not typically warrant a visit to the emergency room, they should be seen by an orthopedic physician as soon as possible (i.e., 1 to 2 days postinjury).

KNEE DISLOCATIONS

Knee dislocations and less-severe multiple-ligament injuries make up about 20% of all Grade III knee ligament injuries. To dislocate the knee, at least three ligaments must be torn. Most often, this involves the ACL, PCL, and one collateral ligament. Although dislocations can occur in any direction, the most common is in an anterior or posterior direction. As with any dislocation, additional damage can occur to other joint structures, including the ligaments, capsular structures, menisci, articular surfaces, tendons, and neurovascular structures. Associated injuries include vascular damage in 20 to 40% and nerve damage in 20 to 30% of all knee dislocations. Posterior knee dislocations are associated with the highest incidence of damage to the popliteal artery.

Signs and Symptoms

Subsequent to a cutting, twisting, or pivoting maneuver, the individual may describe feeling a severe injury to the knee and hearing a loud pop. Deformity of the knee may be present if the knee dislocated and remained unreduced. Unfortunately, knee dislocations often reduce spontaneously, making identification difficult. Swelling occurs within the first few hours, but the swelling may not be large due to an associated capsular injury and extravasation of the hemarthrosis.

Management

This injury is considered a medical emergency. The emergency plan should be activated, including summoning EMS. The coach should not move the individual. While waiting for EMS to arrive, the coach should assess vital signs and treat for shock as necessary.

MENISCAL CONDITIONS

Menisci, which become stiffer and less resilient with age, are injured in a similar manner as ligamentous structures. In addition to compression and tensile forces, shearing forces caused when the femur rotates on a fixed tibia can trap portions of both menisci, leading to some tearing. Tears are classified according to age, location, or axis of orientation. Medial meniscus damage is more common than lateral meniscus damage due to less mobility of the structure.

Longitudinal tears result from a twisting motion when the foot is fixed and the knee flexed (FIG. 15.8A). This action produces compression and torsion on the posterior peripheral attachment. The tear can be partial, affecting only the peripheral segment of the meniscus, or a complete tearing of the inner substance of the meniscus. A "bucket-handle" tear occurs when an entire longitudinal segment is displaced medially toward the center of the tibia (FIG. 15.8B). This tear can lead to locking of the knee at about 10° flexion; however, this occurs in only about 40% of complete meniscal tears.

Horizontal cleavage tears result from degeneration, and often affect the posterior medial portion of the meniscus (FIG. 15.8C). With age, shearing forces from rotational motions tear the inner substance of the meniscus. If

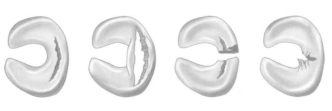

FIGURE 15.8 Meniscal tears. **A**. Longitudinal. **B**. Bucket-handle. **C**. Horizontal. **D**. Parrot-beak.

detached, momentary locking, associated pain, and instability may occur. A parrot-beak tear is two tears that commonly occur in the middle segment of the lateral menisci, leading to the characteristic shape of a parrot's beak. It is seen more frequently in individuals with a history of previous trauma or some cystic pathology that makes the meniscus more fixed at its periphery (FIG. 15.8D).

Signs and Symptoms

Meniscal injuries are difficult to assess because they are not innervated by nociceptors, and only 10 to 30% of the outer border receives direct blood supply. Localized pain and joint-line tenderness near the collateral ligament are probably the most common findings. The individual may experience a clicking sensation accompanied with pain that can lead to the knee buckling or giving way. In addition, the individual has difficulty doing a deep squat or a duck walk.

A chronic degenerative meniscal tear often results from multiple episodes of minimal trauma leading to almost no pain, disability, or swelling, although atrophy of the quadriceps may be present. Painful clicking sensations, as well as recurrent locking, are typical symptoms.

Management

An individual reporting signs and symptoms that suggest a meniscal tear should be referred to a physician for a definitive diagnosis and ongoing treatment. The coach should not permit the individual to continue activity, as doing so could potentially exacerbate the condition. Standard acute treatment including cold and compression can be used to mange pain and swelling.

PATELLAR AND RELATED CONDITIONS

The patellofemoral joint is the region most commonly associated with anterior knee pain. Patellar tracking disorders and instability within the joint, along with obesity, direct trauma, and repetitive motions, all contribute to a variety of injuries. Patellofemoral pain may be classified into mechanical causes (e.g., patellar subluxation or dislocation), inflammatory causes (e.g., prepatellar bursitis or patellar tendinitis), and other causes (e.g., reflex sympathetic dystrophy or tumors).

The main dynamic stabilizer is the quadriceps mechanism (FIG. 15.9). More accurately called the **extensor mechanism**, it is made up of the vastus lateralis, vastus intermedius, VM, and rectus femoris. The VM has two heads, the superior longus head (vastus medialis longus; VML), and the VMO. Although the VMO is incapable of producing knee extension, it provides a dynamic restraint to forces that would laterally displace the patella. Atrophy of this muscle is nearly always evident in patellofemoral dysfunction. The structures that resist medial displacement of the patella (i.e., lateral retinaculum and IT band) are thicker and stronger than the soft tissue structures that resist laterally displacing forces (i.e., medial retinaculum and lateral aspect of femoral sulcus).

Deficiencies in stabilization of the extensor mechanism can be caused by several abnormalities of the patellofemoral region (BOX 15.2), which can lead to anterior knee pain. Each condition can be counterbalanced in a healthy knee

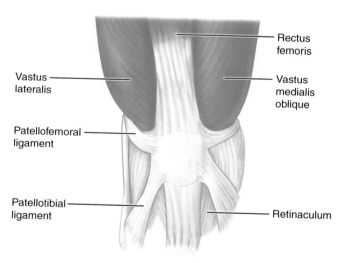

FIGURE 15.9 Extensor mechanism. The extensor mechanism is composed of dynamic and static stabilizers. Working together, they combine rolling and gliding motions to place the femur and patella in specific positions to effect the deceleration mechanism of the patellofemoral articulation and provide stability and function at the knee.

BOX 15.2	**Causes of Patellofemoral Pain**

- **Patellar instability caused by**
  - Abnormally shaped medial patellar facet
  - Shallow patellofemoral (trochlear) groove
  - Variable length and width of the patellar tendon
  - Patella alta (high-riding patella)
  - Weak VMO or VMO dysplasia
- **Hypermobility of the patella caused by:**
  - Muscle atrophy after an injury
  - Tightness of the lateral retinaculum, iliotibial band, and hamstrings

- **Anatomical malalignment caused by**
  - Shallow patellofemoral groove
  - Excessive femoral anteversion or external tibial rotation
  - Genu valgum or genu recurvatum
  - Increased Q-angle
  - Excessive foot pronation

by the triangular shape of the patella, depth of the patellofemoral groove, and limiting action of the static ligamentous structures. Failure of medial structures to restrain the patella in a balanced position or the presence of bony anomalies can result in lateral tilting or lateral excursion of the patella, which can lead to patellofemoral arthralgia, or severe joint pain. In addition, a Q-angle less than 13° or greater than 18° is considered abnormal and can be a predisposing factor to patellar injuries or degeneration.

Patellofemoral Stress Syndrome

Patellofemoral stress syndrome, also called lateral patellar compression syndrome, is pain in the patellofemoral joint without documented instability. The condition often occurs when either the VMO is weak or the lateral retinaculum that holds the patella firmly to the femoral condyle is excessively tight. In either case, the end result is lateral excursion of the patella. The condition is found more commonly in women because of their higher Q-angle.

Signs and Symptoms

The individual may report a dull, aching pain in the anterior knee made worse by squatting, sitting in a tight space with the knee flexed, and descending stairs or slopes. Point tenderness can be located over the lateral facet of the patella, with intense pain and crepitus elicited when the patella is manually compressed into the patellofemoral groove.

Management

Treatment involves standard acute care and NSAIDs. The individual should be referred to a qualified healthcare practitioner for a definitive diagnosis and ongoing treatment options.

Chondromalacia Patellae

Chondromalacia patellae is a true degeneration in the articular cartilage of the patella, which results when compressive forces exceed the normal physical range or when alterations in patellar excursion produce abnormal shear forces that damage the articular surface. Because articular cartilage does not contain nerve endings, chondromalacia should not be considered the true source of anterior knee pain. Chondromalacia is a surgical finding that represents areas of hyaline cartilage trauma or aberrant loading, but is not the cause of pain. The medial and lateral patellar facets are most commonly involved.

Signs and Symptoms

Generalized anterior knee pain and crepitus are present in activities such as walking up and down stairs or doing deep knee bends. Localized pain and tenderness can be palpated on the medial and lateral patellar borders. Pain and crepitus increase with active and resisted knee extension.

Management

Asymptomatic chondromalacia does not require treatment. If symptomatic, treatment involves standard acute care and NSAID as well as referral to a qualified healthcare practitioner for a definitive diagnosis and ongoing treatment options.

Patellar Instability and Dislocations

Patellar instability occurs when the patella has normal or abnormal alignment in the trochlear groove, but is displaced by internal or external forces. Displacement can range from microinstability to subluxation (partial displacement) or gross dislocation (FIG. 15.10). Factors that may lead to congenital extensor mechanism malalignment include VMO dysplasia, vastus lateralis hypertrophy, high and lateral patellar posture, increased Q-angle, and bony deformity.

Signs and Symptoms

Acute patellar subluxations and dislocations appear the same, and generally occur during deceleration with a cutting maneuver. Distinguishing one from the other depends on patient history. In a dislocation, the individual reports that the patella moved and had to be pushed back into place; with a subluxation, the individual reports that the patella slipped out, then went back into place spontaneously. The majority of the medial muscular and retinaculum attachments are torn from the medial aspect of the patella, leading to an audible pop and violent collapse of the knee. The individual reports intense pain as well as localized tenderness along the medial border of the patella. There may also be localized tenderness along the peripheral edge of the lateral femoral condyle where impaction from the patella occurs with flexion of the knee. If the patella remains dislocated (i.e., does not spontaneously reduce), there will be a loss of limb function as the individual will not be able to straighten the knee.

A traumatic displacement has acute effusion associated with a hemarthrosis occurring within the first 2 hours. A dislocation without acute effusion should signal chronic laxity; the tissues are so lax that the patella moves in and out of the groove without traumatizing surrounding tissues. Occasionally, a fracture of the patella or lateral femoral condyle occurs, resulting in a loose, bony fragment in the joint.

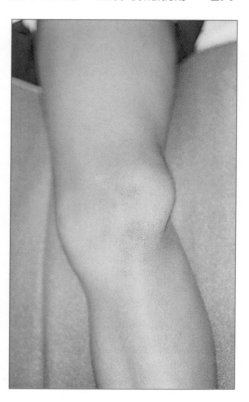

FIGURE 15.10 Dislocated patella. A dislocated patella often displaces laterally and is accompanied by an audible pop and violent collapse of the knee following deceleration involving a cutting maneuver.

Management

Treatment includes ice, elevation, immobilization, and immediate referral to a physician. The coach should not attempt to reduce a dislocated patella.

Patellar Tendinitis (Jumper's Knee)

The patellar tendon frequently becomes inflamed and tender from repetitive or eccentric knee extension activities; these occur in running and sports such as volleyball and basketball in which jumping is a critical action, hence the name "jumper's knee." Extrinsic factors that can lead to the condition include frequency of training, years of play, playing surface, type of training, stretching and warm-up practices, and type of shoe worn. Some intrinsic factors that may have a role in contributing to the condition include lower extremity malalignment, leg-length discrepancies, muscle imbalance, muscle length, and muscle strength.[9]

Signs and Symptoms

Most individuals will complain of chronic anterior knee pain of insidious onset, which might be described as a sharp or aching pain. Initially, pain after activity is concentrated on the inferior pole of the patella or the distal attachment of the patellar tendon on the tibial tubercle. As the condition progresses, pain is present at the beginning of activity, subsides during warm-up, then

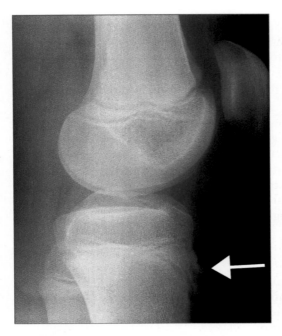

FIGURE 15.11 Patellar tendon traction-type injuries. Patellar tendon traction-type injuries may involve Sinding-Larsen-Johansson disease or Osgood-Schlatter disease. The location of pain typically defines which problem is present.

reappears after activity. Increased pain is often reported while ascending and descending stairs or after prolonged sitting. Eventually, pain is present both during and after activity, and can become too severe for the individual to participate.

Management

Immediate treatment involves standard acute care and NSAIDs. The individual should be referred to a qualified healthcare practitioner for a definitive diagnosis and ongoing treatment options.

Osgood-Schlatter's Disease

OSD is a traction-type injury to the tibial apophysis where the patellar tendon attaches onto the tibial tubercle (FIG. 15.11). OSD typically develops in girls between the ages of 8 and 13 years, and in boys between ages of 10 and 15 years at the beginning of their growth spurt. It is estimated that the condition occurs in 21% of adolescent athletes as compared with 4.5% of age-matched nonathletes.[10] The condition is more common in boys, but the ratio may be equalizing with girls' increased participation in sports.

Signs and Symptoms

Assessment of the condition is usually straightforward. The individual points to the tibial tubercle as the source of pain, and the tubercle appears enlarged and prominent. It is reported that the pain generally occurs during activity and is relieved with rest. Point tenderness can be elicited directly over the tubercle, but ROM is not usually affected. Pain is present at the extremes of knee extension and forced flexion. Severity is rated in three grades depending on the duration of pain:

- Grade 1—Pain after activity that resolves within 24 hours
- Grade 2—Pain during and after activity that does not hinder performance and resolves within 24 hours
- Grade 3—Continuous pain that limits sport performance and daily activities

Management

This individual should be referred to a physician for definitive diagnosis and ongoing treatment. The coach should not permit the individual to continue activity, as doing so could potentially exacerbate the condition.

Sinding-Larsen-Johansson's Disease

A similar condition to OSD is Sinding-Larsen-Johansson's (SLJ) disease. Pain, swelling, and tenderness result from excessive strain on the inferior patellar pole at the origin of the patellar tendon. The condition is usually seen in children 8 to 13 years old.

Signs and Symptoms

The onset of pain over the inferior patellar pole is gradual and seen in children involved in running and jumping sports. The condition is often missed unless the clinician palpates the inferior patellar pole with the individual's knee extended and the patellar tendon relaxed. Repeating the exam with the knee flexed at 90° should reveal diminished tenderness as the patellar tendon becomes taut.

Management

The management is the same as for OSD.

Extensor Tendon Rupture

Extensor tendon ruptures can occur at the superior or inferior pole of the patella, tibial tubercle, or within the patellar tendon itself. Ruptures result from powerful eccentric muscle contractions, or in conjunction with severe ligamentous disruption at the knee. The rupture may be partial or total.

Signs and Symptoms

A partial rupture produces pain and muscle weakness in knee extension. If a total rupture occurs distal to the patella, assessment reveals a high-riding patella, a palpable defect over the tendon, and an inability to perform knee extension or perform a straight-leg raise. If the quadriceps tendon is ruptured from the superior pole of the patella and the extensor retinaculum is still intact, knee extension is still possible, although it is weak and painful.

Management

Treatment involves standard acute care, fitting the individual for crutches, and immediate referral to a physician.

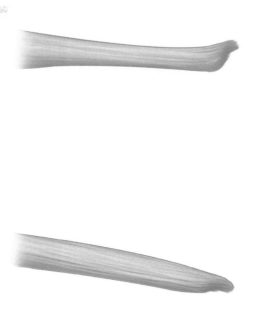

ILIOTIBIAL BAND FRICTION SYNDROME

A condition common in runners, cyclists, weight lifters, and volleyball players is IT band friction syndrome. The band originates on the lateral iliac crest and continues the line of pull from the tensor fasciae latae and gluteus maximus muscle; the deep fibers are associated with the lateral intermuscular septum. The distal fibers become thicker at their attachment on Gerdy's tubercle adjacent to the tibial tubercle on the lateral proximal tibia. The band drops posteriorly behind the lateral femoral epicondyle with knee flexion, and then snaps forward over the epicondyle during extension (FIG. 15.12). Weight-bearing increases compression and friction forces over the greater trochanter and lateral femoral condyle. Individuals with a malalignment problem are predisposed to this condition; see BOX 15.3 for a listing of predisposing factors.

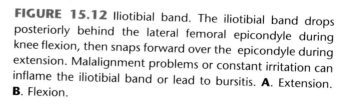

FIGURE 15.12 Iliotibial band. The iliotibial band drops posteriorly behind the lateral femoral epicondyle during knee flexion, then snaps forward over the epicondyle during extension. Malalignment problems or constant irritation can inflame the iliotibial band or lead to bursitis. **A.** Extension. **B.** Flexion.

BOX 15.3 **Predisposing Factors for Iliotibial Band Friction Syndrome**

- Genu varus
- Excessive pronation in feet
- Leg-length discrepancy
- Prominent greater trochanter of femur
- Preexisting iliotibial band tightness
- Muscle weakness in knee extensors, knee flexors, and hip abductors
- Training errors, such as excessive distance in a single run, increasing mileage too quickly, inadequate warm-up, and running on the same side of a crowned road

Signs and Symptoms

Initially, pain is present over the lateral aspect of the knee after running a certain mileage, typically late in the run, but it does not restrict distance or speed. As the condition progresses, the pain begins to occur earlier and earlier, and it does restrict distance and speed. Pain may occur while running uphill and downhill, and while climbing stairs. It is particularly intense on weight bearing from foot strike through midstance. It is during this part of the gait cycle that the IT band is most compressed between the lateral femoral epicondyle and greater trochanter of the femur. With continued activity, the initial lateral ache progresses into a more painful, sharp, and localized discomfort over the lateral femoral condyle just above the lateral joint line, and occasionally radiates distally to the tibial attachment or proximally up the thigh. Flexion and extension of the knee may produce a creaking sound. Eventually pain restricts all running and becomes continuous during activities of daily living.

Management

The immediate treatment should be focused on alleviating inflammation with standard acute care and NSAIDs. This individual should be referred to a physician for definitive diagnosis and ongoing treatment. The coach should not permit the individual to continue activity, as doing so could potentially exacerbate the condition.

FRACTURES AND ASSOCIATED CONDITIONS

Traumatic fractures about the knee area are rare in sports competition, except for high-velocity sports, such as motorcycling and auto racing. These fractures are usually associated with multiple traumas. Other more common fractures and associated bony conditions can occur with regular participation in sport and physical activity. The management for each of the fracture conditions in this section is the same. Specifically, the individual should be referred immediately to a physician. Cold should be applied to the area and, if possible, the individual should be fitted for crutches and instructed to use a non–weight-bearing gait en route to the physician.

Avulsion Fractures

Avulsion fractures are caused by direct trauma, excessive tensile forces from an explosive muscular contraction, repetitive overuse, or a tensile force that pulls a ligament from its bony attachment. For example, getting kicked on the lateral aspect of the knee may avulse a portion of the lateral epicondyle, or the tibial tubercle may be avulsed when the extensor mechanism pulls a fragment away.

Signs and Symptoms

The individual has localized pain and tenderness over the bony site. In some instances, a fragment may be palpated. If a musculotendinous unit is involved, muscle function is limited. When the anterior cruciate is involved, the bony fragment may lodge in the joint, causing the knee to "lock."

Epiphyseal and Apophyseal Fractures

Adolescents in contact sports are particularly susceptible to epiphyseal fractures in the knee region. A shearing force across the cartilaginous growth plate may lead to a disruption of growth and a shortened limb.

Tibial Tubercle Fractures

The tibial tubercle, a common site for apophyseal fractures in boys, may occur as a result of OSD. The typical patient is a muscular, well-developed individual who has almost reached skeletal maturity, and almost always is involved in a jumping sport, most commonly basketball. These fractures usually result from forced flexion of the knee against a straining quadriceps contraction or a violent quadriceps contraction against a fixed foot.

Signs and Symptoms

The individual has pain, ecchymosis, swelling, and tenderness directly over the tubercle. Difficulty going up and down stairs is also reported. When the fracture extends from the tubercle to the tibial epiphysis (type II), or through the secondary epiphysis and into the joint (type III), quadriceps insufficiency makes knee extension painful and weak. In larger fractures involving extensive retinacular damage, the patella rides high, and knee extension is impossible.

Distal Femoral Epiphyseal Fractures

Fractures to the distal femoral epiphysis are 10 times more common than proximal tibial fractures, and are more serious because of possible arterial damage to the growth plate. They may occur at any age, but are often seen in boys aged 10 to 14 years. These fractures occur when a varus or valgus stress is applied on a fixed, weight-bearing foot, as when someone falls on the outer aspect of the knee while the foot is planted.

Signs and Symptoms

The individual complains of pain around the knee and is unable to bear weight on the injured leg.

Stress Fractures

The femoral supracondylar region, medial tibial plateau, and tibia tubercle are common regions for stress fractures. These fractures occur when

- The load on the bone is increased (e.g., jumping or high-impact activity)
- The number of stresses on the bone increase (e.g., changes in training intensity, duration, frequency, or running surface, or unevenly worn shoes)
- The surface area of the bone that receives the load is decreased (i.e., during the normal process of bone repair, certain portions of the bone remain immature and less able to tolerate stress for a period of time).

Signs and Symptoms

The individual complains of localized pain before and after activity that is relieved with rest and nonweight bearing. In a stress fracture of the medial tibial plateau, pain runs along the anteromedial aspect of the proximal tibia just below the joint line. Localized tenderness and edema are present, but initial radiographs of the stress fracture may be negative. As the condition progresses, pain becomes more persistent. Follow-up radiographs 3 weeks postinjury may show periosteal new bone development. Early bone scans are highly recommended.

Chondral and Osteochondral Fractures

A **chondral** fracture is a fracture involving the articular cartilage at a joint. An **osteochondral** fracture involves the articular cartilage and underlying bone (FIG. 15.13). These fractures are the result of compression from a direct blow to the knee causing shearing or forceful rotation. A substantial amount of articular surface on the involved bone can be damaged.

Signs and Symptoms

The individual usually feels a painful "snap" and reports considerable pain and swelling within the first few hours after injury. Displaced fractures can cause locking of the joint and produce crepitation during ROM.

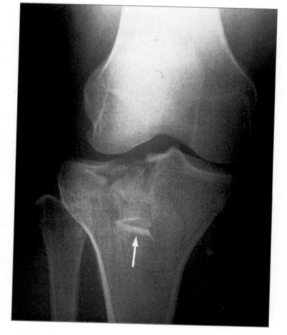

FIGURE 15.13 Osteochondral fracture. This traumatic osteochondral fracture involves the articular cartilage and subchondral bone on the medial epicondyle of the tibia.

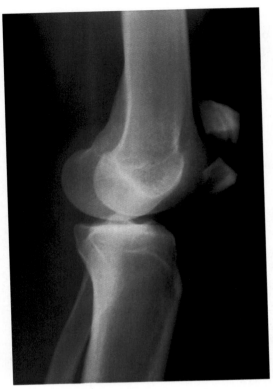

FIGURE 15.14 Traumatic patellar fracture. This radiograph provides a lateral view of a transverse fracture of the patella.

Patellar Fractures

Traumatic fractures of the patella can be transverse, stellate or comminuted, or longitudinal (FIG. 15.14). These fractures occur as a result of a fall onto the knee, a direct blow to the knee, or an eccentric contraction of the quadriceps that overloads the intrinsic tensile strength of the bone, as occurs in jumping activities.

Signs and Symptoms

Diffuse extra-articular swelling on and about the knee is present. A portion of the patella is retracted proximally. There is a visible and palpable defect between the fragments, which are mobile. A straight-leg raise is impossible to perform.

THE COACH AND ON-SITE ASSESSMENT OF A KNEE CONDITION

The lower extremity works as a unit to provide motion. The knee plays a major role in supporting the body during dynamic and static activities. Biomechanical problems at the foot and hip can directly affect strain on the knee. As such, assessment of the knee complex must encompass an overview of the entire lower extremity. It is important for the coach to recognize that while injuries to this region are rarely life-threatening, there are some conditions that will require activation of the emergency plan as they require immediate referral to a physician (Box 15.4).

The assessment begins as the coach approaches the individual or as the individual walks toward the coach. The focus should be on individual's overall presentation, attitude, and general posture. If the person is walking, it is important to determine any abnormal actions (e.g., presence of a limp; walking on the toes). The history component of the exam should focus on the major complaint, mechanism of injury, and presence of any unusual sensations (i.e., pain; sounds; feelings). In particular, location of the pain (e.g., deep in the knee; medial side of the knee; directly over the tibial tubercle), sounds (e.g., pop; click) and feelings (e.g., knee giving way; locking; "shocking," radiating pain) can provide valuable information in determining the potential injury (see APPLICATION STRATEGY 15.2).

BOX 15.4	**Conditions That Necessitate Immediate Referral to a Physician**

- Obvious deformity suggesting a dislocation or fracture
- Significant loss of motion or locking of the knee
- Excessive joint swelling
- Gross joint instability
- Reported sounds, such as popping, snapping, or clicking, or giving way of the knee
- Possible epiphyseal injuries
- Abnormal sensations in the leg or foot
- Any unexplained or chronic pain that disrupts an individual's play or performance

APPLICATION STRATEGY 15.2
On-Site Assessment of an Acute Knee Injury

HISTORY
- Chief complaint
  - What's wrong?
- Mechanism of injury
  - What happened? What were you doing?
  - Was there a direct blow? Was your foot fixed on impact?
  - Were you decelerating, cutting, or pivoting?
  - Did you fall?
  - Are you able to demonstrate how it happened?
- Pain
  - Location
    - Where is the pain?
    - Can you point to a location where it hurts the most?
  - Type—Can you describe the pain (e.g., sharp, shooting, dull, achy, diffuse)?
  - Intensity—What is the level of pain on a scale from 1 to 10?
- Sounds / feelings
  - Did you hear anything when the injury happened (e.g., pop; snap; crack)?
  - Did you feel any unusual sensations (e.g., tearing; knee giving way; locking; cracking) when the injury happened?
- Previous history
  - Have you ever injured your knee before? If so, what happened? What was the injury? Were you treated for it?
- OTHER important/helpful information
  - How old are you? (Remember that many problems are age-related.) Which leg is dominant?
  - Have you made any changes in performance (i.e., technique; intensity; playing surface)?
  - Have you changed your weight training workouts (e.g., increased weight or number of repetitions; added new exercises)?
  - Are you able to perform normal motions/ADLs?
- Is there anything else you would like to tell me about your condition?

OBSERVATION
- General presentation
  - Guarding
  - Moving easily; hesitant to move
- Injury site appearance—deformity; swelling; discoloration; position of patella

PALPATION
The coach should only perform palpation if there is a clear understanding of what is being palpated and why? A productive assessment appropriate to the standard of care of a coach does not necessitate palpation.

TESTING
- Active range of motion (AROM)—bilateral comparison
  - Knee flexion
  - Knee extension
  - Hip motions—flexion; extension; abduction; adduction
- Passive range of motion should not be performed by the coach
- Resistive range of motion
  The coach should only perform resistive range of motion for the muscles that govern the shoulder if
  - Instruction and approval for doing so has been obtained in advance from an appropriate health-care practitioner
  - AROM is normal and pain free as a way to assess strength.
- Activity/sport-specific functional testing
  - Performance of active movements typical of the movements executed by the individual during sport or activity participation (including weight training)
  - Should assess strength, agility, flexibility, joint stability, endurance, coordination, balance, and activity-specific skill performance.

In continuing the observation component, a bilateral comparison should be performed as a means for recognizing any deformity, swelling, discoloration, or alignment abnormalities (e.g., patella position). Again, if the individual is able to walk, an assessment of gait (e.g., favoring one limb, an inability to perform a fluid motion; toe waking) could aid in identifying the structures involved and the seriousness of the condition.

Subsequent to the history and observation components of an assessment, the coach should have established a strong suspicion of the structures that may be damaged. If the coach elects to perform the testing component of the assessment, it should begin with active ROM. Active movements can be performed with the individual in a seated or prone position. Knee extension and knee flexion should be assessed as well as movement of the hip (i.e., flexion, extension, abduction and adduction). If those motions are pain-free, the coach could continue with resisted ROM and, if there are no positive findings, perform functional testing. Otherwise, the assessment should be considered complete.

While the coach should restrict their assessment to on-site injuries, it may be appropriate to initiate the history component of an assessment if an individual reports to an activity with complaints of pain or discomfort. In doing so, the coach can confirm the presence of an acute or chronic/overuse injury and proceed accordingly. When it becomes apparent that an injury is overuse in nature, the coach should refrain from any continued assessment and, instead, refer the individual to an appropriate healthcare practitioner.

SUMMARY

1. The knee (tibiofemoral joint) functions primarily as a modified hinge joint with some lateral and rotational motions allowed.

2. The cruciate ligaments prevent anterior and posterior translation of the tibia on the femur. The ACL is frequently subject to deceleration injuries. The shorter and stronger PCL is considered to be the primary stabilizer of the knee.

3. The collateral ligaments prevent valgus (medial) and varus (lateral) stress at the knee.

4. The menisci aid in lubrication and nutrition of the joint, reduce friction during movement, provide shock absorption by dissipating stress over the articular cartilage, improve weight distribution, and help the capsule and ligaments prevent anterior tibial displacement.

5. Tracking of the patella against the femur is dependent on the direction of the net force produced by the attached quadriceps.

6. Because of its location, the prepatellar bursa is the bursa most commonly injured by compressive forces. The deep infrapatellar bursa is often inflamed by overuse and subsequent friction between the infrapatellar tendon and structures behind it (fat pad and tibia).

7. A straight plane instability implies instability in one of the cardinal planes. A multidirectional instability involves instability in more than one plane.

8. Isolated anterior instability is rare. Instead, an anteromedial or anterolateral laxity usually occurs. The rate of ACL injuries is higher in women, owing partially to a muscle strength imbalance, and both intrinsic and extrinsic factors.

9. Menisci become stiffer and less resilient with age. Tears are classified according to age, location, or axis of orientation, and include longitudinal, bucket-handle, horizontal, and parrot-beak. Because the menisci are not innervated by nociceptors, synovial inflammation and joint effusion may not develop for more than 12 hours after the initial injury.

10. Patellofemoral stress syndrome often occurs when either the VMO is weak or the lateral retinaculum that holds the patella firmly to the femoral condyle is excessively tight. This condition is much more common than chondromalacia patellae, which is a true degeneration in the articular cartilage of the patella.

11. Adolescents are particularly prone to OSD, SLJ disease, and fractures to the distal femoral epiphysis.

12. An individual should be referred to a physician if any of the following conditions are suspected:
   • Obvious deformity suggesting a dislocation or fracture
   • Significant loss of motion or locking of the knee
   • Excessive joint swelling
   • Gross joint instability
   • Reported sounds, such as popping, snapping, or clicking, or giving way of the knee
   • Possible epiphyseal injuries
   • Any unexplained or chronic pain that disrupts an individual's play or performance

APPLICATION QUESTIONS

1. A 16-year-old breaststroke swimmer reports pain in the region of the anteromedial aspect of the proximal tibia just below the knee joint. The pain has been increasing for the past few days. The swimmer recalls no injury. There is little evidence of swelling, no discoloration, and no deformity or other signs of trauma. How should the coach manage this situation? Should the swimmer be permitted to continue swim workouts?

2. A basketball player decelerated and made a cutting maneuver. The player felt a sudden popping sensation and intense pain, and then the knee collapsed. The individual can't point to one specific painful spot, but reports pain deep in the knee. Initial observation reveals no swelling. The coach suspects a tear of the ACL. How should the coach manage the injury? Should EMS be summoned?

3. A 40-year-old apparently healthy female comes to your exercise facility indicating that she has just finished physical therapy following a surgical repair of the medial meniscus. Her physical therapist strongly advises to work on increasing strength of the muscles that govern the knee joint. Demonstrate exercises used to increase strength of the knee musculature.

4. A 12-year-old boy is typically very active during physical education class. The class meets every day and the current unit is soccer. In addition to physical education class, the boy plays recreational soccer one night of the week and on weekends. During the second week of the soccer unit, the boy tells the physical education teacher that his right knee hurts while playing, but he doesn't remember hurting it and wants to keep playing. The physical education teacher begins to pay closer attention to the student and two days later notices that his performance is not as good as it was at the start of the unit. The teacher observes that the tibial tubercle of the right leg appears to be more prominent than the one on the left. What condition should be suspected? How should the physical education teacher manage the situation?

5. A volleyball player fell on the knee and felt an intense anterior knee pain. She reports pain on either side of the patellar tendon, but not directly on the tendon itself. She also reports a "catching" sensation and extreme pain with forced knee extension. What condition should be suspected? How should the injury be managed?

6. You are a personal trainer at a fitness club. As part of rehabilitation for a shoulder injury, one of your clients, a 45-year-old female, is maintaining cardiovascular fitness by using a stationary bike. Cycling has not been a part of her previous fitness workouts. Following 1 week on the bike, the individual complains of pain on the proximal, medial tibia just distal to the knee joint. The pain is particularly evident after her workout. It is painful for her to touch the area. What structure may be inflamed? Are there any factors that may contribute to this condition? What strategies could be implemented to prevent a reoccurrence of the condition?

7. One of your fourth-grade physical education students sustains an acute knee injury during an activity in the gymnasium. The injury occurred with about 20 minutes left in the class period. What questions would you ask in assessing the student's injury? Following the observation component of the assessment, there are no obvious abnormalities,

but the student is complaining of pain and hesitant to move. The school nurse left work for the day is not available. How would you continue to assess the student and manage the situation?

8. Following a twisting-type maneuver, a high school cheerleader on the floor is in obvious pain. In making her way out to the cheerleader, the coach observes the cheerleader semiprone and clearly in a guarded position (i.e., minimal movement of the involved leg). In assessing the individual, the coach finds out that following the twisting maneuver, the cheerleader felt her knee cap move. The coach observes an obvious deformity regarding the position of the involved patella. This particular practice is being held on a Saturday and there are no other schools officials in the building. What condition should be suspected? How should the coach manage the injury?

REFERENCES

1. Adirim TA, and Cheng TL. 2003. Overview of injuries in the young athlete. Sports Med, 33(1):75–81.
2. Rath E, and Richmond JC. 2000. The menisci: basic science and advances in treatment. Br J Sports Med, 34:252–257.
3. Grelsamer RP, and Weinstein CH. 2001. Applied biomechanics of the patella. Clin Orthop, (389):9–14.
4. Mizuno Y, Kumagai M, and Mattessich SM, et al. 2001. Q-angle influences tibiofemoral and patellofemoral kinematics. J Orthop Res, 19(5): 834–840.
5. McClure SK, Adams JE, and Dahm DL. 2005. Common musculoskeletal disorders in women. Mayo Clin Proc, 80(6):796–802.
6. Moul JL. 1998. Differences in selected predictors of anterior cruciate ligament tears between male and female NCAA Division I collegiate basketball players. J Ath Train, 33(2):118–121.
7. Cardon DA, and Tallia AF. 2003. Diagnostic and therapeutic injection of the hip and knee. Am Fam Physician, 67(10):2147–2152.
8. Walsh WM, and Vanicek JJ. Knee injuries. In The team physician's handbook, edited by MB Mellion, et al. Philadelphia, PA: Hanley & Belfus, 2002.
9. Hale SA. 2005. Etiology of patellar tendinopathy in athletes. J Sport Rehabil, 14(3):258–272.
10. Wall EJ. 1998. Osgood-Schlatter's disease: practical treatment for a self-limiting condition. Phys Sportsmed, 26(3):29–34.

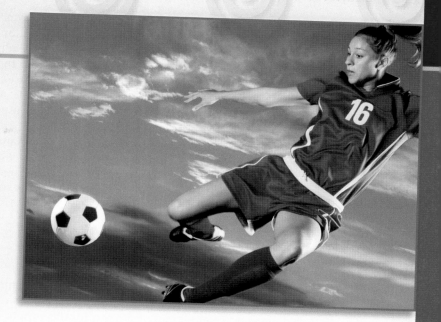

FOOT, ANKLE, AND LOWER LEG CONDITIONS

KEY TERMS

apophysitis

hallus rigidus

hallux

periostitis

pes cavus

pes planus

plantar fascia

sesamoid

turf toe

LEARNING OUTCOMES

1. Describe the major articulations that comprise the foot, ankle, and lower leg.

2. Identify the motions available at the foot and ankle.

3. Explain general principles used to prevent foot, ankle, and lower leg injuries.

4. Describe common injuries and conditions sustained by physically active individuals to the foot, ankle, and lower leg, including their sign, symptoms, and immediate management.

5. Describe an on-site assessment of an acute foot, ankle, and lower leg injury appropriate for use by a coach.

Because of the essential roles played by the lower leg, ankle, and foot during sport and physical activities, injuries to the region are common. Sport participation often places both acute and chronic overloads on the lower extremity, leading to sprains, strains, fractures, and overuse injuries. In particular, basketball, soccer, and football participants sustain a high incidence of injury to this region.[1,2] Lateral ankle sprains are the most common of all sports-related injuries, accounting for about 25% of injuries to the musculoskeletal system.[3] Increasingly, there is recognition that repeated ankle sprains can result in functional instability of the ankle, which predisposes the individual to further injury.[4]

This chapter begins with a review of the anatomy of the elbow, wrist, and hand, followed by an overview of common injuries to the shoulder complex. Information pertaining to mechanism of injury, signs and symptoms, and management by the coach will be provided. Finally, a basic assessment of the region appropriate for coaches is presented.

ANATOMY REVIEW OF THE FOOT, ANKLE, AND LOWER LEG

The foot, ankle, and lower leg comprise numerous bones and articulations (FIG. 16.1). The foot, in particular, has three major regions, namely the forefoot, midfoot, and hindfoot. They provide a foundation of support for the upright body, enabling propulsion through space, adaptation to uneven terrain, and absorption of shock.

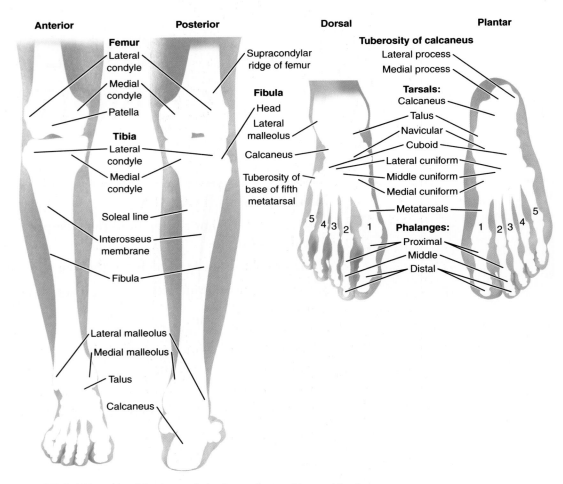

FIGURE 16.1 Skeletal features of the lower leg, ankle, and foot.

Forefoot

The forefoot is composed of five metatarsals and 14 phalanges, along with numerous joints. In conjunction with the midfoot region, the forefoot forms interdependent longitudinal and transverse arches to support and distribute body weight throughout the foot.

Metatarsophalangeal and Interphalangeal Joints

The metatarsophalangeal (MTP) joint is a condyloid joint with a close-packed position in full extension. The proximal interphalangeal (PIP) and distal interphalangeal (DIP) joints are hinge joints with a close-packed position also in full extension. Numerous ligaments reinforce both sets of joints. The toes function to smooth the weight shift to the opposite foot during walking and help maintain stability during weight-bearing by pressing against the ground when necessary. The first digit is referred to as the **hallux**, or "great toe," and is the main body stabilizer during walking or running.

The first MTP joint has two **sesamoid** bones, located on the plantar surface of the joint to share in weight-bearing. The sesamoid bones serve as anatomical pulleys for the flexor hallucis brevis muscle and protect the flexor hallucis longus muscle tendon from weight-bearing trauma as it passes between the two bones.

Tarsometatarsal and Intermetatarsal Joints

The deep transverse metatarsal ligament interconnects the five metatarsals. Both the tarsometatarsal (TM) and intermetatarsal (IM) joints are of the gliding type with the close-packed position in supination. These joints enable the foot to adapt to uneven surfaces during gait.

Midfoot

The midfoot region encompasses the navicular, cuboid, and three cuneiform bones, and their articulations. The navicular, like its counterpart in the wrist, the scaphoid, helps to bridge movements between the hindfoot and forefoot.

Transverse Tarsal Joint

The transverse tarsal (or midtarsal) joint consists of two side-by-side articulations, namely the calcaneocuboid (CC) joint on the lateral side and the talonavicular on the medial side. Collectively, these two joints are called the transverse tarsal joint because they are adjacent and function as a unit.

The CC joint is a saddle-shaped joint with a close-packed position in supination. The joint is nonaxial and permits only limited gliding motion. It is supported by several ligaments (FIG. 16.2). The most important is the long plantar ligament, as it contributes significantly to transverse tarsal joint stability.

Because the talus moves simultaneously on the calcaneus and navicular, the term talocalcaneonavicular joint (TCN) is often used to describe the combined action of the talonavicular and subtalar joint. The TCN is a modified ball-and-socket joint with a close-packed position in supination. Movements at the joint include gliding and rotation. Three ligaments support the joint, namely the plantar calcaneonavicular (spring) ligament inferiorly, deltoid ligament (DL) medially, and the bifurcate ligament laterally (FIG. 16.2).

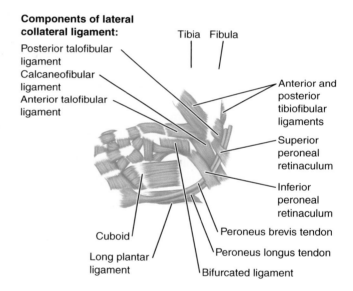

Components of lateral collateral ligament:
Posterior talofibular ligament
Calcaneofibular ligament
Anterior talofibular ligament
Tibia   Fibula
Anterior and posterior tibiofibular ligaments
Superior peroneal retinaculum
Inferior peroneal retinaculum
Peroneus brevis tendon
Peroneus longus tendon
Bifurcated ligament
Cuboid
Long plantar ligament

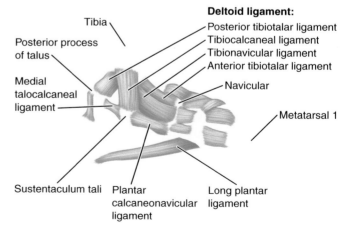

Deltoid ligament:
Posterior tibiotalar ligament
Tibiocalcaneal ligament
Tibionavicular ligament
Anterior tibiotalar ligament
Navicular
Metatarsal 1
Tibia
Posterior process of talus
Medial talocalcaneal ligament
Sustentaculum tali   Plantar calcaneonavicular ligament
Long plantar ligament

FIGURE 16.2 Ligaments supporting the midfoot and hindfoot region. Lateral view (**top**). Medial view (**bottom**).

Because the subtalar joint is mechanically linked to the TCN and transverse tarsal joints, any motion at the subtalar joint produces like motions at the transverse tarsal joints. For example, when the TCN is fully supinated and locked, the midfoot region is supinated and rigid. When the TCN is pronated and loose packed, the midfoot region is mobile and loose.

Other Midtarsal Joints

The remaining joints of the midfoot region include the cuneonavicular, cuboideonavicular, cuneocuboid, and intercuneiform. These joints provide gliding and rotation for the midfoot with a close-packed position in supination.

Hindfoot

The hindfoot includes the calcaneus and talus. The talus is saddle-shaped and serves as the critical link between the foot and ankle. It has several functional articulations, the two most important being the talocrural joint and the subtalar joint. Both serve a unique role in the integrated function of the foot, ankle, and lower leg.

Talocrural Joint

The talocrural (i.e., ankle) joint is a uniaxial, modified synovial hinge joint formed by the talus, tibia, and lateral malleolus of the fibula. The concave end of the weight-bearing tibia mates with the convex superior surface of the talus to form the roof and medial border of the ankle mortise. The fibula assists with weight-bearing, supporting approximately 17% of the load on the leg,[5] serves as a site for muscle and ligamentous attachments, and forms the lateral border of the ankle mortise. The lateral malleolus extends farther distally than the medial malleolus, and, as such, eversion is more seriously limited than inversion. The dome of the talus is wider anteriorly than posteriorly. Therefore, the joint's close-packed position is maximum dorsiflexion.

Although the joint capsule is thin and especially weak anteriorly and posteriorly, a number of strong ligaments cross the ankle and enhance stability. The four separate bands of the medial collateral ligament, more commonly called the DL, cross the ankle medially. The lateral side of the ankle is supported by three ligaments. The anterior talofibular ligament (ATFL) resists inversion during plantar flexion, and limits anterior translation of the talus on the tibia. The calcaneofibular ligament (CFL) is the primary restraint of talar inversion within the midrange of motion. The posterior talofibular ligament limits posterior displacement of the talus on the tibia. The relative weakness of these lateral ligaments as compared with the DL, coupled with the fact of less bony stability laterally than medially, contributes to a higher frequency of lateral ankle sprains.

Subtalar Joint

As the name suggests, the subtalar joint lies beneath the talus, where facets of the talus articulate with the sustentaculum tali on the superior calcaneus. Obliquely crossing the talus and calcaneus is the tarsal canal, a sulcus that allows for the attachment of an intra-articular ligament. Because no muscles attach to the talus, the stability of the subtalar joint is derived from several small ligaments.

The subtalar joint behaves as a flexible structure, with motion only occurring through stretching of ligaments during weight-bearing.[6] Motion at the subtalar joint involves "male" ovoid bone surfaces sliding over reciprocally shaped "female" ovoid bone surfaces.

Tibiofibular Joints

The tibiofibular articulations are supported by the anterior and posterior tibiofibular ligaments, as well as by the crural interosseous tibiofibular ligament. The tibia and fibula are also joined throughout most of their length by the interosseous membrane. This structural arrangement allows for some rotation and slight abduction (spreading) while still maintaining joint integrity. The interosseous membrane is of such strength that strong lateral stresses often fracture the fibula rather than tear the membrane.

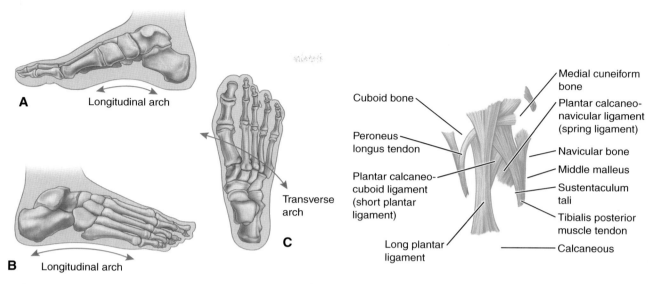

FIGURE 16.3 Arches of the foot. A. Medial view. B. Lateral view. C. Dorsal view.

FIGURE 16.4 Medial longitudinal arch. The medial longitudinal arch is supported by the calcaneonavicular (spring) ligament, short plantar ligament, long plantar ligament, plantar aponeurosis, and tibialis posterior muscle tendon.

Plantar Arches

The bones and supporting ligamentous structures in the tarsal and metatarsal regions of the foot form interdependent longitudinal and transverse arches (FIG. 16.3). They function to support and distribute body weight from the talus through the foot, through changing weight-bearing conditions, and over varying terrain. The longitudinal arch runs from the anterior, inferior calcaneus to the metatarsal heads. Because the arch is higher medially than laterally, the medial side is usually the point of reference, with the navicular bone serving as the point of reference between the anterior and posterior ascending spans.

The transverse arch runs across the anterior tarsals and metatarsals. The foundation of the arch is the medial cuneiform, with the apex of the arch formed by the second metatarsal. The arch is reduced at the level of the metatarsal heads, with all metatarsals aligned parallel to the weight-bearing surface for even distribution of body weight. Structural support is derived from the IM ligaments and the transverse head of the adductor hallucis muscle.

The primary supporting structures of the plantar arches, in order of importance, are the calcaneonavicular (i.e., spring) ligament, long plantar ligament, **plantar fascia** (i.e., plantar aponeurosis), and the short plantar (i.e., plantar CC) ligament (FIG. 16.4). When muscle tension is present, the muscles of the foot, particularly the tibialis posterior, contribute support to the arches and joints as they cross them.

The **plantar fascia**, or plantar aponeurosis, is a specialized, thick, interconnected band of fascia that covers the plantar surface of the foot, providing support for the longitudinal arch (FIG. 16.5). It extends from the posterior medial calcaneus to the proximal phalanx of each toe. During the weight-bearing phase of the gait cycle, the plantar fascia

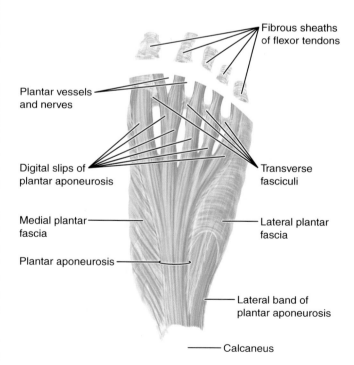

FIGURE 16.5 Plantar fascia. The plantar fascia stores mechanical energy each time the foot deforms during the weight-bearing phase of the gait cycle.

stretches on the order of 9 to 12% of resting length, functioning like a spring to store mechanical energy that is released to help the foot push off from the surface.[7] Stretching the Achilles tendon may elongate the plantar fascia, because both structures attach to the calcaneus.

NERVES AND BLOOD VESSELS OF THE LOWER LEG, ANKLE, AND FOOT

The sciatic nerve and its branches provide primary innervation for the lower leg, ankle, and foot (see FIG. 14.5). Just proximal to the popliteal fossa on the posterior leg, the sciatic nerve branches into smaller nerves. The major branches are the tibial nerve that innervates the posterior aspect of the leg and the common peroneal nerve that spawns the deep and superficial peroneal nerves, which innervate muscles in the anterior and lateral compartments, respectively.

The blood supply to the lower leg, ankle, and foot enters the lower extremity as the femoral artery. The femoral artery becomes the popliteal artery proximal and posterior to the knee, and then branches into the anterior and posterior tibial arteries just distal to the knee (FIG. 16.6). The anterior tibial artery becomes the dorsalis pedis artery to supply the dorsum of the foot. The posterior tibial artery gives off several branches that supply the posterior and lateral compartments as well as the plantar region of the foot.

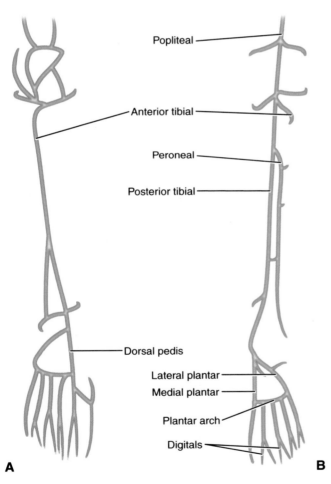

Popliteal

Anterior tibial

Peroneal

Posterior tibial

Dorsal pedis

Lateral plantar
Medial plantar

Plantar arch

Digitals

A   **B**

FIGURE 16.6 Blood supply to the leg, ankle, and foot region. **A.** The dorsalis pedis artery is easily palpated in the midfoot region between the second and third tendons of the extensor digitorum longus. **B.** The posterior tibial artery can be palpated just posterior of the medial malleolus.

KINEMATICS AND MAJOR MUSCLE ACTIONS OF THE FOOT, ANKLE, AND LOWER LEG

Evaluation of the kinematics of gait during walking and running can provide important clues for the likelihood of injuries. This section describes the kinematics of the lower leg, ankle, and foot, and identifies muscles responsible for specific movements (FIGS. 16.7 and 16.8).

The Gait Cycle

The gait cycle requires a set of coordinated, sequential joint actions of the lower extremity. Despite variation in individual gait patterns, enough commonality exists in human gaits that one can describe as the typical gait cycle (FIG. 16.9). The gait cycle begins with a period of single-leg support in which body weight is supported by one leg, while the other leg swings forward. The swing phase can be divided into the initial swing, midswing, and terminal swing. The period of double support begins with the contact of the swing leg with the ground or floor. As body weight transfers from the support leg to the swing leg, the swing leg undergoes a loading response and becomes the new support leg. A new period of single support then begins as the swing leg loses ground contact. The time through which body weight is balanced over the support leg is referred to as midstance. As the body's center of gravity shifts forward, the terminal stance phase of the support leg coincides with the terminal swing phase of the opposite leg.

Differences in running gait have been documented based on both gender and age. Among recreational runners, females appear to have greater hip adduction, hip internal rotation, and knee abduction compared to males.[8]

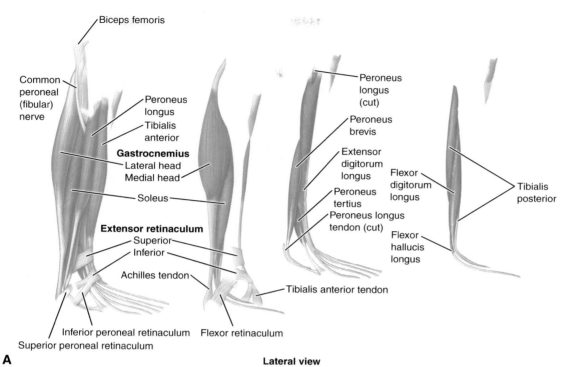

A   **Lateral view**

B   **Posterior view**

FIGURE 16.7 Muscles of the lower leg and foot. **A**. Lateral and medial view. **B**. Posterior view.

A study of elite master sprinters showed an age-related decline in running speed related to reduction in stride length and increase in ground contact time.[9]

Toe Flexion and Extension

Several muscles contribute to flexion of the second through fifth toes. These include the flexor digitorum longus, flexor digitorum brevis, quadratus plantae, lumbricals, and interossei. The flexor hallucis longus and brevis produce flexion of the hallux. Conversely, the extensor hallucis longus, extensor digitorum longus, and extensor digitorum brevis are responsible for extension and overextension of the toes.

Dorsiflexion and Plantar Flexion

Motion at the ankle occurs primarily in the sagittal plane, with ankle flexion and extension being termed dorsiflexion and plantar flexion, respectively (FIG. 16.10A). The medial and lateral malleoli serve as pulleys to channel the tendons of the leg muscles either posterior or anterior to the axis of rotation, and, in doing so, enabling their contributions to either plantar flexion or dorsiflexion. Muscles with tendons passing anterior to the malleoli (i.e., the tibialis anterior, extensor digitorum longus, and peroneus tertius) are dorsiflexors. Those with tendinous attachments running posterior to the malleoli contribute to plantar flexion. The major plantar flexors are the soleus, gastrocnemius, plantaris, and flexor hallucis longus, with assistance provided by the peroneal longus and brevis, and the tibialis posterior.

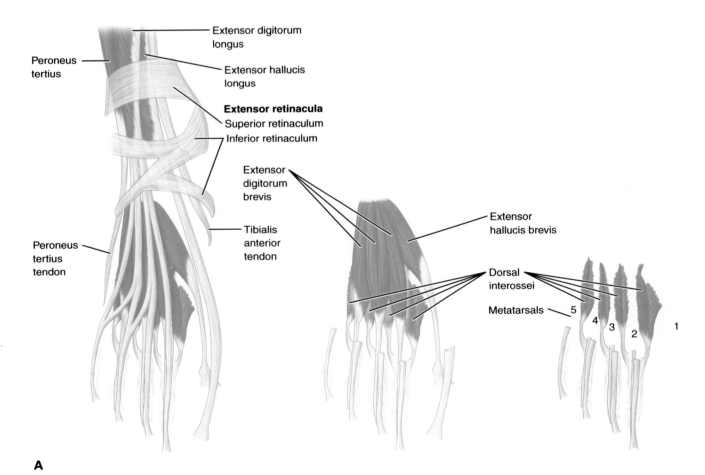

A

FIGURE 16.8 Intrinsic muscles of the foot. **A.** Dorsal view. (*continued*)

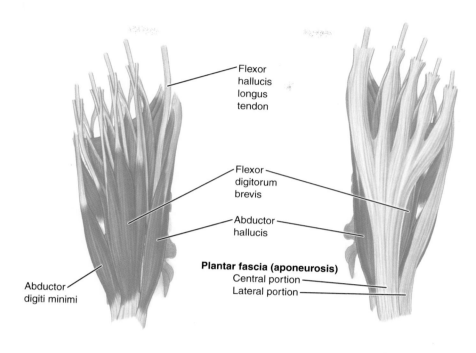

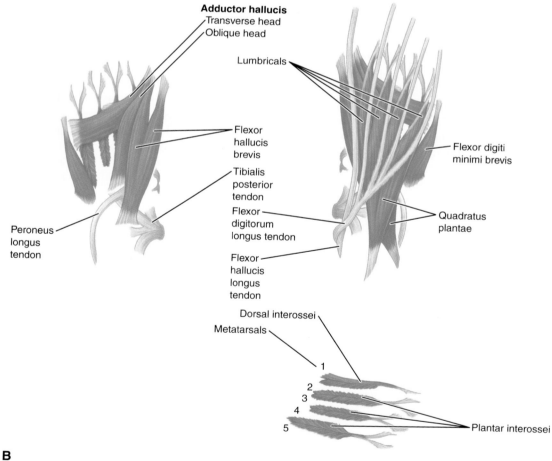

B

FIGURE 16.8 (continued) **B**. Plantar view.

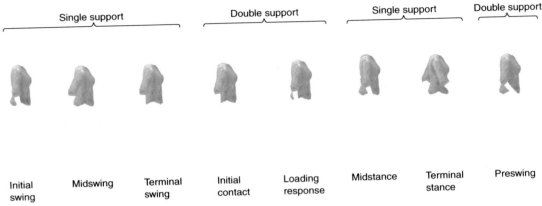

Single support   Double support   Single support   Double support

Initial swing   Midswing   Terminal swing   Initial contact   Loading response   Midstance   Terminal stance   Preswing

FIGURE 16.9 Gait. The gait cycle consists of alternating periods of single leg support and double leg support.

Inversion and Eversion

Rotations of the foot in the medial and lateral directions are termed inversion and eversion, respectively (FIG. 16.10B). These movements occur primarily at the subtalar joint, with secondary contributions from gliding movements at the intertarsal and TM joints. The tibialis posterior is the major inverter, with the tibialis anterior providing a minor contribution. Peroneus longus and peroneus brevis, with tendons passing behind the lateral malleolus, are primarily responsible for eversion, with assistance provided by the peroneus tertius.

Pronation and Supination

The lower extremity moves through a cyclical sequence of movements during gait. Among these, the action at the subtalar joint during weight-bearing has the most significant implications for lower extremity injury potential. During heel contact, the hindfoot is typically somewhat inverted. As the foot rolls forward and the forefoot initially contacts the ground, the foot is plantar flexed. This combination of calcaneal inversion, foot adduction, and plantar flexion is known as supination. During weight-bearing at midstance, calcaneal eversion and foot abduction tend to occur, as the foot moves into dorsiflexion. These movements are collectively known as pronation. Supination of the subtalar joint also results in external rotation of the tibia, with pronation linked to internal tibial rotation (FIG. 16.10C).

Although a normal amount of pronation is useful in reducing the peak forces sustained during impact, excessive or prolonged pronation can lead to several overuse injuries, including

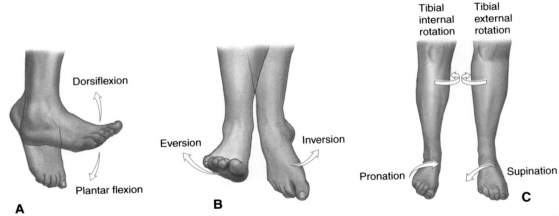

FIGURE 16.10 Motions of the foot and ankle. **A.** Dorsiflexion and plantar flexion. **B.** Eversion and inversion. **C.** Supination of the subtalar joint results in external rotation of the tibia; pronation is linked with internal rotation of the tibia.

stress fractures of the second metatarsal and irritation of the sesamoid bones, plantar fasciitis, Achilles tendinitis, and medial tibial stress syndrome.[10] Normal walking gait typically involves about 6° to 8° pronation.

PREVENTION OF FOOT, ANKLE, AND LOWER LEG CONDITIONS

Several steps can reduce the incidence or severity of injury. These include the use of appropriate protective equipment, footwear, and physical conditioning.

Physical Conditioning

Physical conditioning is one of the strongest defenses against injury. Unfortunately, the foot and lower leg are often neglected. Lack of flexibility can predispose an individual to certain injuries. For example, a tight Achilles tendon has been shown to predispose an individual to plantar fasciitis, Achilles tendinitis, and lateral ankle sprains. Exercises should focus on ensuring normal range of motion, and may be performed alone or with a partner.

Strengthening exercises for the intrinsic and extrinsic muscles of the region are essential in injury prevention. Foot strength can be improved by picking up marbles or dice with the toes and placing them in a container close to the foot, or placing a tennis ball between the soles of the feet and rolling the ball back and forth from the heel to the forefoot. The lower leg muscles can be strengthened by securing a weight or piece of elastic tubing around the forefoot, and moving through the ranges of motion for three sets of 10 to 15 repetitions. Bilateral toe raises and heel raises may also be incorporated. APPLICATION STRATEGY 16.1 demonstrates several exercises that can be used to prevent injuries to the lower leg, ankle, and foot.

Protective Equipment

Shin pads can protect the anterior tibial area from direct impact by a ball, bat, stick, or a kick from a foot. Commercial ankle braces used to prevent or support a postinjury ankle sprain come in three categories: lace-up brace, semirigid orthosis, or air bladder brace. A lace-up brace can limit all ankle motions, whereas semirigid orthoses and air bladder braces limit only inversion and eversion. In general, ankle braces are more effective than taping the ankle to reduce injuries, are easier for the wearer to apply independently, do not produce some of the skin irritation associated with adhesive tape, provide better comfort and fit, and are more cost-effective and comfortable to wear. Specific foot conditions can be padded and supported with a variety of products, including innersoles, semirigid orthotics, rigid orthotics, antishock heel lifts, heel cups, or commercially available pads and devices. Adhesive felt (e.g., Moleskin), felt, and foam can also be cut to construct similar pads to protect specific areas.

Footwear

The demands of a particular activity require adaptations in shoe design and selection. In field sports, shoes may have a flat-sole, long cleat, short cleat, or a multicleated design. Cleats should be positioned under the major weight-bearing joints of the foot, and should not be felt through the sole of the shoe. In individuals with arch problems, the shoe should include adequate forefoot, arch, and heel support. In all cases, individuals should select shoes based on the demands of the activity.

TOE AND FOOT CONDITIONS

Many individuals are at risk for toe and foot problems because of a leg-length discrepancy, postural deviation, muscle dysfunction (e.g., muscle imbalance), or a malalignment syndrome (e.g., **pes cavus, pes planus,** and hammer or claw toes). Typically, when compared to a man's foot, a

APPLICATION STRATEGY 16.1

Exercises to Prevent Injury to the Lower Leg

FOOT INTRINSIC MUSCLE EXERCISES

- Plantar fascia stretch—Place a towel around the toes, and slowly overextend the toes. Dorsiflex the ankle to stretch the Achilles tendon.
- Towel crunches—Place a towel between the plantar surfaces of the toes and feet. Push the toes and feet together, crunching the towel between the toes.
- Toe curls—With the foot resting on a towel, slowly curl the toes under, bunching the towel beneath the foot. Variation: Use two feet or a book or small weight on the towel for added resistance.
- Picking up objects—Pick up small objects such as marbles or dice with the toes, and place in a nearby container, or use therapeutic putty to work the toe flexors.
- Shin curls—Slide the plantar surface of the foot up the opposite shin, moving distal to proximal.
- Unilateral balance activities—Stand on uneven surfaces with the eyes first open, then closed.
- BAPS (biomechanical ankle platform system) board—Seated position: Roll the board slowly clockwise, then counterclockwise 20 times.

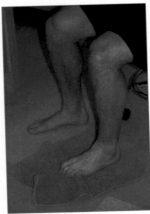

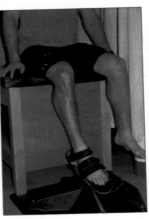

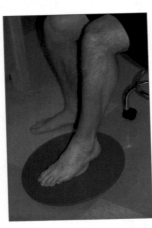

ANKLE/LOWER LEG MUSCLE EXERCISES

- Ankle alphabet—Using the ankle and foot only, trace the letters of the alphabet from A to Z, three times with capital letters, and three times with lowercase.
- Triceps surae stretch—Keeping the back leg straight and heel on the floor, lean against a wall until tension is felt in the calf muscles (1). To isolate the soleus, bend both knees (2). Point the toes outward, straight ahead, and inward to stretch the various fibers of the Achilles tendon.
- Thera-Band or surgical tubing exercises—Secure the Thera-Band or tubing around a table leg, and do resisted dorsiflexion, plantar flexion, inversion, and eversion.
- Unilateral balance exercises—Balance on the opposite leg while doing Thera-Band exercises.
- BAPS board—Standing position: Balance on the involved foot and repeat the process. Additional challenges, such as using no support, or dribbling with a basketball while balancing, can be added.

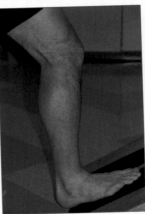

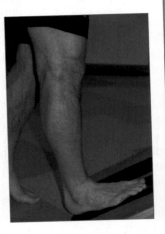

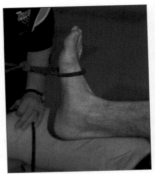

woman's foot has a narrower hindfoot, a relatively increased forefoot-to-hindfoot width, and increased pronation. Also, due to fashion trends and societal pressures, women tend to wear shoes that are narrower than the women's feet and have narrow toe boxes. High heels shift the forefoot forward into the toe box, causing crowding of the toes and a tight heel cord. Consequently, women tend to be more prone to hallux valgus deformities, bunionettes, hammer toes, and neuromas.[11]

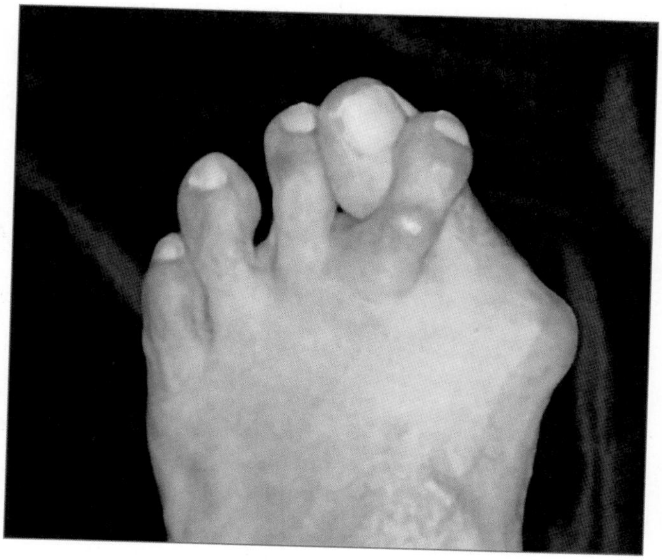

Toe Deformities

Most toe deformities are minor and can be treated conservatively. A few deformities require surgical intervention to correct serious structural malalignment. Common deformities are explained in this section. In each case, the management requires physician referral for an accurate diagnosis and treatment options.

Hallus Rigidus

Degenerative arthritis in the first MTP joint, associated with pain and limited motion, is known as **hallus rigidus.** Activities that involve running and jumping may predispose an individual to this condition due to degenerative changes resulting from direct injury, a hyperextension injury, or varus/valgus stress.[12]

Signs and Symptoms

The individual presents with a tender, enlarged first MTP joint, loss of motion, and difficulty wearing shoes with an elevated heel. A hallmark sign is restricted toe extension (dorsiflexion) variably less than 60° owing to a ridge of osteophytes that can be palpated easily along the dorsal aspect of the metatarsal head.

Hallus Valgus

Prolonged pressure against the medial aspect of the first MTP joint can lead to thickening of the medial capsule and bursa (i.e., bunion), resulting in a severe valgus deformity of the great toe (FIG. 16.11). The condition may be caused by heredity, metatarsus primus varus, pes planus, rheumatoid arthritis, and neurologic disorders. The most common cause is wearing poorly fitted shoes with a narrow toe box.

Signs and Symptoms

Many individuals with the deformity are asymptomatic. Those with symptoms complain of pain over the MTP joint, and have difficulty wearing shoes because of the medial prominence and associated overlapping toe deformity. The condition may also cause the second metatarsal to bear more weight leading to a callus under the second metatarsal head.

Claw, Hammer, and Mallet Toe

Other lesser toe deformities may be congenital, but more often develop because of improperly fitted shoes, neuromuscular disease, arthritis, or trauma. A hammertoe is extended at the MTP joint, flexed at the PIP joint, and hyperextended at the DIP joint (FIG. 16.12). Claw toe involves hyperextension of the MTP joint and flexion of the DIP and PIP joints. A mallet toe is in neutral position at the MTP and PIP joints, but flexed at the DIP joint.

Signs and Symptoms

Each condition can lead to painful callus formation on the dorsum of the IP joints. This pressure against the shoe and under the metatarsal head, particularly the second toe, is caused by the retrograde pressure on the long toe.

FIGURE 16.11 Hallus valgus. Hallux valgus is an abnormality in which the great toe is deviated laterally and may overlap the second toe. An enlarged, painful, inflamed bursa (bunion) may form on the medial side.

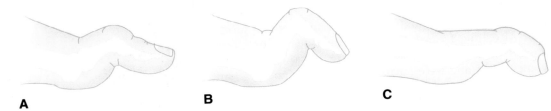

FIGURE 16.12 Toe deformities. **A**. Hammer toe. **B**. Claw toe. **C**. Mallet toe.

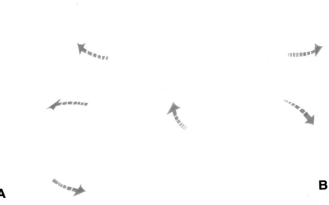

FIGURE 16.13 Common foot deformities. **A**. Pes cavus. **B**. Pes planus.

Pes Cavus and Pes Planus

Pes cavus is an excessively high arch that does not flatten during weight-bearing. The deformity can involve the forefoot, mid, hindfoot, or combination of those areas (FIG. 16.13). The potential cause of pes cavus varies. While some causes are idiopathic, other potential etiologies include heredity, muscle imbalances, and an underlying neuromuscular problem (e.g., muscular dystrophy). In most cases, pes cavus is associated with a rigid foot.

Pes planus is the opposite of pes cavus. The condition, referred to as flat foot, is the consequence of the arch or instep of the foot collapsing and contacting the ground. In most cases, pes planus is an acquired deformity resulting from injury or trauma involving the soft tissue structures that maintain the normal integrity of the arch. Pes planus typically results in a mobile foot.

Pes cavus and pes planus can occur at any age. While both conditions can be asymptomatic, they are often associated with several common injuries (BOX 16.1).

CONTUSIONS

Contusions of the foot and leg result from direct trauma, such as dropping a weight on the foot, or being stepped on, kicked, or hit by a speeding ball or implement. Many of these injuries are minor and easily treated with standard acute care. However, a few injuries can result in complications, such as excessive hemorrhage, periosteal irritation, nerve damage, or damage to tendon sheaths, leading to tenosynovitis.

BOX 16.1	Common Injuries Associated with Foot Deformities

PES CAVUS	PES PLANUS
• Plantar fasciitis metatarsalgia	• Tibialis posterior tendinitis
• Stress fractures of the tarsals and metatarsals	• Achilles tendinitis plantar fasciitis sesamoid disorders
• Peroneal tendonitis	• Medial tibial stress syndrome
• Sesamoid disorders	• Patellofemoral pain
• Iliotibial band friction syndrome	

Foot Contusions

Midfoot Trauma

Compression on the midfoot can be painful, and can damage the extensor tendons or lead to a fracture of the metatarsals or phalanges. During weight-bearing, contusions of the plantar aspect of the forefoot may result from a loose cleat or spike irritating the ball of the foot.

Signs and Symptoms

The area is painful to touch and, as such, it can be painful with walking.

Management

Standard acute care involving the application should reduce swelling and pain. In addition, if the trauma is due to a problem with the shoe, eliminating the mechanism by repairing or replacing the shoe would aid in preventing re-injury. If the condition does not improve within 3 to 4 days, the individual should be referred to a physician.

Heel Contusion

A contusion to the hindfoot, called a heel bruise, can be a serious injury. Elastic adipose tissue lies between the thick skin and the plantar aspect of the calcaneus to cushion and protect the inferior portion of the calcaneus from trauma. It is constantly subjected to extreme stress in running, jumping, and changing directions. Excessive body weight, age, poorly cushioned or worn-out running shoes, increases in training, and hard, uneven training surfaces can predispose an individual to this condition.

Signs and Symptoms

Severe pain and inability to bear weight on the heel are typical symptoms. Walking barefoot is particularly painful.

Management

Application of cold to minimize pain and inflammation, followed by regular use of a heel cup or doughnut pad, can minimize the condition. The individual should be referred to a qualified healthcare practitioner for a definitive diagnosis and treatment options. Despite excellent care, the condition may persist for months.

Lower Leg Contusions

Gastrocnemius Contusion

A compression mechanism, such as a kick, or blow from a thrown ball, can result in a severe injury.

Signs and Symptoms

Contusions to the gastrocnemius result in immediate pain, weakness, and partial loss of motion. Hemorrhage and muscle spasm quickly lead to a tender, firm mass that is easily palpable.

Management

Ice should be applied the area. In doing so, the muscle should be kept on stretch to decrease muscle spasm. If the condition does not improve in 2 to 3 days, the individual should be referred to a physician for an accurate diagnosis, including the potential for conditions resulting from the swelling and hemorrhage associated with the injury.

Tibial Contusion

A contusion to the tibia, commonly called a shin bruise, may occur in soccer, field hockey, baseball, softball, football, or activities in which the lower leg is subjected to high-impact forces. The shin is particularly void of natural subcutaneous fat, and is vulnerable to direct blows that irritate the periosteal tissue around the tibia.

Signs and Symptoms

Pain and swelling are the primary symptoms. Unless there is repeated trauma to the area, the condition typically resolves within a couple of days.

Management

Participants should always wear appropriate shin guards to protect this highly vulnerable area. Although painful, the condition can be managed effectively with ice, compression, elevation, and rest. A doughnut pad over the area and additional shin protection can allow the individual to participate within pain tolerance levels.

Acute Compartment Syndrome

An acute compartment syndrome occurs when there is a rapid increase in tissue pressure within a nonyielding anatomical space that leads to increased local venous pressure and obstructs the neurovascular network. In the lower leg, it tends to be caused by a direct blow to the anterolateral aspect of the tibia, or a tibial fracture. The anterior compartment is particularly at risk, because it is bounded by the tibia medially, the interosseous membrane posteriorly, the fibula laterally, and a tough fascial sheath anteriorly. Although an acute compartment syndrome occurs less frequently than the more common chronic compartment syndrome, the acute syndrome is considered a medical and surgical emergency because of the compromised neurovascular functions.

Signs and Symptoms

Signs and symptoms include a recent history of trauma, excessive exercise, a vascular injury, or prolonged, externally applied pressure. The increasing severe pain and swelling appear to be out of proportion to the clinical situation. A firm mass, tight skin (because it has been stretched to its limits), loss of sensation on the dorsal aspect between the great toe and second toe, and diminished pulse at the dorsalis pedis are delayed and dangerous signs. However, a normal pulse does not rule out the syndrome. Acute compartment syndrome can produce functional abnormalities within 30 minutes of onset of hemorrhage. Immediate action is necessary because irreversible damage can occur within 12 to 24 hours.

Management

Immediate care involves ice and total rest. Compression is not recommended because the compartment is already unduly compressed and additional external compression only hastens the deterioration. In addition, the limb must not be elevated, because this decreases arterial pressure and further compromises capillary filling. This condition requires activation of the emergency plan. It will necessitate either immediate referral to an emergency room or summoning of EMS (dependent upon the symptoms and the length of time it would take to transport the individual to an emergency room using private transportation).

FOOT AND ANKLE SPRAIN

Sprains to the foot and ankle region are common in sports, particularly for those individuals who play on badly maintained fields. In many sports, cleated shoes become fixed to the ground, while the limb continues to rotate around it. In addition, the very nature of changing directions places an inordinate amount of strain on the ankle region. Other methods of injury include stepping in a hole, stepping off a curb, stepping on an opponent's foot, or rolling the foot off the surface.

Toe and Foot Sprains and Dislocations

The toes and feet can be common sites for sprains particularly during an activity in which there is minimal support for the foot. The management for these conditions involves standard acute care as well as referral to a qualified healthcare practitioner for an accurate diagnosis and treatment options.

MP and IP Joints

Sprains and dislocations to the MP and IP joints of the toes may occur by tripping or stubbing the toe. Varus and valgus forces more commonly affect the first and fifth toes, rather than the middle three.

Signs and Symptoms

Pain, dysfunction, immediate swelling, and, if dislocated, gross deformity are evident.

Midfoot

Midfoot sprains often result from severe dorsiflexion, plantar flexion, or pronation. Although the condition is seen in basketball and soccer players, it is more frequent in activities where the foot is unsupported, such as in gymnastics or dance in which slippers are typically worn, or in track athletes who wear running flats.

Signs and Symptoms

Pain and swelling is deep on the medial aspect of the foot, and weight-bearing may be painful.

Turf Toe

Turf toe, a sprain of the plantar capsular ligament of the first MTP joint, results from forced hyperextension or hyperflexion of the great toe (i.e., jamming the toe into the end of the shoe). Repetitive overload can also lead to injury, particularly when associated with a valgus stress.

Signs and Symptoms

The individual has pain, tenderness, and swelling on the plantar aspect of the MTP joint of the great toe. Extension of the great toe is extremely painful. This condition has the potential to persist for weeks or months.

Because the sesamoid bones are located in the tendons of the flexor hallucis brevis, this condition sometimes is associated with tearing of the flexor tendons, fracture of the sesamoid bones, bone bruises, and osteochondral fractures in the metatarsal head.

Ankle Sprains

Ankle sprains are the most common injury in recreational and competitive sports. They are classified as Grade I (first degree), Grade II (second degree), and Grade III (third degree), based on the progression of anatomical structures damaged and the subsequent disability (TABLE 16.1). In basketball, ankle sprains comprise more than 45% of all injuries, and in soccer, up to 31% of all injuries are ankle sprains.[13]

TABLE 16.1	Mechanisms of Common Ankle Sprains and Resulting Ligament Damage		
MECHANISM	FIRST (MILD)	SECOND (MODERATE)	THIRD (SEVERE)
Inversion and plantar flexion	Anterior talofibular stretched	Partial tear of anterior talofibular, with calcaneofibular stretched	Rupture of anterior talofibular and calcaneofibular, with posterior talofibular and tibiofibular torn
Inversion	Calcaneofibular stretched	Calcaneofibular torn, and anterior talofibular stretched	Rupture of calcaneofibular, and anterior talofibular with posterior talofibular stretched
Dorsiflexion eversion	Tibiofibular stretched, deltoid stretched, or an avulsion fracture of medial malleolus	Partial tear of tibiofibular, partial tear of deltoid and tibiofibular	Rupture of tibiofibular, rupture of deltoid, and interosseous membrane with possible fibular fracture above syndesmosis

Medial   Lateral

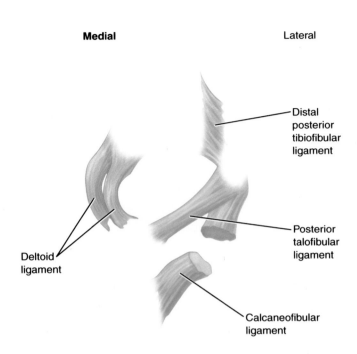

Distal
posterior
tibiofibular
ligament

Posterior
talofibular
ligament

Deltoid
ligament

Calcaneofibular
ligament

FIGURE 16.14 Inversion ankle sprain. During inversion, the medial malleolus acts as a fulcrum to further invert the talus, leading to stretching or tearing of the calcaneofibular ligament.

Inversion Ankle Sprains

Excessive supination of the foot (i.e., adduction, inversion, and plantar flexion) results when the plantar aspect of the foot is turned inward toward the midline of the body, commonly referred to as an inversion sprain (FIG. 16.14). Acute inversion (i.e., lateral) sprains often occur while changing directions rapidly. Interestingly, injury typically involves the unloaded foot and ankle (or, more accurately, just at the moment of loading) with a plantar flexion and inversion force.

In plantar flexion, the ATFL is taut and the CFL is relatively loose, whereas in dorsiflexion, the opposite is true. The medial and lateral malleoli project downward over the talus to form a mortise-tenon joint. The lateral malleolus projects farther downward than the medial, thus limiting lateral talar shifts. As stress is initially applied to the ankle during plantar flexion and inversion, the ATFL first stretches. If the strain continues, the ankle loses ligamentous stability in its neutral position. The medial malleolus acts as a fulcrum to further the inversion, and stretches or ruptures the CFL.

Signs and Symptoms

In a Grade I injury, the individual reports pain, but can typically bear weight immediately after injury. In a Grade II injury, the individual reports a "pop" suggesting the tearing of a ligament (i.e., the ATF)L. Rapid swelling and tenderness are localized over the ATFL and may extend over the CFL, and the individual can bear some weight, but definitely walks with a limp. A Grade III injury mimics a Grade II injury, except that the person is unable to bear weight as there is a functional instability.

Management

Initial treatment should consist of standard acute care (i.e., cold, compression, elevation, and protected rest) and restricted activity. Crutches should be used if the individual is unable to bear weight.

Because lateral ankle sprains are common, there may be a tendency to view all injuries around the ankle as "ankle sprains." The coach should not simply dismiss an ankle injury as a sprain. Referral to a physician is warranted for accurate diagnosis and ongoing treatment. A moderate to severe sprain requires immediate referral to a physician.

Eversion Ankle Sprains

Excessive pronation (i.e., abduction, eversion, and dorsiflexion) results when the plantar aspect of the foot is turned laterally, referred to as an eversion sprain (FIG. 16.15). Eversion (i.e., medial) ankle sprains involve injury to the medial, deltoid-shaped talocrural ligaments (Dl). Although an isolated injury to the DL may result from forced dorsiflexion and eversion, such as landing from a long jump with the foot abducted or landing on another player's foot. These account for less than 10% of all injuries.[13] Most injuries to the DL are associated with a fibula fracture, syndesmotic injury, or severe lateral ankle sprain. Individuals with pronated or hypermobile feet tend to be at a greater risk for eversion injuries.

The talar dome is wider anteriorly than posteriorly. During dorsiflexion, the talus fits more firmly in the mortise supported by the distal anterior tibiofibular ligament. During excessive dorsiflexion and eversion, the talus is thrust laterally against the longer fibula, resulting in either a mild sprain to the DL or, if the force is great enough, a lateral malleolar fracture. If the force continues after the fracture occurs, the deltoid ligament may be ruptured, or may remain intact, avulsing a small bony fragment from the medial malleolus and leading to a bimalleolar fracture. In either case, the distal anterior tibiofibular ligament and interosseous membrane may be torn, producing total instability of the ankle joint and eventual degeneration.

Signs and Symptoms

Signs and symptoms of an isolated eversion sprain depend on the severity of injury. In mild to moderate injuries, the individual is often unable to recall the mechanism of injury. There may be some initial pain at the ankle when it was everted and dorsiflexed, but as the ankle returns to its normal anatomical position, pain often subsides and the individual continues to be active. In attempts to run or put pressure on the area, pain intensifies but the individual may not make the connection between the pain and the earlier injury. Swelling may not be as evident as a lateral sprain because hemorrhage occurs deep in the leg and is not readily visible. Swelling may occur just posterior to the lateral malleolus, between it and the Achilles tendon. Point tenderness can be elicited over the DL.

Management

The management is the same as for an inversion ankle sprain.

Syndesmosis Sprain

Injury to the distal tibiofibular syndesmosis (i.e., a "high" ankle sprain) often goes undetected, resulting in a longer recovery time and greater disability than the more frequent lateral ankle sprain. The incidence of injury is reported between 1 and 11% of all ankle injuries.[14] The mechanism of injury differs from that of an inversion sprain. Often, the foot is dorsiflexed and externally rotated. External rotation injures the structures of the syndesmosis by widening the ankle mortis.

Signs and Symptoms

The area of maximum point tenderness is usually over the anterolateral tibiofibular joint. The degree of pain and swelling can be significant. The individual will have difficulty bearing weight on the injured ankle. The most commonly injured ligament, and a source of anterolateral ankle impingement, is the anterior inferior tibiofibular ligament; the least injured ligament is the posterior inferior tibiofibular ligament, although the interosseous ligament may also be variably injured.[15]

Management

The management is the same as for an inversion ankle sprain. This sprain typically takes longer to heal than an inversion or eversion sprain. Participation in sports and physical activity may be delayed for up to 3 months after the initial treatment begins.

Subtalar Dislocation

A serious sprain that involves the subtalar joint results from a fall from a height (as in basketball or volleyball). The foot lands in inversion, disrupting the interosseous talocalcaneal and talonavicular ligaments. If the foot lands in dorsiflexion and inversion, the CFL is also ruptured. When the dislocation occurs, the injury is better known as "basketball foot."

Signs and Symptoms

Extreme pain and total loss of function is present. Gross deformity at the subtalar joint may not be clearly visible. The foot may appear pale and feel cold to the touch if neurovascular damage is present. The individual may show signs of shock.

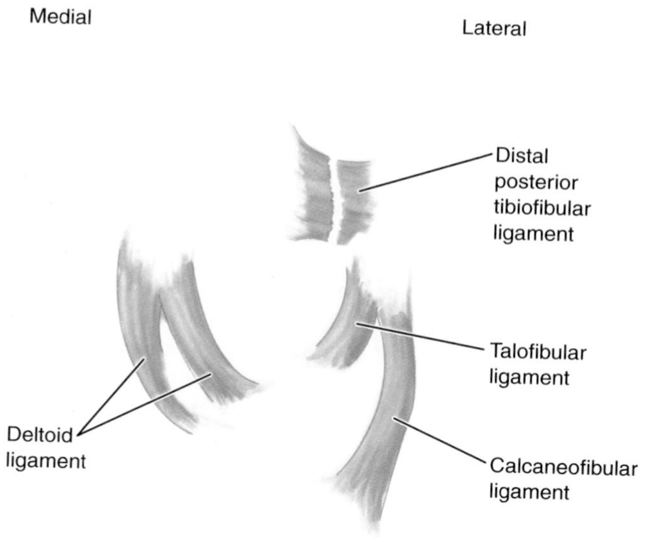

FIGURE 16.15 Eversion ankle sprain. During a severe eversion ankle sprain, the lateral malleolus can fracture, the deltoid ligament can avulse the medial malleolus, and the distal tibiofibular joint can be disrupted.

Management

Because of the potential for peroneal tendon entrapment and neurovascular damage, leading to reduced blood supply to the foot, this dislocation is considered a medical emergency. The coach should activate the emergency action plan, including summoning of EMS. While waiting for EMS to arrive, the coach should monitor the individual for shock and treat as necessary.

TENDINOPATHIES OF THE FOOT AND LOWER LEG

Tendinopathies of the foot and lower leg are relatively common and encompass a wide spectrum of conditions ranging from tendinitis to tenosynovitis to partial and complete ruptures. The tendons most often involved in the foot and ankle include the Achilles, posterior tibialis, peroneal brevis, and peroneal longus tendons. In contrast to acute traumatic tendinous injury, these injuries most involve repetitive submaximal loading of the tissues, resulting in repetitive microtraumas.

Strains and Tendinitis

Muscle strains seldom occur in the lower extremity, except in the gastrocnemius-soleus complex. Instead, injury occurs to the musculotendinous junction or the tendon itself. Most of the tendons in the lower leg have a synovial sheath surrounding the tendon, except the Achilles tendon, which has a peritendon sheath that is not synovial. Several factors can predispose an individual to tendinitis (Box 16.2). Common sites for tendon injuries include

- The Achilles tendon just proximal to its insertion into the calcaneus
- The tibialis posterior just behind the medial malleolus
- The tibialis anterior on the dorsum of the foot just under the extensor retinaculum
- Peroneal tendons just behind the lateral malleolus and at the distal attachment on the base of the fifth metatarsal

Signs and Symptoms

Common signs and symptoms include a history of stiffness following a period of inactivity (e.g., morning stiffness), localized tenderness over the tendon, possible swelling or thickness in the tendon and peritendon tissues, pain with passive stretching, and pain with active and resisted motion.

BOX 16.2   Predisposing Factors for Tendinitis in the Lower Leg

Training errors that include
- Lack of flexibility in the gastrocnemius-soleus muscles
- Poor training surface or sudden change from soft to hard surface or vice versa
- Sudden changes in training intensity or program (e.g., adding hills, sprints, or distance)
- Inadequate work-rest ratio that may lead to early muscle fatigue
- Returning to participation too quickly following injury
- Direct trauma
- Infection from a penetrating wound into the tendon
- Abnormal foot mechanics producing friction among shoe, tendon, and bony structure
- Poor footwear that is not properly fitted to foot

Management

In assessing these conditions, it should become apparent to the coach during the history component that the injury is overuse in nature and, as such, the coach should refrain from continuing assessment. Rather, the coach should refer this individual to a physician for accurate diagnosis and treatment options. The coach should not permit the individual to continue activity, as doing so could potentially exacerbate the condition. In addition, the coach could suggest the application of cold to the area to decrease pain and potential spasm.

Gastrocnemius Muscle Strain

Strains to the medial head of the gastrocnemius are often seen in tennis players over 40, hence the nickname "tennis leg." Common mechanisms are forced dorsiflexion, while the knee is extended; forced knee extension, while the foot is dorsiflexed; and muscular fatigue with fluid-electrolyte depletion and muscle cramping. If related to muscle cramping, the strain is commonly attributed to dehydration (particularly in the heat), electrolyte imbalance, or prolonged muscle fatigue that stimulates cramping followed by an actual tear in the muscle fibers.

Signs and Symptoms

In an acute strain, the individual experiences a sudden, painful tearing sensation in the calf muscles, primarily at the musculotendinous junction between the muscles and Achilles tendon or in the medial head of the gastrocnemius muscle (FIG. 16.16). Immediate pain, swelling, loss of function, and stiffness are common. Later, ecchymosis progresses down the leg into the foot and ankle.

Management

Initial treatment should consist of standard acute care (i.e., cold, compression, elevation, and protected rest) and restricted activity. Crutches should be used if the individual is unable to bear weight. If an apparently mild injury does not significantly improve in 3 to 4 days or if the injury is considered moderate to severe, immediate referral to a physician is necessary.

Achilles Tendon Rupture

Acute rupture of the Achilles tendon is probably the most severe acute muscular problem in the lower leg. It is more commonly seen in individuals 30 to 50 years old.[16] The usual mechanism is a push-off of the forefoot while the knee is extending, a common move in many propulsive activities. Tendinous ruptures usually occur 1 to 2 inches proximal to the distal attachment of the tendon on the calcaneus (FIG. 16.17).

Signs and Symptoms

The individual hears and feels a characteristic "pop" in the posterior ankle and reports a feeling of being shot or kicked in the heel. Clinical signs and symptoms include a visible defect in the tendon, inability to stand on tiptoes or even balance on the affected leg, swelling and bruising around the malleoli, and excessive passive dorsiflexion. Because the peroneal longus, peroneal brevis, and muscles in the deep posterior compartment are still intact, the individual may limp or walk with the foot and leg externally rotated, since this does not require push-off with the superficial calf muscles.

Management

A compression wrap should be applied from the toes to the knee. The individual should be referred immediately to a physician. While this situation does not normally warrant summoning EMS, it can require immediate transport to an emergency care facility.

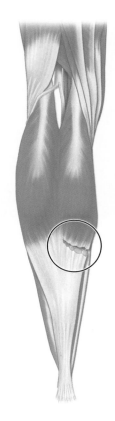

FIGURE 16.16 Gastrocnemius muscle strain. The medial head of the gastrocnemius muscle commonly is strained in individuals older than 40 years.

OVERUSE CONDITIONS

Repetitive microscopic injury to tendinous structures can lead to chronic inflammation that overwhelms the tissue's ability to repair itself. Other factors, such as faulty biomechanics, poor

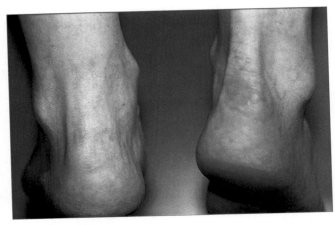

FIGURE 16.17 Achilles tendon rupture. The Achilles tendon often is ruptured 1 to 2 inches proximal to its distal attachment. This patient's ruptured left Achilles tendon appears to be thickened and less distinct than that on the normal right side, and the patient is unable to plantar flex the left foot.

cushioning or stiff-soled shoes, or excessive downhill running, can also inflame the tendons. Several overuse conditions are common in specific sports, such as plantar fasciitis in running; medial tibial stress syndrome in football, dance, or running; and exertional compartment syndrome in soccer or distance running. Many individuals complain of vague leg pain, but have no history of a specific injury that caused the pain, differentiating these conditions from an acute muscle strain. A common complaint is pain caused by activity.

Plantar Fasciitis

Plantar fasciitis is the most common hind foot problem in runners, affecting approximately 10% of runners.[17] Extrinsic factors that increase the incidence of the condition include training errors, improper footwear, and participating on unyielding surfaces. Intrinsic factors include pes cavus or pes planus, decreased planar flexion strength, reduced flexibility of the plantar flexor muscles (e.g., Achilles tendon), excessive or prolonged pronation and torsional malalignment. These factors can overload the plantar fascia's origin on the anteromedial aspect of the calcaneus during weight-bearing activities.

Signs and Symptoms

The individual reports pain on the plantar, medial heel that is relieved with activity, but recurs after rest. Pain increases with weight-bearing. It is particularly severe with the first few steps in the morning, particularly in the proximal, plantar, medial heel, but diminishes within 5 to 10 minutes. Pain and stiffness are related to muscle spasm and splinting of the fascia secondary to inflammation. Pain can radiate up the medial side of the heel, and occasionally across the lateral side of the foot. Normal muscle length is not easily attained, and it leads to additional pain and irritation. Point tenderness is elicited over or just distal to the medial tubercle of the calcaneus, and increases with passive toe extension. Passive extension of the great toe and dorsiflexion of the ankle will increase pain and discomfort.

Management

The coach should refer this individual to a physician for accurate diagnosis and treatment options. The coach should not permit the individual to continue activity, as doing so could potentially exacerbate the condition. In addition, the coach could suggest the application of cold to the area to decrease pain and potential spasm.

Medial Tibial Stress Syndrome

Medial tibial stress syndrome (MTSS) is a **periostitis** along the posteromedial tibial border, usually in the distal third, not associated with a stress fracture or compartment syndrome. Although originally thought to be related to stress along the posterior tibialis muscle and tendon causing myositis, fasciitis, and periostitis, it is now believed to be related to periostitis of the soleus insertion along the posterior medial tibial border. The soleus makes up the medial third of the heel cord as it inserts into the calcaneus. Excessive pronation or prolonged pronation of the foot causes an eccentric contraction of the soleus, resulting in the periostitis that produces the pain. Other contributing factors include recent changes in running distance, speed, form, stretching, footwear, or running surface.

Signs and Symptoms

Typically seen in runners or jumpers, the pain can occur at any point during a workout and is typically characterized as a dull ache, although it occasionally can be sharp and penetrating. As activity progresses, pain diminishes, only to recur hours after activity has ceased. In later stages, pain is present before, during, and after activity, and may restrict performance. Point tenderness is elicited in a 3- to 6-cm area along the distal posteromedial tibial border. Pain is aggravated by resisted plantar flexion or standing on tiptoe. There is often an associated varus alignment of the lower extremity, including a greater Achilles tendon angle.

Management

The coach should refer this individual to a physician for accurate diagnosis and treatment options. The coach should not permit the individual to continue activity, as doing so could potentially exacerbate the condition. In addition, the coach could suggest the application of cold to the area to decrease pain and potential spasm.

Exertional Compartment Syndrome

Exertional compartment syndrome (ECS) is characterized by exercise-induced pain and swelling that is relieved by rest. The compartments most frequently affected are the anterior (50 to 60%) and deep posterior (20 to 30%). The remaining 10 to 20% are divided evenly among the lateral, superficial posterior, and the "fifth" compartment around the tibialis posterior muscle.[18] Whereas acute ECS generally occurs in relatively sedentary people who undertake strenuous exercise, chronic ECS usually is seen in well-conditioned individuals younger than 40.[19]

Signs and Symptoms

The typical history of chronic ECS is exercise-induced pain that is often described as a tight, cramp-like, or squeezing ache and a sense of fullness, both over the involved compartment. The condition often affects both legs. Symptoms are almost always relieved with rest, usually within 20 minutes of exercise, only to recur if exercise is resumed. Activity-related pain begins at a predictable time after starting exercise or after reaching a certain level of intensity and increases if the training persists. Many individuals with anterior compartment involvement describe mild foot drop or paresthesia (or both) on the dorsum of the foot, and demonstrate fascial defects or hernias, usually in the distal third of the leg over the intramuscular septum.

Management

The immediate management involves ceasing activity. Ultimately, the individual needs to be assessed by a qualified healthcare practitioner. Assessment should include both extrinsic factors (e.g., training patterns, technique, shoe design, and training surface) and intrinsic factors (e.g., foot alignment, especially hindfoot pronation, muscle imbalance, and flexibility).

FRACTURES

Fractures in the foot and lower leg region seldom result from a single traumatic episode. Often, repetitive microtraumas lead to apophyseal or stress fractures. Tensile forces associated with severe ankle sprains can lead to avulsion fractures of the fifth metatarsal, or severe twisting can lead to displaced and undisplaced fractures in the foot, ankle, or lower leg. A combination of forces can lead to a traumatic fracture-dislocation.

The management for the conditions in this section is the same for each, unless otherwise noted. If a fracture is suspected, immediate referral to a physician is warranted. The application of cold and gentle compression to minimize pain and swelling can be advantageous. Crutches should be used if the individual is unable to bear weight.

Freiberg's Disease

Freiberg's disease is a painful avascular necrosis of the second, or rarely, third metatarsal head, often seen in active adolescents aged 14 to 18 years before closure of the epiphysis.

Signs and Symptoms

The condition can lead to diffuse pain in the forefoot region.

BOX 16.3 | **Conditions Associated with Heel Pain in Physically Active Young Individuals**

- **Plantar fasciitis**
- **Heel fat pad syndrome**
- **Achilles tendinitis/strain**
- **Retrocalcaneal bursitis**
- **Calcaneal stress fracture**

- **Calcaneal exostosis**
- **Contusion**
- **Infection**
- **Tarsal coalition**
- **Tarsal tunnel syndrome**

Sever's Disease

Sever's disease, or calcaneal **apophysitis**, is frequently seen in 7- to 10-year-olds. It is associated with growth spurts, decreased heel cord and hamstring flexibility, and other biomechanical abnormalities contributing to poor shock absorption (e.g., forefoot varus, hallux valgus, pes cavus, pes planus, and more commonly, forefoot pronation). Because the apophyseal plate is vertically oriented, it is particularly susceptible to shearing stresses from the gastrocnemius. Hard surfaces, poor-quality or worn-out athletic shoes, being kicked in the region, or landing off-balance may also precipitate the condition.

Signs and Symptoms

The individual complains of unilateral or bilateral, intermittent or continuous, posterior heel pain that occurs shortly after beginning a new sport or season. Pain tends to be worse during and after activity, but improves with rest. Although gait may be normal, the child may walk with a limp or exhibit a forceful heel strike. Point tenderness can be elicited at or just anterior to the insertion of the Achilles tendon along the posterior border of the calcaneus. Standing on the tiptoes can elicit pain. Other conditions that may also lead to heel pain should be ruled out prior to determining the treatment plan (BOX 16.3).

Stress Fractures

Stress fractures are often seen in running and jumping, particularly after a significant increase in training mileage, or a change in surface, intensity, or shoe type. Women with amenorrhea of longer than 6 months duration and oligomenorrhea have a higher incidence of stress fractures of the foot and leg during sport activity; however, women who use oral contraceptives tend to have significantly fewer stress fractures than do nonusers.[12,20]

Stress fractures can be generally classified as noncritical and critical. Noncritical stress fractures of the lower leg, foot, and ankle include the medial tibia, fibula, and metatarsals 2, 3, and 4. The neck of the second metatarsal is the most common location for a stress fracture, although it is also seen on the fourth and fifth metatarsals. Treatment usually requires relative rest. Physically active individuals may benefit from a short period of immobilization in a walking boot for up to 3 weeks, or in the case of metatarsal stress fractures, from a stiff sole shoe or steel insert. Return to activity is generally seen in 6 to 8 weeks.

Critical stress fractures require special attention due to a higher rate of nonunion. Common sites include the anterior tibia, medial malleolus, talus, navicular, fifth metatarsal, and sesamoids.

Stress fractures of the tibia and fibula result from repetitive stress to the leg leading to muscle fatigue. The resulting loss in shock absorption increases stress on the bone and periosteum. In the tibia, most stress fractures occur at the junction of the middle and distal thirds (most common site), the posterior medial tibial plateau, or just distal to the tibial tuberosity. Fibular stress fractures usually occur in the distal metadiaphyseal region. Because the fibula has a minimal role in weight bearing, it is believed that fibular stress fractures result from muscle traction and torsional forces.[21]

Signs and Symptoms

Pain from a stress fracture begins insidiously, increasing with activity and decreasing with rest; pain is usually limited to the fracture site.

Avulsion Fractures

Avulsion fractures may occur at the site of any ligamentous or tendinous attachment. Severe eversion ankle sprains may cause the deltoid ligament to avulse a portion of the distal medial malleolus rather than tearing the ligament. Inversion ankle sprains can provide sufficient overload to cause the plantar aponeurosis or peroneus brevis tendon to be pulled from the bone, avulsing the base of the fifth metatarsal, the so-called dancer's fracture (FIG. 16.18A).

A much more complicated avulsion fracture seen in sprinters and jumpers involves a transverse fracture into the proximal shaft of the fifth metatarsal at the junction of the diaphysis and metaphysis, called a Jones fracture (FIG. 16.18B). It is often overlooked in conjunction with a severe ankle sprain that involves plantar flexion and a strong adduction force to the forefoot.

Displaced Fractures and Fracture Dislocations

Severe fractures result from direct compression in acute trauma (e.g., falling from a height or being stepped on), or combined compression and shearing forces, as occurs during a severe twisting action. Because of the proximity of major blood vessels and nerves, many displaced and undisplaced fractures necessitate immediate immobilization and referral to the nearest trauma center. Because shock is possible in serious traumatic fractures, the emergency action plan should be activated. In some settings, this will include summoning of EMS to immobilize and transport the individual to the nearest medical facility.

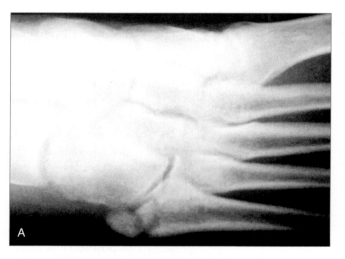

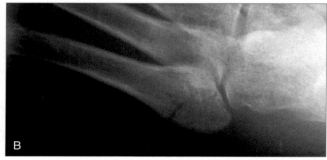

FIGURE 16.18 Avulsion fractures. **A.** A type I transverse fracture into the proximal shaft of the fifth metatarsal often is overlooked in cases of an inversion ankle sprain, resulting in a nonunion fracture. **B.** A type II fracture involves the styloid process of the fifth metatarsal.

Forefoot Fractures

Phalangeal fractures are caused by an axial load (e.g., jamming the toe into an immovable object) or direct trauma (e.g., crushing injury). Most are minor injuries, with the exception of a fracture to the great toe.

Signs and Symptoms

Swelling, ecchymosis, and pain are present. The individual is able to walk, but may have problems with footwear.

Metatarsal fractures are classified according to their anatomical location (i.e., neck, shaft, or base).

Signs and Symptoms

A single fracture tends to be minimally displaced because of the restraining forces of the IM ligaments. Swelling and pain are localized over the fracture site; pain increases with weight-bearing.

Tibia-Fibula Fractures

Nearly 60% of tibial fractures involve the middle and lower third of the tibia. The majority are closed.[22] Whether open or closed, this fracture is associated with complications, such as delayed union, nonunion, or malunion. The most common cause of an isolated tibial fracture is torsional force, resulting in either a spiral or an oblique fracture of the lower third of the tibia.

Signs and Symptoms

Gross deformity, gross bone motion at the suspected fracture site, crepitus, immediate swelling, extreme pain, or pain with motion should signal immediate action.

Ankle Fracture-Dislocations

Fracture-dislocations usually are caused by landing from a height with the foot in excessive eversion or inversion or by being kicked from behind while the foot is firmly planted on the ground.

Signs and Symptoms

Typically, the foot is displaced laterally at a gross angle to the lower leg and extreme pain is present. This position can compromise the posterior tibial artery and nerve.

Management

Because of the traumatic nature of this condition, the emergency plan should be activated, including summoning EMS. While waiting for EMS to arrive, the coach should monitor and treat the individual for shock as necessary.

THE COACH AND ON-SITE ASSESSMENT OF A FOOT, ANKLE, LOWER LEG CONDITION

Although pain, discomfort, or weakness may occur at a specific site, the lower extremities work as a unit to provide a foundation of support for the upright body, propulsion through space, absorption of shock, and adaptation to varying terrain. As such, assessment must include the entire lower extremity. While the coach should restrict their assessment to on-site injuries, it may be appropriate to initiate the history component of an assessment if an individual reports to an activity with complaints of pain or discomfort. In doing so, the coach can confirm the presence of an acute or chronic/overuse injury and proceed accordingly. When it becomes apparent that an injury is overuse in nature, the coach should refrain from any continued assessment and, instead, refer the individual to an appropriate healthcare practitioner.

It is important for the coach to recognize that many injuries to this region are rarely life-threatening. However, there are some conditions that will require activation of the emergency plan as they require immediate referral to a physician (Box 16.4).

BOX 16.4	**Conditions that Warrant Immediate Referral to a Physician**

- **Obvious deformity suggesting a dislocation, fracture, or ruptured Achilles tendon**
- **Significant loss of motion or muscle weakness**
- **Excessive joint swelling**
- **Possible epiphyseal or apophyseal injuries**
- **Abnormal sensation, or absent or weak pulse**
- **Gross joint instability**
- **Any unexplained pain that affects normal function**

The assessment begins as the coach approaches the individual or as the individual walks toward the coach. The focus should be on individual's overall presentation, attitude, and general posture. If the person is walking, it is important to determine any abnormal actions (e.g., presence of a limp; walking on the toes; walking on the heel). The history component of the exam should focus on the major complaint, mechanism of injury, and presence of any unusual sensations (i.e., pain; sounds; feelings). The location and onset of pain should be noted. An acute onset should lead one to suspect bony trauma or an acute ankle sprain until ruled out. A gradual onset of pain may signal inflammation from overuse of a muscle or the plantar fascia or the development of a stress fracture (see APPLICATION STRATEGY 16.2).

In continuing the observation component, a bilateral comparison should be performed as a means for recognizing any deformity, swelling, discoloration, or alignment abnormalities. Again, if the individual is able to walk, an assessment of gait (e.g., favoring one limb, an inability to perform a fluid motion; toe walking) could aid in identifying the structures involved and the seriousness of the condition.

Subsequent to the history and observation components of an assessment, the coach should have established a strong suspicion of the structures that may be damaged. If the coach elects to perform the testing component of the assessment, it should begin with active range of motion. Active movements can be performed with the individual in a seated or prone position. The motions should include

- Dorsiflexion of the ankle
- Plantar flexion of the ankle
- Pronation
- Supination
- Toe extension
- Toe flexion
- Toe abduction and adduction

If those motions are pain-free, the coach could continue with resisted range of motion and, if there are no positive findings, perform functional testing. Otherwise, the assessment should be considered complete.

APPLICATION STRATEGY 16.2

On-site Assessment of an Acute Foot, Ankle, Lower Leg Injury

HISTORY
- Chief complaint
  - What's wrong?
- Mechanism of injury
  - What happened? What were you doing?
  - Was there a direct blow?
  - What was the position of the foot and leg when the injury occurred?
  - Are you able to demonstrate how it happened?
- Pain
  - Location
    - Where is the pain?
    - Did the pain come on suddenly (acute) or gradually (overuse)?
    - Can you point to a location where it hurts the most?

- Type—Can you describe the pain (e.g., sharp, shooting, dull, achy, diffuse)?
- Intensity
  - What is the level of pain on a scale from 1 to 10?
  - Can you bear weight on the leg or balance on the leg?
- Sounds/feelings
  - Did you hear anything when the injury happened (e.g., pop; snap; crack)?
  - Did you feel any unusual sensations (e.g., tearing; knee giving way; locking; cracking) when the injury happened?
- Previous history
  - Have you ever injured your knee before? If so, what happened? What was the injury? Were you treated for it?

continued on page 316

APPLICATION STRATEGY 16.2 *continued*

On-site Assessment of an Acute Foot, Ankle, Lower Leg Injury

- OTHER important/helpful information
  - How old are you? (Remember that many problems are age-related.)
  - Have you made any changes in performance (i.e., technique; intensity; playing surface)?
  - Have you changed your training workouts (e.g., increased running distance; increased running intensity)?
  - Are you able to perform normal motions/ADLs?
- Is there anything else you would like to tell me about your condition?

OBSERVATION
- General presentation
  - Guarding
  - Moving easily; hesitant to move
  - Walking on toes; walking on heel
- Injury site appearance—deformity; swelling; discoloration; position of patella

PALPATION
The coach should only perform palpation if there is a clear understanding of what is being palpated and why? A productive assessment appropriate to the standard of care of a coach does not necessitate palpation.

TESTING
- Active Range of Motion (AROM)—bilateral comparison

- Dorsiflexion of the ankle
- Plantar flexion of the ankle
- Pronation
- Supination
- Toe extension
- Toe flexion
- Toe abduction and adduction
- Knee flexion (gastrocnemius)
- Passive range of motion should not be performed by the coach
  - Resistive range of motion
    The coach should only perform resistive range of motion for the muscles that govern the foot, ankle, and lower leg if
  - Instruction and approval for doing so has been obtained in advance from an appropriate healthcare practitioner
  - AROM is normal and pain-free as a way to assess strength
- Activity/sport-specific functional testing
  - Performance of active movements typical of the movements executed by the individual during sport or activity participation (including weight training)
  - Should assess strength, agility, flexibility, joint stability, endurance, coordination, balance, and activity-specific skill performance

SUMMARY

1. The true ankle (talocrural) joint is between the tibia, fibula, and talus. Plantar flexion and dorsiflexion occur at this joint. Motion at the subtalar joint involves inversion and eversion. The combination of calcaneal inversion, foot adduction, and plantar flexion is known as supination; calcaneal eversion is called foot abduction, and dorsiflexion is known as pronation.

2. The primary supporting structures of the plantar arches are the spring (calcaneonavicular) ligament, long plantar ligament, plantar fascia (plantar aponeurosis), and the short plantar (plantar CC) ligament. In addition, the tibialis posterior provides some support.

3. Congenital abnormalities, leg length discrepancy, muscle dysfunction (e.g., muscle imbalance), or a malalignment syndrome (e.g., pes cavus, pes

planus, pes equinus, and hammer or claw toes) can predispose an individual to several chronic injuries.

4. Generalized forefoot pain may result from intrinsic factors (e.g., excessive body weight, limited flexibility of the Achilles tendon, pronation, valgus heel, hammer toes, fallen metatarsal arch, pes planus, or pes cavus) or extrinsic factors (e.g., narrow toe box, improperly placed shoe cleats, repetitive jumping or running, or landing poorly from a height).

5. An acute anterior compartment syndrome is a medical emergency. Signs and symptoms include a recent history of trauma, a palpable firm mass in the anterior compartment, tight skin, and a diminished dorsalis pedis pulse.

6. Ankle sprains are classified as Grade I, II, or III based on the progression of anatomical structures damaged and the subsequent disability. Incersion sprains involve plantar flexion and inversion, the ATFL is torn first, followed by the calcaneal fibular ligament. In eversion ankle sprains, the deltoid ligament is injured; there may also be an associated avulsion fracture of one or both malleoli.

7. Common sites for tendon injuries include the Achilles tendon just proximal to its insertion into the calcaneus, the tibialis posterior just behind the medial malleolus, the tibialis anterior just under the extensor retinaculum, and the peroneal tendons behind the lateral malleolus or at the distal attachment on the styloid process of the fifth metatarsal.

8. Risk factors for Achilles tendinitis include a tight heel cord, foot malalignment deformities, a recent change in shoes or running surface, a sudden increase in workload (e.g., distance or intensity), or changes in the exercise environment (e.g., changing footwear, or excessive hill climbing or impact-loading activities, such as jumping).

9. Medial tibial stress syndrome is a periostitis along the posteromedial tibial border, usually in the distal third, not associated with a stress fracture or compartment syndrome. Signs and symptoms include point tenderness in a 3- to 6-cm area along the distal posteromedial tibial border, and pain and weakness with resisted plantar flexion or standing on tiptoe.

10. Exertional compartment syndrome is characterized by exercise-induced pain and swelling that are relieved by rest. The anterior compartment is most frequently affected, and if so, mild foot drop or paresthesia (or both) may be present. Fascial defects or hernias also may be present in the distal third of the leg over the anterior intramuscular septum.

11. Fractures of the lower leg, ankle, and foot may involve
    • Freiberg's disease (i.e., avascular necrosis of the second metatarsal head)
    • Sever's disease (i.e., calcaneal apophysis)
    • Stress fractures (neck of the second metatarsal is most common)
    • Avulsion fractures (e.g., styloid process of the fifth metatarsal, and medial and lateral malleoli)
    • Displaced fractures or fracture-dislocations

12. Conditions that warrant special attention include
    • Obvious deformity suggesting a dislocation, fracture, or ruptured Achilles tendon
    • Significant loss of motion or weakness in a myotome
    • Excessive joint swelling
    • Possible epiphyseal or apophyseal injuries
    • Abnormal reflexes or sensation, or absent or weak pulse
    • Gross joint instability
    • Any unexplained pain

APPLICATION QUESTIONS

1. The defensive back on a high school football team reports to the coach that he is experiencing throbbing pain on the plantar side of the great toe of the right foot. The pain has been present for the last 2 days. The athlete does not recall a specific mechanism or time of onset. The pain increases significantly when the athlete pushes off the right foot to block an opponent. For the past 3 days, the team was forced to practice indoors on a composite-type floor. What injury should be suspected? Why? How should the coach manage this situation?

2. During a physical education class, a 16 year old was kicked in the anterolateral aspect of the lower leg during a soccer game. The student continued to play the remaining 10 minutes of the game. The last 20 minutes of the class was used to provide verbal instructions and demonstrations. The student was not physically active during that time. By the end of the instructional session, the student began to experience severe pain to the injured area. In observing the leg, the physical education teacher noted a firm mass and tight skin over the injured site. What condition should be suspected? What further assessment should be performed by the physical education teacher? How should the physical education teacher manage this condition?

3. A 30-year-old client at a fitness club sustained an ankle injury while playing basketball. The assessment by the fitness specialist suggested a moderate to severe ankle inversion sprain. How should the fitness specialist mange the situation?

_____

_____

4. One of your clients at a fitness club is a slightly overweight novice runner and is in the third week of training for a 10 K run. Prior to the start of a training session, he reports the following symptoms: excruciating pain in the anteromedial hindfoot upon arising in the morning, which disappears within 5 to 10 minutes; point tenderness just distal to the medial calcaneal tubercle; and pain that increases with weight bearing. What condition may be present? How should this injury be managed? Should the individual be permitted to continue his normal workout?

_____

_____

5. A fifth-grade school physical education teacher is conducting a 4-week unit on physical fitness. The class, which meets for 50 minutes every day, involves a variety of activities, which include running, jumping, and pivoting/cutting type maneuvers. In anticipation of the potential injuries, what conditions should be familiar to the physical education teacher because they could lead to heel pain in young individuals (e.g., fifth grade students)?

_____

_____

6. A 40-year-old apparently healthy male comes to your exercise facility indicating that he has just finished physical therapy following a Grade III inversion ankle sprain. His physical therapist strongly advises him to work on increasing strength of the muscles that govern of the foot, ankle, and lower leg. Demonstrate exercises used to increase strength of the those muscles.

_____

_____

7. A high school cross country runner reports to the coach that he has been experiencing lower leg pain for the past two weeks. In completing the history component of an assessment, the coach learns the following: pain is near the distal 1/3 of the medial aspect of the tibia; the pain is usually a dull ache, but there are times when it can be sharp and penetrating. In the last 2 days, the pain has been present before, during, and after activity. The runner indicates that the pain is starting to have an impact on his performance. How should the coach mange this condition? Why?

_____

_____

8. A 16-year-old participant on a recreational basketball team falls after jumping for a rebound. The individual is immediately in severe pain. In reaching the individual, the coach does not observe a gross deformity, but a total loss of function is evident. How should the coach mange this situation? Why?

_____

_____

REFERENCES

1. Puffer JC. 2001. The sprained ankle. Clin Cornerstone, 3(5):38–49.
2. McKay GD, Goldie PA, Payne WR, and Oakes BW. 2001. Ankle injuries in basketball: injury rate and risk factors. Br J Sports Med, 35(2):103–108.
3. Cohen RS, and Balcom TA. 2003. Current treatment options for ankle injuries: lateral ankle sprain, Achilles tendonitis, and Achilles rupture. Curr Sports Med Reports, 2(5):251–261.
4. Caulfield B, and Garrett M. 2004. Changes in ground reaction force during jump landing in subjects with functional instability of the ankle joint. Clin Biomech, 19(6):617–621.
5. Wang Q, Whittle M, Cunningham J, Kenwright J, 1997. Fibula and its ligaments in load transmission and ankle joint stability. Clin Orthop, (330):261–270.

6. Leardini A, Stagni R, and O'Connor JJ. 2001. Mobility of the subtalar joint in the intact ankle complex. J Biomech, 34(6):805–809.

7. Gefen A. 2003. The in vivo elastic properties of the plantar fascia during the contact phase of walking. Foot Ankle Int, 24(3):238–244.

8. Ferber R, Davis IM, and Williams DS. 2003. Gender differences in lower extremity mechanics during running. Clin Biomech, 18(4):350–357.

9. Korhonen MT, Mero A, and Suominen H. 2003. Age-related differences in 100-m sprint performances in male and female master runners. Med Sci Sports Exerc, 35(8):1419–1428.

10. O'Connor KM, and Hamill J. 2004. The role of selected extrinsic foot muscles during running. Clin Biomech, 19(1):71–77.

11. McClure SK, Adams JE, and Dahn DL. 2005. Common musculoskeletal disorder in women. Mayo Clin Proc, 80(6):796–802.

12. McBryde AM, and Hoffman JL. 2004. Injuries to the foot and ankle in athletes. South Med J, 97(8):738–741.

13. Clanton TO, and Porter DA. 1997. Primary care of foot and ankle injuries in the athlete. Clin Sports Med, 16(3):435–466.

14. Norkus SA, and Floyd RT. 2001. The anatomy and mechanisms of syndesmotic ankle sprains. J Ath Train, 36(1):68–73.

15. Smith AH, and Bach BR Jr. 2004. High ankle sprains. Phys Sportsmed, 32(12):39–43.

16. Brown DE. Ankle and leg injuries. In The team physician's handbook, edited by MB Mellion, et al. Philadelphia, PA: Hanley & Belfus, 2002.

17. Harmon KG, and Rubin A. 2002. Plantar fasciitis: prescribing effective treatments. Phys Sportsmed, 30(7):21–25.

18. Davey JR, Rorabeck CH, and Fowler PJ. 1984. The tibialis posterior muscle compartment: an unrecognized cause of exertional compartmental syndrome. Am J Sports Med, 12(5):391–397.

19. Edwards P, and Myerson MS. 1996. Exertional compartment syndrome of the leg: steps for expedient return to activity. Phys Sportsmed, 24(4):31–46.

20. Blue JM, and Matthews LS. 1997. Leg injuries. Clin Sports Med, 16(3):467–478.

21. Wilder RP, and Sethi S. 2004. Overuse injuries: tendinopathies, stress fractures, compartment syndrome and shin splints. Clin Sports Med, 23(1):55–81.

22. Garl TC, Alexander L, Ahlfeld SK, Rink L, et al. 1997. Tibial fracture in a basketball player: treatment dilemmas and complications. Phys Sportsmed, 25(6):41–53.

Special Considerations

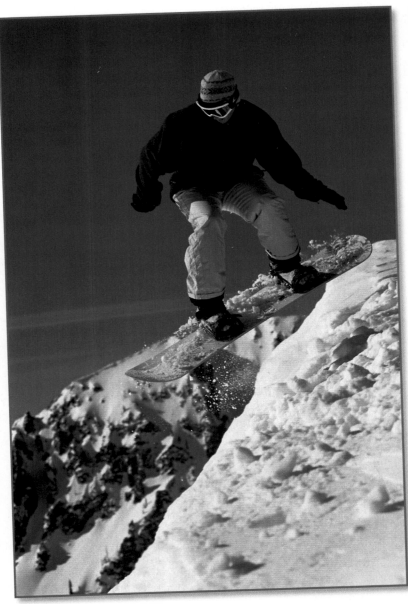

17

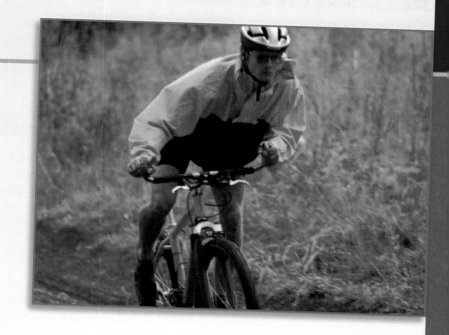

ENVIRONMENTAL CONDITIONS

KEY TERMS

acclimatization

apnea

cold diuresis

diuretics

homeostasis

hyperhydrate

hyperthermia

hypothalamus

hypothermia

relative humidity

Raynaud's syndrome

thermoregulation

urticaria

LEARNING OUTCOMES

1. Describe the activation of heat-regulating mechanisms in the body, including the methods used to generate heat via internal and external sources.

2. Explain methods used to prevent heat illness.

3. Identify the signs and symptoms of heat-related conditions.

4. Describe the appropriate management of heat-related conditions.

5. Differentiate between frostbite and systemic cooling, and describe the appropriate management of each condition.

6. Explain the dangers of lightening, and list lightening-safety guidelines for sport and exercise participation.

Environmental conditions affect even the best-conditioned individuals. Participation in physical activity on hot, humid days or on cold, windy days predisposes individuals to **hyperthermia** and **hypothermia**, respectively. In addition, exercising during thunderstorms that produce lightning can be extremely dangerous. These environmental conditions are discussed in this chapter.

HEAT-RELATED CONDITIONS

The process by which the body maintains body temperature is called **thermoregulation**. It is controlled primarily by the **hypothalamus**, which is a region of the diencephalon forming the floor of the third ventricle of the brain. **Hyperthermia**, or elevated body temperature, occurs when internal heat production exceeds external heat loss. The hypothalamus is a gland that maintains **homeostasis**, or a state of equilibrium within the body, by initiating cooling or heat-retention mechanisms to achieve a relatively constant body core temperature between 36.1 and 37.8°C (97 to 100°F). The body core encompasses the skull, thoracic, and abdominal area.

Internal Heat Regulation

During exercise, the body gains heat either from external sources (i.e., environmental temperatures) or from internal processes (FIG. 17.1). Much of the internal heat is generated during muscular activity through energy metabolism. The act of shivering can increase the total metabolic rate by three- to five-fold. During sustained, vigorous exercise, the metabolic rate can increase by 20- to 25-fold above the resting level. Theoretically, such a rate can increase core temperature by approximately 1°C (1.8°F) every 5 to 7 minutes.

During exercise, the circulatory system must deliver oxygen to the working muscles and heated blood from deep tissues (i.e., core) to the periphery (i.e., shell) for dissipation. The increased blood flow to the muscles and skin is made possible by increasing cardiac output and redistributing regional blood flow (i.e., blood flow to the visceral organs is reduced).

As exercise begins, heart rate and cardiac output increase, while superficial venous and arterial blood vessels dilate to divert warm blood to the skin surface. Heat is dissipated when the warm blood flushes into skin capillaries. This is evident when the face becomes flushed and reddened on a hot day or after exercise. When the individual is in a resting state and the air temperature is less than 30.6°C (87°F), approximately two-thirds of the body's normal heat loss results from conduction, convection, and radiation (BOX 17.1). As air temperature approaches skin temperature and exceeds 30.6°C, evaporation becomes the predominant means of heat dissipation.

Relative humidity is the most important factor in determining the effectiveness of evaporative heat loss. Relative humidity is the ratio of water in the ambient air to the total quantity of moisture that can be carried in air at a particular ambient temperature. It is expressed as a percentage. For example, 65% relative humidity means that ambient air contains 65% of the air's moisture-carrying capability at the specific temperature. When humidity is high, the

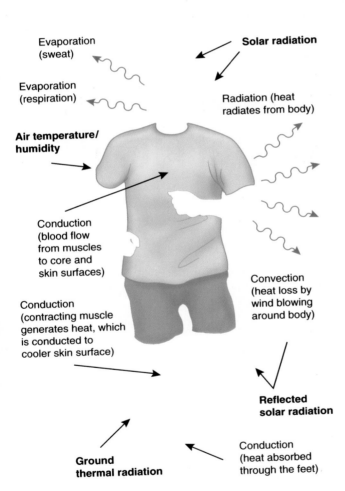

FIGURE 17.1 Heat gain and loss. Heat produced within working muscles is transferred to the body's core and skin. During exercise, body heat is dissipated into the surrounding environment by radiation, conduction, convection, and evaporation. Straight lines represent heat gain, and wavy lines indicate heat loss.

BOX 17.1   Methods of Heat Exchange

- **Radiation**—The loss of heat from a warmer object to a cooler object in the form of infrared waves (thermal energy) without physical contact. For example, when temperatures of surrounding objects in the environment, such as the sun or hot artificial turf, exceed skin temperature, radiant heat is absorbed by the body.

- **Conduction**—The direct transfer of heat through a liquid, solid, or gas from a warm object to a cooler object. For example, a football player can absorb heat through the feet simply by standing on hot artificial turf.

- **Convection**—Transfer of heat depends on conduction from the skin to the water or air next to it. The effectiveness of heat loss depends on how fast the air (or water) next to the body is exchanged once it becomes warmer. If air movement is slow, air molecules next to the skin are warmed and act as insulation. In contrast, if warmer air molecules are continually replaced by cooler air molecules, as occurs on a breezy day or in a room with a fan, heat loss

increases as the air currents carry heat away. In water, the body loses heat more rapidly by convection while swimming than while lying motionless.

- **Evaporation**—The most effective heat-loss mechanism used to cool the body. Sweat evaporates when molecules in the water absorb heat from the environment and become energetic enough to escape as a gas. As core temperature rises during exercise or illness, peripheral blood vessels dilate and sweat glands are stimulated to produce noticeable sweat, which can amount to a loss of 1.5 to 2.5 liters of body water in 1 hour. On a hot, dry day, sweating is responsible for more than 80% of heat loss. The total sweat vaporized from the skin depends on three factors:
  - The skin surface exposed to the environment
  - The temperature and relative humidity of the ambient air
  - The convective air currents around the body

---

ambient vapor pressure approaches that of the moist skin, and evaporation is greatly reduced. Therefore, this avenue for heat loss is closed, even though large quantities of sweat bead on the skin, eventually, roll off. In this form, sweating represents a useless water loss that can lead to a dangerous state of dehydration and overheating. When temperature and relative humidity are combined, the values can be charted on the heat index to determine the risk of potential heat illness (FIG. 17.2).

In addition to heat loss through sweating, a basal level of body heat loss exists because of the continuous evaporation of water from the lungs, from the mucosa of the mouth, and through the skin. This averages approximately 350 mL of water as it seeps through the skin every day, as well as another 300 mL of water vaporized from mucous membranes in the respiratory passages and mouth. The latter is illustrated when you "see your breath" in very cold weather. In total, it is not uncommon for an individual to lose 1.5 to 2.5 L/hour of water during exercise. This translates into a loss of 3 to 6 pounds of body weight per hour. During a 2- to 3-hour workout, an individual could lose from 6 to 12 pounds of body weight. Although an individual may continually drink water throughout an exercise bout, less than 50% of the fluid lost is replenished. This "voluntary dehydration" was recognized long ago and continues to be characterized by researchers.[1] Accordingly, a physically active individual should drink as much fluid as possible before exercise and

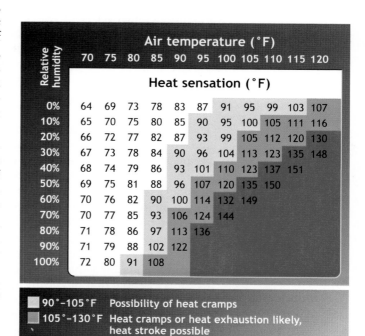

FIGURE 17.2 The heat stress index. If the relative humidity and ambient air temperature are known, the heat stress index can be consulted to determine the relative degree of heat stress.

BOX 17.2	**Physiologic Changes Seen After 10 Days of Heat Exposure**

- **Heart rate and body temperature decrease**
- **Peripheral blood flow and plasma volume increase**
- **Sweating capacity nearly doubles**
- **Sweat becomes more diluted (i.e., less salt is lost)**
- **Sweat is distributed more evenly over the skin surface**
- **The increased perspiration rate is sustained over a longer period of time**

before thirst is perceived during exercise. It is critical to drink beyond the perception of satisfying one's thirst to **hyperhydrate** the body to prevent voluntary dehydration.

Factors that Modify Heat Tolerance

Several factors can affect an individual's tolerance to heat. **Acclimatization** and proper hydration are among the most critical in preventing heat illness.

Acclimatization

Exercising moderately during repeated heat exposures can result in physiologic adaptation to a hot environment, which can improve performance and heat tolerance (Box 17.2). In general, the major acclimatization occurs during the first week of heat exposure and is complete after 10 to 14 days. Only 2 to 4 hours of daily heat exposure is required. The first several exercise sessions should be light and last approximately 15 to 20 minutes. Thereafter, exercise sessions can progressively increase in duration and intensity. Well-acclimatized individuals should train for 1 to 2 hours under the same heat conditions that will be present during their competitive event.[2] Proper hydration is essential for the acclimatization process to be effective.

Heat acclimatization is lost rapidly, however. As a general rule, 1 day of heat acclimatization is lost over 2 to 3 days without heat exposure, with the major benefits being lost within 2 to 3 weeks after returning to a more temperate environment.

Fluid Rehydration

The primary objective of fluid replacement is to maintain plasma volume so that circulation and sweating occur at optimal levels. Dehydration progressively decreases plasma volume, peripheral blood flow, sweating, and stroke volume (i.e., the quantity of blood ejected with each heartbeat), and it leads to a compensatory increase in heart rate. The general deterioration in circulatory and thermoregulatory efficiency increases the risk of heat illness, impairs physiologic functions, and decreases physical performance.

Thirst is not an adequate indicator of water needs during exercise. Physically active individuals may not become thirsty until systemic water loss equals 2% of body weight.[3] Rather, thirst develops in response to increases in osmolality and blood sodium concentrations and decreases in plasma volume caused by dehydration.

It is essential that physically active individuals begin an exercise session when they are well hydrated and have ready access to adequate water replacement throughout the exercise session to prevent dehydration. Pre-exercise hydration should involve 17 to 20 oz of water or a sports drink 2 to 3 hours before exercise and 7 to 10 oz of water or a sports drink 10 to 20 minutes after exercise.[4] Cold liquids, especially water, empty from the stomach and small intestines significantly faster than warm fluids do. Fluid replacement during exercise should approximate the losses of sweat and urine, resulting in a loss of body weight no greater than 2% weight. This generally requires 7 to 10 oz of fluid every 10 to 20 minutes.[4] Postexercise hydration should be completed within 2 hours of the exercise bout. This should include water, carbohydrates to replenish glycogen stores, and electrolytes to speed rehydration. Several steps can be taken to

BOX 17.3   **Strategies to Reduce the Risk of Dehydration**

HEALTHY POPULATION

- Drink 8 to 12 cups (8 oz/cup) of fluid at least 24 hours before an event.
- Drink at least 16 oz of fluid 2 hours before exercise and again approximately 20 minutes before exercise.
- When exercising for 1 hour or more, drink at least 5 to 10 oz of fluid every 15 to 20 minutes. Drink beyond satisfying thirst.
- Drink cool fluids containing less than 8% carbohydrates.
- Use individual water bottles to accurately measure fluid consumption.

- Freeze fluid in plastic bottles before exercise; the bottles will thaw and stay cool during exercise sessions.
- Record pre- and post-exercise weight to determine if excessive and unsafe weight loss has occurred.
- Replenish lost fluid with at least 24 oz of fluid for every pound of body weight lost.
- Avoid caffeine, alcohol, and carbonated beverages.

CHILDREN (IN ADDITION TO ABOVE)

- Allow 10 to 14 days of acclimatization.
- Reduce intensity of prolonged exercise.

ensure adequate hydration before, during, and after exercise (Box 17.3). In order to prevent dehydration, fluids must be ingested and absorbed by the body. Running through sprinklers or pouring water over the head may feel cool and satisfying, but it does not prevent dehydration. A standard rule is to drink until thirst is quenched—and then drink a few more ounces.

An easy method to determine if enough fluids are being consumed is to monitor the color and volume of the urine. An average adult's urine amounts to 1.2 quarts in a 24-hour period. Urination of a full bladder usually occurs four times each day. Within 60 minutes of exercise, passing light-colored urine of normal to above-normal volume is a good indicator of adequate hydration. If the urine is dark yellow in color, of a small volume, and of strong odor, the individual needs to continue drinking. Ingesting vitamin supplements often can result in a dark-yellow urine; as such, urine color, volume, and odor must all be considered when determining hydration status.[1,3]

Electrolyte Replacement

The minerals sodium, chloride, magnesium, and potassium are called electrolytes, because they are dissolved in the body as electrically charged particles called ions. Electrolytes regulate fluid balance, nerve conduction, and muscle contractions. Sweat contains high levels of sodium and chloride but little potassium, calcium, or magnesium. Ionic concentrations in sweat are greatly influenced by the rate of perspiration and acclimatization. 4 L of perspiration equals an approximately 5.8% loss of body weight. Such a loss can lower the body's content of sodium and chloride by 5 to 7% and of potassium by less than 1.2%.[5] Because the body loses more water than electrolytes, the ionic concentration of these minerals in the body fluids rises. Accordingly, during periods of heavy perspiration, the need to replace body water is greater than the need to replace electrolytes. Lost electrolytes are readily replenished by adding a slight amount of salt to food or by eating potassium-rich foods, such as citrus fruits and bananas. A glass of orange or tomato juice replaces almost all the potassium, calcium, and magnesium excreted in approximately 3 L of sweat.

Electrolyte solutions are unnecessary for individuals with normal diets. Individuals demanding peak performance in competitions of greater than 1 hour or during intense intermittent exercise, however, may benefit from carbohydrate drinks.[4,6] Commercial drinks may be used but should be cooler than ambient temperature (10 to 15°C [50 to 59°F]), flavored to enhance palatability, range between 4 and 8% of multiple transportable carbohydrate, and contain a small amount of sodium chloride.[4,6,7] Electrolyte drinks should be consumed during the pre-exercise hydration session (2 to 3 hours pre-exercise) and 30 minutes before exercise. During exercise, 1 L of a 6% carbohydrate drink is recommended every hour. Fruit juices, carbohydrate gels, sodas, and some sports drinks have carbohydrate concentrations of greater than 8% and are not recommended during an exercise session as the sole beverage.[4] While maintaining hydration, the participant should avoid **diuretics**, such as excessive amounts of protein, caffeinated drinks (e.g., soda, tea, and coffee), chocolate, and alcoholic beverages.

Clothing

Light-colored, lightweight, porous clothing is preferred to dark, heavyweight, nonporous material. Clothing made of 100% cotton is not recommended, especially in hot climates, because moisture in sweat-soaked cotton does not evaporate easily. Evaporative heat loss occurs only when clothing is thoroughly wet and perspiration can evaporate. Changing into a dry shirt simply prolongs the time between sweating and cooling. Heavy sweat suits or rubberized plastic suits produce high relative humidity close to the skin and retard evaporation, severely increasing the risk of heat illness. Even when wearing only football helmets and loose-fitting, porous jerseys and shorts, 50% of the body surface of football players can be sealed and evaporative cooling limited. The increased metabolic rate that is needed to carry the weight of the equipment and the increased temperature on artificial surfaces also can increase the risk of heat illness. As such, football players should initially practice in t-shirts, shorts, and low-cut socks. On hot, humid days, uniforms should not be worn, and if possible, shoulder pads and helmets should be removed often to allow radiation and evaporative cooling. Because much of the body's heat escapes through the head, helmets used in noncontact sports (e.g., cycling) should allow adequate airflow and evaporation.

Age

Children have a lower sweating capacity and a higher core temperature during exposure to heat as compared to adolescents and adults. This occurs even though children have a higher number of heat-activated sweat glands per unit of skin. Sweat composition in children also differs. Children excrete higher concentrations of sodium and chlorine and lower concentrations of lactate and potassium. Therefore, children do not benefit from electrolyte beverages and should use only cool water for fluid replacement.[8] In addition, children require a longer time to acclimatize to heat as compared to adolescents and young adults.

In general, middle-aged and older men and women are less tolerant to exercising in heat. When compared to younger men and women, older men and women develop higher heart rates, higher skin and core temperatures, and lower sweat rates during exercise in heat. Aging can lead to a limited peripheral vascular response that can impair local vasodilation. Onset of sweating also appears to be delayed with advancing age, and the sweating response appears to be blunted. This may result from either a limitation in sweat gland output or a dehydration-limited sweat output if fluid replacement is insufficient. In addition, older individuals do not recover from dehydration as effectively as younger individuals do, which may be related to a blunted thirst drive. This may make older individuals more prone to dehydration that could adversely affect the thermoregulatory capacity.[9]

Sex

The general consensus is that women can tolerate the physiologic and thermal stress of exercise at least as well as men of comparable fitness and level of acclimatization. Both sexes can acclimatize to a similar degree; however, sweating does differ. Although women possess more heat-activated sweat glands per unit of skin area as compared to men, women sweat less than men do. Compared with men, women begin to sweat at higher skin and core temperatures, produce less sweat for a comparable heat-exercise load, yet show an equivalent heat tolerance. Women probably rely more on circulatory mechanisms for heat dissipation, whereas men rely on evaporative cooling. The production of less sweat to maintain thermal balance can provide women with significant protection from dehydration during exercise at a high ambient temperature.

Diuretics, Supplements, and Medications

Individuals taking diuretics or laxatives should be carefully observed for dehydration. These agents increase fluid loss, reduce plasma volume, and may adversely affect thermoregulation and cardiovascular function. Substances used to induce vomiting and diarrhea also leads to dehydration and may cause excessive electrolyte loss with accompanying muscle weakness. Some nutritional supplements, such as creatine phosphate, require additional fluids to decrease the risk of heat cramps and other associated heat illnesses. Medications, such as β-adrenergics, anticholinergics, antihistamines, β-blockers, calcium channel blockers, and tricyclic antidepressants can impair the body's normal mechanisms of dissipating heat, which may result in a dangerously high core temperature.[10] Before taking supplements or medications, an individual should be fully informed regarding the proper use and possible side-effects of the substances.

Practice Schedules

On hot, humid days, workouts, practices, and competitions should be scheduled during early morning or evening hours to avoid the worst heat of the day (i.e., 11:00 AM to 3:00 PM). It also may be necessary to allow frequent water breaks (i.e., 10 minutes every half an hour), shorten practices, and lessen the exercise intensity. Whenever possible, participants should be moved out of direct sunlight (e.g., shade trees and tents), and restrictive equipment (e.g., pads and helmets) should be removed frequently.

Weight Charts

Measuring pre- and post-exercise weight can decrease the risk of heat illness. A fluid loss equivalent to as little as 1% of body mass is associated with a significant increase in rectal temperature. For each liter of sweat-loss dehydration, the heart rate can increase by approximately eight beats per minute, with a corresponding decrease in cardiac output. When water loss reaches 4 to 5% of body mass, a definite impairment is noted in physical work capacity, physiologic function, and thermoregulation. A rule of thumb is that for every pound of water lost, 24 oz (i.e., three cups) of fluid should be ingested, meaning that 150% of the fluid loss during exercise is replenished.[5]

In addition to fluids, carbohydrates also should be ingested within 30 minutes postexercise, especially those with high water content (e.g., melons or tomatoes). Even under the best circumstances, 24 hours is needed to fully restore the fluids and muscle glycogen that are used during just 2 hours of strenuous exercise. Before the next exercise period, the individual should ingest 3.5 to 4.5 g of carbohydrates per pound of body weight. Alcohol should be avoided. Lost fluid should be replaced and weight normalized before the next episode of exercise.

Identifying Individuals at Risk

Healthy individuals at risk for heat illness include those who are poorly acclimated or conditioned, those who are inexperienced with heat illness, those with large muscle mass, children, wheelchair athletes, Special Olympians, and elderly people. Others who are at risk are listed in Box 17.4.

Heat Illnesses

If the signs and symptoms of heat stress (e.g., thirst, fatigue, lethargy, flushed skin, headache, and visual disturbances) are not treated, cardiovascular compensation begins to fail, and a series of progressive complications, termed as heat illness, can result. The various forms of heat illness, in order of severity, include exercise-associated muscle (heat) cramps, exercise (heat) exhaustion, and exertional heat stroke. Although symptoms often overlap between the conditions, failure to take immediate action can result in severe dehydration and possible death.

Exercise-Associated Muscle (Heat) Cramps

Heat cramps are painful, involuntary muscle spasms caused by excessive water and electrolyte loss during and after intense exercise in the heat. Paradoxically, the condition most frequently occurs in well-conditioned, acclimatized, physically active individuals who have overexerted themselves in hot weather and rehydrated only with water. Predisposing factors include lack of acclimatization, use of diuretics or laxatives, and sodium depletion in the normal diet. The condition can be prevented by ingesting copious amounts of water and increasing the daily intake of salt through a normal diet several days before the period of heat stress.

| BOX 17.4 | **Individuals at Risk for Heat Illness** |

HEALTHY INDIVIDUALS

- Age extremes (children, elderly persons)
- Excessive muscle mass, large, or obese
- Poorly acclimatized or conditioned
- Previous history of heat illness
- Salt or water depletion
- Sleep deprived

THOSE WITH ACUTE ILLNESSES

- Illnesses that involve fever
- Gastrointestinal illnesses

THOSE WITH CHRONIC ILLNESSES

- Alcoholism and substance abuse (e.g., amphetamines, cocaine, hallucinogens, laxatives, diuretics, narcotics)
- Cardiac disease

- Certain nutritional supplements (e.g., creatine phosphate)
- Cystic fibrosis
- Eating disorders
- Medications (e.g., anticholinergics, antidepressants, antihistamines, diuretics, neuroleptics, β-blockers)
- Skin problems with impaired sweating (e.g., miliaria rubra or miliaria profunda)
- Uncontrolled diabetes mellitus or hypertension
- Using oil- or gel-based sunscreens that block evaporative cooling

WHEELCHAIR ATHLETES WHO

- Have a spinal cord injury (alters thermoregulation)
- Limit water intake to avoid going to the bathroom

Signs and Symptoms

Exercise-associated muscle cramps commonly occur in the calf and abdominal muscles, but they also may involve the muscles of the upper extremity. Signs and symptoms mimic dehydration and include thirst, sweating, transient muscle cramps, and fatigue. Body temperature is not usually elevated, and the skin remains moist and cool. Pulse and respiration may be normal or slightly elevated. Dizziness may be present.

Management

The coach should require the individual to stop activity, provide fluids (if available, fluids containing sodium), and begin mild, passive stretching of the involved muscle(s) and ice massage over the affected area. The individual should ingest enough fluids to drink beyond the point of satisfying thirst. A recumbent position may allow more rapid redistribution of blood flow to cramping leg muscles.[2] The individual should be watched carefully, because this condition may precipitate heat exhaustion or heat stroke.

Exercise (Heat) Exhaustion

Exercise (heat) exhaustion usually occurs in unacclimatized individuals during the first few intense exercise sessions on a hot day. Those who wear protective equipment or heavy uniforms also are at greater risk, because evaporation through the material may be retarded. It is a "functional" illness and is not associated with organ damage. Heat exhaustion is caused by ineffective circulatory adjustments compounded by a depletion of extracellular fluid, especially plasma volume, as a result of excessive sweating. Blood pools in the dilated peripheral vessels, which dramatically reduces the central blood volume necessary to maintain cardiac output.

Signs and Symptoms

Thirst, headache, dizziness, light-headedness, mild anxiety, fatigue, profuse sweating, weak and rapid pulse, and low blood pressure in the upright position are common signs and symptoms (FIG. 17.3A). The individual may appear to be ashen and gray, with cool, clammy skin. An uncoordinated gait often is present. Sweating may be reduced if the person is dehydrated, but

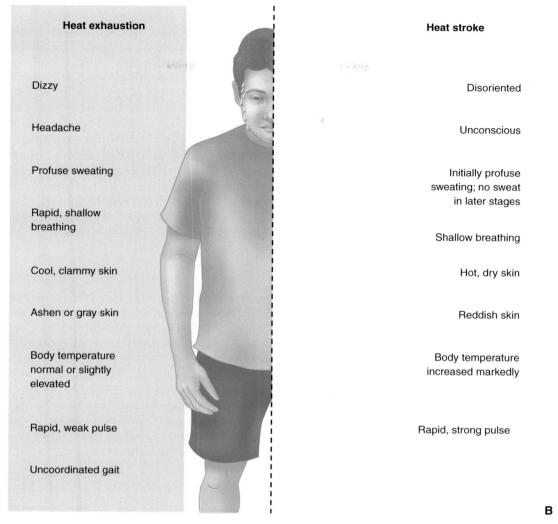

Heat exhaustion

Dizzy

Headache

Profuse sweating

Rapid, shallow
breathing

Cool, clammy skin

Ashen or gray skin

Body temperature
normal or slightly
elevated

Rapid, weak pulse

Uncoordinated gait

Heat stroke

Disoriented

Unconscious

Initially profuse
sweating; no sweat
in later stages

Shallow breathing

Hot, dry skin

Reddish skin

Body temperature
increased markedly

Rapid, strong pulse

A

B

FIGURE 17.3 Signs and symptoms of heat exhaustion and heat stroke. **A.** Heat exhaustion. **B.** Heat stroke.

body temperature generally does not exceed 39.5°C (103°F). The individual may have an urge to defecate or may experience diarrhea. Significant neurological impairment is absent.

Management

The individual should be moved immediately to a cool place. All equipment and unnecessary clothing should be removed. Rapid cooling of the body should be initiated. Two effective cooling methods are evaporative cooling and ice immersion. Evaporative cooling involves spraying copious amounts of tap water over the individual's skin with air fanning. Ice immersion involves placing the individual into a pool or tub of cold water (~1 to 15°C [35 to 59°F]).[2,11] Circulation of the water may enhance cooling. If immersion in ice water is not available, other cooling methods should be used. These may include wrapping in cool, wet, iced towels; using fans; and applying crushed-ice packs to the neck, axilla, and groin. Fans and cool-mist machines, however, have limited use during humid conditions. It is essential to administer copious amounts of cool fluids with a diluted electrolyte solution as quickly as possible.

Elevating the legs to reduce postural hypotension also can be effective. If recovery is not rapid and uneventful, the individual should be transported to the closest medical facility; intravenous fluids may need to be administered. Some individuals, particularly endurance athletes exercising in the heat, may require as much as 4 L of fluid replacement.[12] Physical activity should not be resumed until the individual has returned to the pre-dehydrated state and been cleared by a physician.

Exertional Heat Stroke

Exertional heat stroke is the least common, but most serious, heat-related illness. In football, heat stroke is second only to head injuries as the most frequent cause of death. The condition also is seen in dehydrated distance runners and wrestlers. Heat stroke almost always is preceded by prolonged, strenuous physical exercise in individuals who are poorly acclimatized or seen in situations during which evaporation of perspiration is blocked.

During exercise, metabolic heat continues to rise. Decreased blood plasma volume causes the heart to beat faster and work harder to pump blood through the circulatory system. The thermoregulatory system is overloaded, and the body's cooling mechanisms fail to dissipate the rising core temperature. The hypothalamus shuts down all heat-control mechanisms, including the sweat glands in an effort to conserve water loss. A vicious circle is created in which, as temperature increases, the metabolic rate increases, which in turn increases heat production. The skin becomes hot and dry. As the temperature continues to rise, permanent brain damage may occur. Core temperature can rise to 40.6°C (105°F), and it has been known to reach 41.7 to 42.2°C (107 to 108°F). If untreated, death is imminent. Mortality is directly related to the magnitude and duration of the hyperthermia.

Signs and Symptoms

By definition, the condition occurs when body temperature is elevated to a level that causes characteristic clinical and pathological damage to body tissues and affects multiple organs. Initial symptoms include a feeling of burning up, confusion, disorientation, irrational behavior, agitation, profuse sweating, and an unsteady gait. As the condition deteriorates, sweating ceases. The skin is hot and dry and appears to be reddened or flushed (FIG. 17.3B). The individual hyperventilates or breathes deeply and has dilated pupils, giving the appearance of a glassy stare. As core temperature rises, the pulse becomes rapid and strong (as high as 150 to 170 beats per minute). The individual may become hysterical or delirious. Tissue damage by excessive body heat leads to vasomotor collapse, shallow breathing, decreased blood pressure, and a rapid and weak pulse. Muscle twitching, vomiting, or seizures may occur just before the individual lapses into a coma.

Management

The emergency plan, including summoning emergency medical services (EMS), should be activated. Mortality and organ damage appear to be directly proportional to the length of time between elevation of core body temperature and initiation of cooling therapy. As such, while waiting for EMS to arrive, the individual should be moved immediately to a cool place. All equipment and unnecessary clothing should be removed, and rapid cooling of the body should be initiated. Physical activity should not be resumed until the individual has returned to the pre-dehydrated state and been cleared by a physician.

COLD-RELATED CONDITIONS

Hypothermia, or reduced body temperature, occurs when the body is unable to maintain a constant core temperature. In cold weather, three primary heat-promoting mechanisms attempt to maintain or increase core temperature. The initial response is cutaneous vasoconstriction to prevent blood from shunting to the skin. Because the skin is insulated with a layer of subcutaneous fat, heat loss is reduced. The second response is to increase metabolic heat production by shivering, which is an involuntary contraction of skeletal muscle, or to increase physical activity. During vigorous exercise, skeletal muscles can produce 30- to 40-fold the amount of heat produced at rest. During gradual, seasonal changes, an increased amount of the hormone thyroxine is released by the thyroid gland, which serves as the third avenue to increase metabolic rate.

Because of their larger ratio of surface area to body mass and smaller amount of subcutaneous fat, children are more prone to heat loss during cold exposure than adults are. Cold exposure also increases the risk for exercise-induced bronchospasm, which is seen increasingly in children. Women are less able to produce heat through exercise or shivering because of their lower percentage of lean body mass, although the additional subcutaneous fat does provide

---

BOX 17.5   Predisposing Factors for Cold-Related Injuries

- Inadequate insulation from cold and/or wind
- Restrictive clothing or arterial disease that prevents peripheral circulation, especially in the feet
- Diet lacking adequate carbohydrates or fat
- Presence of chronic metabolic disorders
- Spinal cord injury (cannot vasoconstrict peripheral arterioles in the skin and has a blunted shivering response to cold)
- Pre-existing fatigue or general weakness
- Use of alcohol, tobacco products (especially smoking tobacco), and other medications, such as barbiturates, phenothiazines, reserpine, and narcotics
- Age (very young or old)
- Decreased circulation

---

more tissue insulation. Men tend to maintain lower heart rate, higher stroke volume, and higher mean arterial blood pressure than women do, but no distinct differences are seen in cold tolerance when genders are matched for aerobic fitness at the same relative workload. Elderly people, however, have a decreased capacity for metabolic heat production and vasoconstriction. Alcohol dulls mental awareness of cold and inhibits shivering, perhaps by causing hypoglycemia.[9]

Preventing Cold-Related Injuries

During cold weather, body heat is lost through respiration, radiation, conduction, convection, and evaporation. Although the body attempts to generate heat through heat-producing mechanisms, this may be inadequate to maintain a constant core temperature. Box 17.5 lists predisposing factors that contribute to cold-related injuries.

Several steps that can be taken to prevent heat loss are summarized in Box 17.6. The "layered principle" of clothing allows several (i.e., three or more) thin layers of insulation rather

---

BOX 17.6   Reducing the Risk of Cold-Related Injuries

- Monitor weather conditions, and consider possible deterioration
- Closely observe individuals who may be susceptible to cold
- Dress in several light layers
- Wear windproof, dry, well-insulated clothing that allows water evaporation; wool, polypropylene, or polyesters (e.g., Capilene, Thermastat) are recommended
- Carry windproof pants and jacket if conditions warrant; keep your back to the wind
- Wear well-insulated, windproof mittens, gloves, hats, and scarves
- Wear well-insulated footwear that keeps the feet dry

- Avoid dehydration. Do not drink alcoholic beverages or eat snow, because these worsen hypothermia
- Carry nutritious snacks that contain predominantly carbohydrates
- Eat small amounts of food frequently
- Do not stand in one position for extended periods of time. Wiggle your toes, and keep moving to bring warm blood to various areas of the body
- Stay dry by wearing appropriate rain gear or protective clothing. Wet clothing should be changed as soon as possible
- Breathe through your nose, rather than your mouth, to minimize heat and fluid loss
- Observe the face, ears, and fingers for signs of frostbite

than one or two thick ones. Fabrics should be light yet porous enough to allow free exchange of perspiration, and they should not restrict movement. Fabrics may include wool, wool/synthetic blends, polypropylene, treated polyesters (e.g., Capilene), and hollow polyesters (e.g., Thermastat).[13] Cotton has poor insulating ability that is markedly decreased when saturated with perspiration. Pile garments that contain down (e.g., Dacron, Hollofil, Thinsulate, or Quallofil) are more useful when worn during warm-up, time-outs, or cool-down periods following exercise. Jackets with a hood and drawstring as well as pants made of wind-resistant material (e.g., Gore-Tex, nylon, or 60/40 cloth) can protect against the wind. A ski cap, face mask, and neck warmer can protect the face and ears from frostbite. Ski goggles can protect the eyes; goggles must be well ventilated to prevent fogging and be treated with antifog preparations. Polypropylene gloves or, in extreme temperatures, woolen mittens can be worn with windproof outer mittens of Gore-Tex or nylon. Athletic shoes should be large enough to accommodate an outer pair of heavy wool socks.

It is important to avoid getting wet, because heat loss can be increased by evaporation. The insulating ability of clothing can be decreased by as much as 90% when saturated either with external moisture or with condensation from perspiration. If weather conditions are bad enough, it is better to cancel the practice or event for the day.

Cold Conditions

People tend to adapt less readily to cold than to heat. Even inhabitants of cold regions show only limited evidence of adaptation, such as a higher metabolic rate. Like heat illness, cold-related injuries range from minor problems, such as **Raynaud's syndrome**, cold-induced bronchospasm, or frostbite, to the more severe, general systemic cooling, or hypothermia, which can be life-threatening. Cold emergencies occur in two ways. In one, the core temperature remains relatively constant, but the shell temperature decreases. This results in localized injuries from frostbite. In the other, both core temperature and shell temperature decrease, leading to general body cooling. All body processes slow down, and systemic hypothermia results. If left unabated, death is imminent.

Raynaud's Syndrome

Raynaud's syndrome is seen in young individuals, especially females, and is characterized by bilateral episodes of spasms of the digital blood vessels in response to emotion or cold exposure. It can be caused by an underlying disease or anatomical abnormality, and can be a long-term complication of frostbite. However, its source is usually unknown. Initially, during the ischemic phase, the affected digits (usually the fingers) become cold, pale, and numb. This is followed by **hyperemia** with redness, throbbing pain, and swelling. The condition is treated by warming the affected extremity. A physician should evaluate the individual to rule out an underlying condition. Cigarette smoking should be avoided, because it compromises circulation.

Cold-Induced Bronchospasm

Cold-induced bronchospasm is a condition seen frequently in young people. It is brought on by exposure to cold, dry air during cold-weather sports. Linked to exercise-induced bronchospasm, the individual experiences difficulty in breathing, as manifested by shortness of breath, coughing, chest tightness, and wheezing. Attacks can be prevented by the use of bronchodilators or cromolyn sodium. Salmeterol, a more recent, long-acting bronchodilator, administered 30 to 60 minutes before exercise appears to protect many individuals for up to 12 hours.[13]

Frostbite Injuries

Frostbite is caused by the freezing of soft tissue. Individuals who have cold **urticaria** (cold allergy) or **Raynaud's syndrome** are at higher risk for frostbite. Frostbite is classified on a continuum of three degrees (BOX 17.7). First-degree, or superficial, frostbite involves the skin and underlying tissues, but the deeper tissues are soft and pliable. If damage extends into the subcutaneous tissues, it is classified as second-degree frostbite. Third-degree, or deep, frostbite involves the tissues deep to the subcutaneous layers and may result in complete destruction of the injured tissue, including damage to bones, joints, and tendons.[14] Damage depends on the

BOX 17.7	Signs and Symptoms of Frostbite

- **First degree**—skin is soft to the touch and appears initially red, then white, and usually is painless. The condition typically is noticed by others first.
- **Second degree**—skin is firm to the touch, but tissue beneath is soft and initially appears red and swollen. Diffuse numbness may be preceded by an itchy or prickly sensation. White or waxy skin color may appear later.
- **Third degree**—skin is hard to the touch, totally numb, and appears blotchy white to yellow-gray or blue-gray.

depth of cold penetration that results from the duration of exposure, temperature, and wind velocity. Areas commonly affected are the fingertips, toes (especially when wearing constricting footwear), earlobes, and tip of the nose.

Signs and Symptoms

In superficial frostbite, the area may feel firm to the touch, but the tissue beneath is soft and resilient. The skin initially appears red and swollen, and the individual complains of diffuse numbness that may or may not be preceded by an itchy or prickly sensation. If the frostbite extends into the subcutaneous or deep layers, the skin feels hard, because it actually is frozen tissue. The area then turns white, with a yellow or blue tint that looks waxy.

Management

A person with superficial frostbite should be removed from the cold and taken indoors immediately, then treated with careful, rapid warming of the area. Clothing, jewelry, or rings should be removed and the injured area immersed in water heated to between 39 and 45°C (102 to 113°F) for 30 to 45 minutes.[15] A basin large enough to prevent the skin from touching the sides of the container should be used. Hot water should be avoided, because it may cause burns. If frostbite is superficial, rewarmed skin may have clear blisters, whereas with deep frostbite, the rewarmed skin has hemorrhagic blisters.[14] The involved area should be dried and a sterile dressing applied. If fingers or toes are involved, sterile dressings should be placed between the digits before covering. The entire area can be covered with towels or a blanket to keep it warm, and the individual should be transported to the nearest medical center, with the affected limb slightly elevated.

Deep frostbite is best rewarmed under controlled conditions in a hospital. The emergency plan, including summoning EMS, should be activated. During transport, the individual should be kept warm, but active rewarming of the frozen part should not occur. If the frostbite is severe, hemorrhagic blisters may form over the area, and gangrene may develop within 2 to 3 weeks. Throbbing, aching pain as well as burning sensations may last for weeks. The skin may remain permanently red, tender, and sensitive to re-exposure to cold.

Systemic Body Cooling (Hypothermia)

Hypothermia is more of a danger to individuals who are exposed to cold for long periods of time, such as long-distance runners and Nordic ski racers, especially those who are slowing down late in a race because of fatigue or injury. Any injured or ill individual who has been exposed to cold weather or cold water should be suspected of having hypothermia until proved otherwise.

Most of the body heat is lost through radiation involving the exposed surfaces on the hands, face, head, and neck. When the temperature is 4.4°C (40°F), more than half the body's generated heat can be lost from an uncovered head. If the temperature is −315°C (5°F), up to 75% of the body's heat is lost through the head. Air movement coupled with cold produces a wind-chill factor that causes heat loss from the body much faster than occurs in still air. The faster the wind, the higher the wind-chill factor (FIG. 17.4).

									Temperature (°F)										
Calm	40	35	30	25	20	15	10	5	0	-5	-10	-15	-20	-25	-30	-35	-40	-45
5	36	31	25	19	13	7	1	-5	-11	-16	-22	-28	-34	-40	-46	-52	-57	-63
10	34	27	21	15	9	3	-4	-10	-16	-22	-28	-35	-41	-47	-53	-59	-66	-72
15	32	25	19	13	6	0	-7	-13	-19	-26	-32	-39	-45	-51	-58	-64	-71	-77
20	30	24	17	11	4	-2	-9	-15	-22	-29	-35	-42	-48	-55	-61	-68	-74	-81
25	29	23	16	9	3	-4	-11	-17	-24	-31	-37	-44	-51	-58	-64	-71	-78	-84
30	28	22	15	8	1	-5	-12	-19	-26	-33	-39	-46	-53	-60	-67	-73	-80	-87
35	28	21	14	7	0	-7	-14	-21	-27	-34	-41	-48	-55	-62	-69	-76	-82	-89
40	27	20	13	6	-1	-8	-15	-22	-29	-36	-43	-50	-57	-64	-71	-78	-84	-91
45	26	19	12	5	-2	-9	-16	-23	-30	-37	-44	-51	-58	-65	-72	-79	-86	-93
50	26	19	12	4	-3	-10	-17	-24	-31	-38	-45	-52	-60	-67	-74	-81	-88	-95
55	25	18	11	4	-3	-11	-18	-25	-32	39	-46	-54	-61	-68	-75	-82	-89	-97
60	25	17	10	3	-4	-11	-19	-26	-33	-40	-48	-55	-62	-69	-76	-84	-91	-98

Wind speed (mph)

Wind Chill (°F) = 35.74 + 0.6215 T - 35.75 (V$^{0.16}$) + 0.4275 T (V$^{0.16}$)
Where, T = Air Temperature (°F); V = Wind Speed (mph)

☐ Little Danger   Frostbite Times: ☐ 30 minutes ☐ 10 minutes ☐ 5 minutes

FIGURE 17.4 Wind-chill index.

When core temperature falls below 34.4°C (94°F), essential biochemical processes begin to slow. Heart and respiration rates slow, cardiac output and blood pressure fall, and, as the skin and muscles cool, shivering increases violently. Numbness sets in, and even the simplest task becomes difficult to perform. If core temperature continues to drop below 32°C (90°F), shivering ceases and muscles become cold and stiff. **Cold diuresis** (polyuria) occurs as blood is shunted away from the shell to the core in an effort to maintain vascular volume. This leads to excessive excretion of urine by the kidneys. If intervention is not initiated, death is imminent.

Signs and Symptoms

In mild hypothermia, the individual is still shivering. The individual may appear clumsy, apathetic, or confused and may slur speech, stumble, and drop things. In more severe cases, an individual does not feel any sensation or pain, and shivering ceases to occur. Movements become jerky, and the individual becomes unaware of his or her surroundings.

Management

With mild hypothermia, EMS should be activated immediately while the individual is carefully moved into a warm shelter. Rewarming of the individual can be accomplished by allowing him or her to shiver until warm inside a sleeping bag, or by using external rewarming devices, such as hot water bottles or heating pads. Hot tubs can be used if available. The water should be approximately 43°C (110°F). Hot (preferably noncaffeinated) drinks may be useful after the individual is partly rewarmed and able to swallow. The individual should continue to be rewarmed en route to the nearest medical facility.

EXERCISING IN THUNDERSTORMS

Another environmental threat is inclement weather conditions, such as rain, lightning, and thunderstorms. Most organized outdoor sport practices and competitions are held between 3:00 PM and 9:00 PM, which are peak periods for the development of thunderstorms and lightning. If the lightning (flash) to thunder (bang) occurs within 30 seconds, all outdoor activities should end, and all participants should seek shelter, preferably in a sturdy building.

Lightening Injuries

Lightning strikes claim the lives of approximately 100 people each year.[16] Lightning poses a triple threat of injury—namely, burns from the high temperature of the lightning strike, injury caused by the elicited mechanical forces activated by the intense levels of electricity (electromechanical forces), and the resulting concussive forces that can propel objects through the air, causing blunt trauma (e.g., fracture and concussion). Lightning injuries usually are the result of five different mechanisms[17]:

- Direct strike
- Contact injury
- Side flash (splash)
- Ground current (step voltage)
- Blunt trauma

Signs and Symptoms

The most common burn from lightning is a Lichtenberg Figure, which resembles a feathering pattern on the skin. A Lichtenberg Figure is not actually a burn; rather, it is a pattern on the skin from the electron avalanche that strikes the body hit by lightning, causing an inflammatory dermal response.[18] The pattern is transient and fades after 24 hours.

Direct strikes are the most deadly, particularly when the person is in contact with metal (e.g., golf club, shoe cleats, belt buckle, bra clips, watch band, or metal bleachers), with the burn normally appearing where the person's body is in contact with that metal object. Additional symptoms are cardiac asystole (cardiac standstill) and respiratory arrest. Fortunately, the heart is likely to restart spontaneously if the victim is not experiencing respiratory arrest.

The most critical factor in determining morbidity and mortality associated with a lightning strike is the duration of **apnea** rather than cardiac asystole. It is not uncommon for a person to become unconscious or confused or to develop amnesia following a lightning strike. Other medical conditions that have been reported include blunt trauma, including fractures and internal organ damage; brain lesions because of hypoxia caused by cardiac asystole; ruptured tympanic membranes; ocular problems, including hyphemas as well as fixed and dilated pupils; seizures; subdural and epidural hematomas; anterior compartment syndromes; and transitory lower extremity paralysis.[18]

Management

If the person is conscious and has normal cardiorespiratory function, a secondary assessment should be conducted to determine if burns, fractures, or other trauma have been sustained. If an individual is not breathing and is in cardiac arrest, the emergency plan, including summoning EMS, should be activated. The coach should perform rescue breathing and cardiopulmonary resuscitation. Unless ruled out, a cervical spine injury should always be suspected, and treatment should proceed accordingly. Any person struck by lightning should be immediately transported to the nearest medical facility.

Lightning Safety Policy

As mentioned, most organized outdoor sport practices and competitions are conducted between the hours of 3:00 PM and 9:00 PM, when risk of thunderstorms is greatest; 70% of all lightning injuries and fatalities occur in the afternoon.[19] Thunderstorms can become threatening within 30 minutes of the first sign of thunder. Coaches and physically active individuals should understand the development of thunderstorms and lightning strikes. Organizations or institutions should develop a policy within guidelines that can be implemented when conditions are favorable for thunderstorm and lightning activity.[20] This lightning safety policy can decrease the risk of injury and death as well as protect the organization or institution from litigation if the policy is referred to and heeded.

SUMMARY

1. The body generates heat by cutaneous vasoconstriction, increasing the metabolic heat production by shivering or physical activity, and the increase of the hormone thyroxine during gradual, seasonal changes. The body loses heat through respiration, radiation, conduction, convection, and evaporation.

2. During exercise, the body gains heat from external sources (e.g., environmental temperatures) or internal processes (e.g., muscle activity).

3. During rest, approximately two-thirds of the body's normal heat loss results from conduction, convection, and radiation. As air temperature approaches skin temperature and exceeds 30.6°C (87°F), evaporation becomes the primary means of heat dissipation.

4. Sweating places a high demand on the body's fluid reserves and can create a relative state of dehydration. If sweating is excessive and fluids are not continually replaced, plasma volume falls, and core temperature may rise to lethal levels.

5. Acclimatization and proper hydration are among the most critical factors in preventing heat illness. Minerals lost through sweating generally can be replaced through the diet. During prolonged exercise, a small amount of electrolytes added to a rehydration beverage replaces fluids more effectively than drinking plain water.

6. Fluids must be ingested and absorbed by the body to prevent dehydration. Cold liquids, especially water, empty from the stomach and small intestines faster than warm fluids do.

7. Exercise-associated muscle (heat) cramps are caused by excessive loss of water and electrolytes during and after intense exercise in the heat. Treatment involves passive stretching of the involved muscles and ice massage over the affected area. The individual also should drink fluids containing an electrolyte solution to beyond the point of satisfying thirst.

8. Exercise (heat) exhaustion is a functional illness and is not associated with organ damage. Treatment involves moving the individual to a cool place and rapidly cooling the body. The individual also should drink fluids containing an electrolyte solution to beyond the point of satisfying thirst. Intravenous fluids may need to be administered if the dehydrated state is moderate to severe.

9. Exertional heat stroke signifies a significantly elevated core temperature and dehydration. The emergency plan, including summoning EMS, should be activated, because the individual may require airway management, intravenous fluids, and in severe cases, circulatory support. While waiting for EMS to arrive, the individual should be moved to a cool place, and efforts should be made to rapidly cool the body.

10. In the prevention of cold-related injuries, the principle of layering clothing has proven to be effective through providing several thin layers of insulation. In addition, a ski cap, face mask, and neck warmer can protect the face and ears from frostbite.

11. Frostbite occurs when the core temperature remains relatively constant, but the shell temperature decreases. Superficial frostbite is treated by moving the individual indoors and rapidly rewarming the involved body part in water heated to between 39 to 42°C (102 to 108°F) for 30 to 45 minutes. Deep frostbite is best rewarmed under controlled conditions in a hospital. The emergency medical plan should be activated.

12. Hypothermia occurs when both core and shell temperatures decrease, leading to general body cooling. If hypothermia is mild, the individual can be rewarmed; if hypothermia is moderate to severe, on-site rewarming should not be attempted. The emergency plan, including summoning EMS, should be activated.

13. Lightning poses a double threat of injury—namely, burns from the high temperature of the lightning strike and concussive injuries caused by the elicited electromechanical forces.

14. Most thunderstorms occur between 3:00 PM and 9:00 PM. Schools and sport organizations should have a detailed lightning safety policy to prevent injury or death from storms.

APPLICATION QUESTIONS

1. A high school field hockey team is scheduled to practice for this afternoon. The U.S. Weather Bureau is forecasting 90°F (air temperature), with a relative humidity of 80% during the practice time. Based on this information, what measures should the coach take to reduce the risk of heat-related illness?

2. The weather for a scheduled high school soccer game is forecast to be in the low 40s, with winds gusting up to 25 miles per hour. What measures should the coach take to prevent cold-related conditions?

3. The threat exists for thunderstorms to pass through the area during a scheduled afternoon lacrosse game. Based on this information, what actions should be taken by the coach before the game? How should a decision to suspend the game be determined?

4. Your fitness facility offered a cross-country skiing trip to adult members participating in an aerobic fitness program. During the experience, one of the participants complains of pain and numbness in the fingers and toes. In assessing the condition, the fitness specialist observes red and swollen toes and fingers; palpation finds the areas to be cold to touch. What condition should be suspected by the fitness specialist? What is the management for this condition?

5. You are the new athletic director at a high school. One day, you observe members of the wrestling team wearing rubberized sweat suits during running and conditioning exercises. Is there a problem with this practice? If yes, what is the problem?

6. A 30-year-old male recreational soccer player is having problems with muscular cramps during competition. The cramps are most likely related to dehydration. What actions can this athlete take to decrease the risk of heat cramps?

REFERENCES

1. Murray R. 1996. Dehydration, hyperthermia, and athletes: science and practice. J Athl Train, 31(3):248–252.
2. Binkely HM, Beckett J, Casa DJ, et al. 2002. National Athletic Trainers' Association position statement: exertional heat illnesses. J Athl Train, 347(3):329–343.
3. Mellion MB, and Shelton GL. Safe exercise in the head and heat injuries. In The team physician's handbook, edited by MB Mellion et al. Philadelphia, PA: Hanley & Belfus, 2002.
4. Casa DJ, Armstrong LE, Hillman SK. 2000. National Athletic Trainers' Association position statement: fluid replacement for athletes. J Athl Train, 35(2):212–224.
5. Gatorade Sports Science Institute. Dehydration & heat injuries: identification, treatment, and prevention. Chicago: Gatorade, 1997.
6. Shi X, and Gisolfi CV. 1998. Fluid and carbohydrate replacement during intermittent exercise. Sports Med, 25(3):157–172.
7. American College of Sports Medicine. 1996. Position stand on exercise and fluid replacement. Med Sci Sports Exerc, 28(1):i–vii.

8. Myer F, Bar-Or D, MacDougall D, and Heigenhauser G. 1995. Drink composition and electrolyte balance of children exercising in the heat. Med Sci Sport Exerc, 27(6):882–887.

9. Moran DS. 2001. Potential applications of heat and cold stress indices to sporting event. Sports Med, 31(13):909–917.

10. Wexler RK. 2002. Evaluation and treatment of heat-related illnesses. Am Fam Physician, 65 (11):2307–2314.

11. Armstrong LE, Crago LE, Adams AE, et al. 1996. Whole-body cooling of hyperthermic runners: comparison of two filed therapies. Am J Emerg Med, 14(4):355–358.

12. Coris EE, Ramirez AM, and Van Durme DJ. 2004. Heat illness in athletes: the dangerous combination of heat, humidity and exercise. Sports Med, 34(1):9–16.

13. Bowman WD. Safe exercise in the cold and cold injuries. In The team physician's handbook, edited by MB Mellion et al. Philadelphia, PA: Hanley & Belfus, 2002.

14. Biem J, Koehncke N, Classen D, and Dosman J. 2003. Out of the cold: management of hypothermia and frostbite. CMAJ, 168(3): 305–311.

15. McCullough L, and Arora S. 2004. Diagnosis and treatment of hypothermia. Am Fam Physician, 70(12):2325–2332.

16. Cherington M, Yarnell P, and Wappes JR. 1997. Lightning strikes: how to lower your risk. Phys Sportsmed, 25(5):129–130.

17. Whitcomb D, Martinez JA, and Daberkow D. 2002. Lightning injuries. South Med J, 95(11): 1331–1334.

18. Walsh KM, Hanley MJ, Graner SJ, et al. 1997. A survey of lightning policy in selected Division I colleges. J Athl Train, 32(3):206–210.

19. Uman MA. All about lightning. New York, NY: Dover, 1996.

20. Bennett BL. 1997. A model lightning safety policy for athletics. J Athl Train, 32(3):251–253.

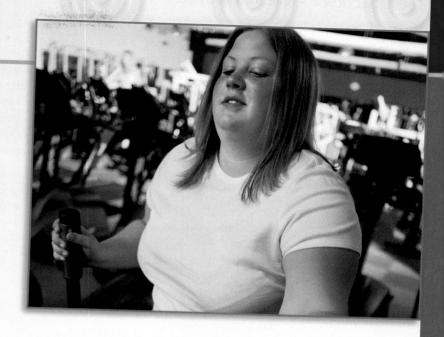

SYSTEMIC CONDITIONS

KEY TERMS

asthma
bronchitis
bronchospasm
diabetes mellitus
hyperglycemia
hypoglycemia
ketoacidosis
polyphagia
polyuria

LEARNING OUTCOMES

1. Identify the signs and symptoms of bronchial asthma and exercise-induced bronchial asthma. Describe the management of both conditions.

2. Explain the physiologic basis of diabetes.

3. Describe Type 1 and Type 2 diabetes mellitus.

4. Describe the signs and symptoms of insulin shock and diabetic coma. Explain the management of both conditions.

5. Explain the nutritional recommendations and identify physical activities that are indicated for physically active individuals with Type 1 and Type 2 diabetes.

6. Identify the causes of epilepsy.

7. List the types of generalized and partial seizures.

8. Describe the characteristics and management of common seizures.

9. Explain the exercise guidelines for individuals with controlled seizures.

A systemic condition affects the body as a whole rather than a particular part of the body. An understanding of systemic disorders is essential in ensuring the health and well-being of an individual with a systemic disorder during their participation in sport and physical activity.

This chapter will provide a basic overview of some common systemic conditions, namely bronchial **asthma**, exercise-induced asthma, diabetes, and epilepsy. Information pertaining to signs and symptoms, management by the coach, and physical activity guidelines will be provided.

BRONCHIAL ASTHMA

Asthma is caused by a constriction of bronchial smooth muscles (**bronchospasm**), increased bronchial secretions, and mucosal swelling, all leading to an inadequate airflow during respiration (especially expiration) (FIG. 18.1). The condition is classified as intermittent, seasonal, or chronic. Intermittent asthma usually is of relatively short duration, occurring less than 5 days per month with extended, symptom-free periods. Symptoms of seasonal asthma occur for prolonged periods as a result of exposure to seasonal inhalant allergens. Chronic asthma occurs daily or near daily, with an absence of extended, symptom-free periods.

Signs and Symptoms

Wheezing is a common sign that results from air squeezing past the narrowed airways. Because the airways cannot fill or empty adequately, the diaphragm tends to flatten, and the accessory muscles must work harder to enlarge the chest during inspiration. This increased workload leads to a rapid onset of fatigue when the individual can no longer hyperventilate enough to meet the increased oxygen need. Acute attacks may occur spontaneously, but they often are provoked by a viral infection. As dyspnea continues, anxiety, loud wheezing, sweating, rapid heart rate, and labored breathing develop. In severe cases, respiratory failure may be indicated by cyanosis, decreased wheezing, and decreased levels of consciousness.

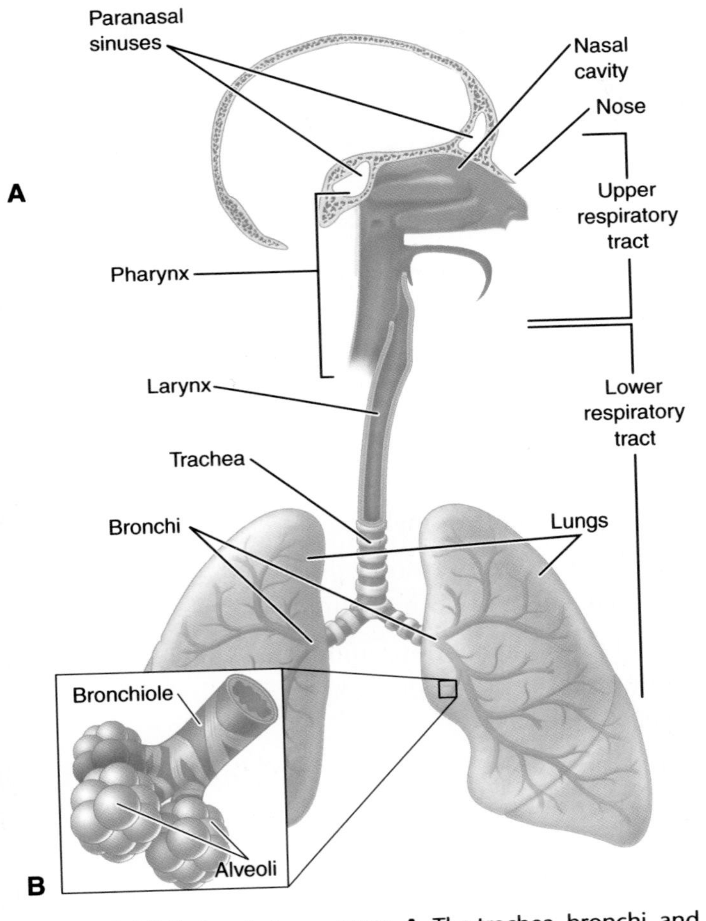

Management

Individuals who are diagnosed with asthma typically carry medication that is delivered by a compressor-driven nebulizer or inhaler to alleviate the attack. As such, the coach should be certain that an individual's medication is readily available (e.g., an inhaler identified for use by a specific individual is stored in the first aid kit). The occurrence of a severe asthma attack can be life-threatening. In those situations, the emergency plan should be activated, including summoning of EMS.

EXERCISE-INDUCED BRONCHOSPASM

Exercise-induced bronchospasm (EIB) affects up to 90% of those with asthma and up to 35% of those without known asthma. Factors contributing to the severity of EIB include ambient air conditions (e.g., cold air, low humidity, and pollutants); duration, type, and intensity of exercise; exposure to allergens in sensitized individuals; overall control of asthma; poor physical conditioning; respiratory infections; time since the last episode of EIB; and any underlying bronchial hyperreactivity.[1]

FIGURE 18.1 Respiratory system. **A**. The trachea, bronchi, and lungs. **B**. The terminal ends of the bronchial tree are alveolar sacs, where oxygen and carbon dioxide are exchanged.

Paranasal sinuses
Nasal cavity
Nose
Upper respiratory tract
Pharynx
Larynx
Lower respiratory tract
Trachea
Bronchi
Lungs
Bronchiole
Alveoli

Individuals suffering from allergies, sinus disease, or hyperventilation may be at increased risk for EIB, and symptoms can be exacerbated for those with **bronchitis**, emphysema, and other diseases affecting the bronchial tubes.

Despite the prevalence of EIB, the precise mechanisms that are responsible for it remain unknown. Theories include hyperventilation resulting in airway heat and water loss, carbon dioxide loss with hyperventilation, and release of chemical mediators causing bronchospasm; however, these theories have not been substantiated. It is thought that breathing dry, cold air through the mouth stimulates bronchospasm. As such, breathing through the nose or covering the nose and mouth when exercising in cold weather can warm and humidify the air and lessen the onset of symptoms. Swimming in an indoor pool, where the air typically is warm and humid, also may prevent the onset of symptoms. Regardless of the mechanism, the amount of ventilation and the temperature of the inspired air both during and after exercise are important factors in determining the severity of EIB. The greater the ventilations (i.e., volume of air inspired) in cold, dry, air, the greater the risk of EIB, and the more strenuous the exercise, the greater the ventilations.

Signs and Symptoms

EIB occurs in three distinct phases. In the first phase, symptoms peak 5 to 10 minutes after exercise begins, and they last for 30 to 60 minutes. Common signs and symptoms of EIB include chest pain, chest tightness, or a burning sensation with or without wheezing; a regular, dry cough; shortness of breath shortly after or during exercise; and stomach cramps after exercise.

Approximately 50% of individuals with EIB experience the second phase of the condition, a "refractory" period. This phase starts 30 minutes to 4 hours after exercise begins and is associated with limited to no bronchospasm. During this period, it may be possible to exercise longer and more strenuously without difficulty.

The final phase involves symptoms similar to those experienced during the first phase, but these symptoms are less severe. Symptoms recur 12 to 16 hours after exercise is completed and usually remit within 24 hours.[2-4]

APPLICATION STRATEGY 18.1

Management Algorithm for Exercise-Induced Bronchospasm

GENERAL RECOMMENDATIONS
- Consult a physician before beginning an exercise program
- Take medication for asthma as prescribed to achieve overall control of asthmatic symptoms, including those caused by exercise and airborne allergens
- Use a peak flowmeter as directed by a physician
- Avoid exposure to air pollutants and allergens whenever possible
- Avoid exercise during the early morning hours, when the concentration of ragweed is highest

EXERCISE ROUTINE
- Use a bronchodilator before exercise
- Perform a 5- to 10-minute warm-up period of moderate stretching, and work out slowly for another 10 to 15 minutes, keeping the pulse rate below 60% of maximum heart rate

- Increase the time and intensity of the workout as tolerated, especially if the activity is new
- Breathing:
  - Breathe slowly through the nose to warm and humidify the air. Exercise in a warm, humid environment, such as a heated swimming pool.
  - In cold, dry environments, breathe through a mask or a scarf. Alternatively, consider different locations and types of exercise during winter months, such as swimming, running, or cycling indoors.
- Perform a gradual 10- to 30-minute cool-down period after a vigorous workout:
  - This avoids rapid thermal changes in the airways.
  - This can be achieved by slowing to a less-intense pace while jogging, cycling, swimming, and stretching.

Management

Management includes medications used in regular asthma treatment. Competitive athletes, however, should consult with the appropriate governing sport body to ensure the medication is legal for competition.

Children and young adults who have asthma, are physically fit, and are free of significant airway obstruction respond to exercise similar to individuals without asthma. Many strenuous physical activities are well tolerated when preceded by a 10- to 15-minute warm-up period at 60% of maximum heart rate performed a half-hour before the more intense activity. Following the warm-up period, a short-acting inhaler should be used to protect against an attack for 2 to 6 hours. Using an inhaler by itself does not always allow a full dose of medication to be delivered to the lungs; as such, adjunct medications can be used with metered-dose inhalers to enhance the delivery and more evenly distribute the medication to the bronchial tubes and lungs. Following activity, a cooldown period allows a gradual rewarming of the airways and makes postactivity symptoms less likely.[3] APPLICATION STRATEGY 18.1 presents a management algorithm for individuals with EIB.

DIABETES MELLITUS

Diabetes mellitus (DM) is a chronic metabolic disorder characterized by a near or absolute lack of the hormone insulin, insulin resistance, or both. The disease affects approximately 15 million Americans and ranks fifth among the leading causes of death in the United States. It is estimated that approximately 2.7 million or 11.4% of African-Americans aged 20 years or older have diabetes. The most life-threatening consequences of diabetes are heart disease and stroke, which strike people with diabetes more than twice as often as they do those without the disorder.[5] Several factors increase the risk and severity of diabetes, including heredity, increasing age, minority ethnicity, obesity, female gender, stress, infection, a sedentary lifestyle, and a diet high in carbohydrates and fat.

Physiologic Basis of Diabetes

Carbohydrates in human nutrition supply the body's cells with glucose to deliver energy to the body's systems. Eating causes the blood glucose (BG) to rise, stimulating the pancreas to release insulin. Under normal conditions, BG ranges between 80 and 120 mg/dL. The main effect of insulin is lowered blood sugar levels, but it also stimulates amino acid uptake, fat metabolism, and protein synthesis in muscle tissue. Insulin lowers blood sugar by enhancing membrane transport of glucose and other simple sugars from the blood into body cells, especially the skeletal and cardiac muscles (FIG. 18.2). It does not accelerate the entry of glucose into liver, kidney, and brain tissue, all of which have easy access to BG regardless of insulin levels. After glucose enters the target cells, insulin

- Promotes the oxidation of glucose for adenosine triphosphate production.
- Joins glucose together to form glycogen.
- Converts glucose to fat for storage, particularly in adipose tissue.

As a general rule, energy needs are met first, and then liver and muscle cells can assemble the excess single glucose cells into long, branching chains of glycogen for storage. The liver cells also are able to convert excess glucose to fat for export to other cells. High BG levels return to normal as excess glucose is stored as glycogen, which can be converted back to glucose, and as fat, which cannot be converted back to glucose.

When BG falls, as occurs between meals, other special cells of the pancreas respond by secreting glucagon into the blood. Glucagon raises BG by stimulating the liver to dismantle its glycogen stores and release glucose into the blood for use by the body's cells. Epinephrine, another hormone, also can stimulate the liver cells to return glucose to the blood from liver glycogen. This "fight-or-flight" response often is triggered when a person experiences stress.

When insulin activity is absent or deficient, as in those with diabetes, the level of blood sugar remains high after a meal. Glucose is unable to move into most tissue cells, causing BG levels to increase to abnormally high levels. Increased osmotic blood pressure drives fluid from the cells into the vascular system, leading to cell dehydration. The excess glucose is passed into

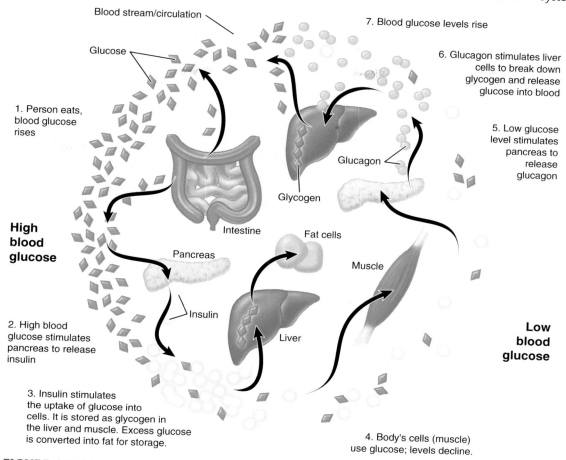

FIGURE 18.2 Maintaining a balance of BG. Insulin must be available to stimulate uptake of BG into the body's cells. As the cells use glucose, blood levels decline, and the liver responds by releasing glucagon into the bloodstream. Glucagon stimulates liver cells to break down stored glycogen and releases glucose into the blood and, in doing so, raises BG to normal levels.

the kidneys, resulting in **polyuria**, a huge urine output of water and electrolytes that leads to decreased blood volume and further dehydration. Serious electrolyte losses also occur as the body rids itself of excess ketones. Because ketones are negatively charged ions, they carry positive ions out with them; as a result, sodium and potassium ions are lost. An electrolyte imbalance leads to abdominal pains, possible vomiting, and the stress reaction spirals. Dehydration stimulates the hypothalamic thirst centers, causing polydipsia, or excessive thirst. In response, the body shifts from carbohydrate metabolism to fat metabolism for energy. The final cardinal sign, **polyphagia**, refers to excessive hunger and food consumption—a sign that the person is "starving." As such, although plenty of glucose is available, it cannot be used. In severe cases, blood levels of fatty acids and their metabolites rise dramatically, producing an excess of ketoacids that, in turn, results in acidosis. Acetone, formed as a by-product of fat metabolism, is volatile and blown off during expiration, which gives the breath a sweet or fruity odor. If the condition is not rectified with insulin injection, further dehydration and **ketoacidosis** result as the ketones begin to spill into the urine (i.e., ketonuria). If untreated, ketoacidosis disrupts virtually all physiologic processes, including heart activity and oxygen transport. Severe depression of the nervous system leads to confusion, drowsiness, coma, and finally, death.

Types of Diabetes

The National Diabetes Data Group and the World Health Organization recognize four types of DM: Type 1, Type 2, gestational DM, and diabetes secondary to other conditions. Each group

BOX 18.1	**Comparison of Type 1 and Type 2 Diabetes Mellitus**	
	TYPE 1	**TYPE 2**
Former names	Juvenile-onset diabetes Insulin-dependent diabetes mellitus	Adult-onset diabetes Non-insulin-dependent diabetes mellitus
Age of onset	Usually before 30 years	Usually after 30 years
Type of onse	Abrupt (i.e., days to weeks)	Usually gradual (i.e., weeks to months)
Nutritional status	Almost always lean	Usually obese
Insulin production	Negligible to absent	Present, but may be in excess and ineffective because of obesity
Insulin	Needed for all patients	Necessary in only 20 to 30% of patients
Diet	Mandatory, along with insulin for control of BG	Diet alone frequently is sufficient to control BG
High incidence	White population	Women with a history of gestational diabetes, Blacks, Native Americans, Hispanics
Family history	Minor	Common link

is characterized by high BG levels or **hyperglycemia**. Because physical educators, exercise specialists, and coaches will most likely encounter physically active individuals with Type 1 or Type 2 DM, these conditions will be discussed in detail, and are compared in Box 18.1.

Type 1 Diabetes Mellitus

In Type 1, the pancreas cannot synthesize insulin. As such, the individual must obtain insulin to assist the cells in taking up the needed fuels from the blood. Formerly called insulin-dependent diabetes or juvenile diabetes, Type I DM is considered an autoimmune disorder and is one of the most frequent chronic childhood diseases. The onset is usually acute, developing over a period of a few days to weeks. Over 95% of individuals who develop Type 1 DM are under 25 years of age, with equal incidence in both sexes and an increased prevalence in the white population.[6] Individuals generally have a more severe time balancing glucose levels, the effects of exercise on the metabolic state are more pronounced, and the management of exercise-related problems is more difficult.

Type 2 Diabetes Mellitus

Formerly called non-insulin-dependent diabetes or adult-onset diabetes, Type 2 DM is the most common form of diabetes (90 to 95% of all cases).[7,8] It is highly associated with a family history of diabetes, older age, obesity, and lack of exercise. It is also more common in women who have a history of gestational diabetes and in African Americans, Native Americans, and Hispanics.[6] Although the exact cause of Type 2 DM is unknown, high BG and insulin resistance are major contributing factors.

Onset is typically after an age of 40 years, but this disease is also seen in obese children. Obesity, a major factor in adults, affects nearly 90% of adults with Type 2 DM. Compared with normal-weight individuals, obese people require much more insulin to maintain normal BG. More insulin is produced, but as body fat increases, the number of insulin receptors and their ability to function decreases. Consequently, insulin resistance increases, and adipose and muscle tissues become less able to take up glucose. At some point, the body cannot supply enough insulin to keep up, and Type 2 DM develops.

Complications of Diabetes Mellitus

In Types 1 and 2 DM, glucose fails to enter into the cells; instead, it accumulates in the blood, which can lead to both acute and chronic complications. Chronically elevated BG levels can damage the blood vessels and nerves, leading to circulatory and neural damage. Failure to adequately balance nutrition, exercise, insulin injections, and BG levels can also cause a physically active individual to experience insulin shock or diabetic coma.

Hypoglycemia

Hypoglycemia, which is common in those with Type 1 insulin-treated diabetes, can range from very mild, lower levels of glucose (60 to 70 mg/dL) with minimal or no symptoms to severe hypoglycemia with very low levels of glucose (<40 mg/dL) and neurologic impairment. Although hypoglycemia can occur with any individual, it is critical in a person with Type 1 DM, because the ability to recover from it is limited. Recovery is mediated by the release of epinephrine, norepinephrine, and glucagon.[9] In a person with diabetes, hypoglycemia associated with insulin therapy may be related to errors in dosage, delayed or skipped meals, exercise, intensity of BG control, variation in absorption of insulin from subcutaneous injection sites, variability of insulin binding, impairment of counter-regulation, and possibly, use of human insulin.[7] When left untreated, this condition can lead to insulin shock.

Insulin Shock

Exercise lowers blood sugar; as such, any exercise must be counterbalanced with increased food intake or decreased amounts of insulin. Hypoglycemia results if BG falls below normal levels. Although any individual can experience hypoglycemia, it is particularly critical for the physically active person with diabetes to address the situation immediately.

Signs and Symptoms

Contrary to the slow onset of a diabetic coma, hypoglycemia has a rapid onset. Signs and symptoms include dizziness; headache; intense hunger; aggressive behavior; pale, cold, and clammy skin; profuse perspiration; salivation; drooling; and tingling in the face, tongue, and lips. Other observable signs may include a staggering gait, clumsy movements, confusion, and a general decrease in performance.

Management

Because glucose levels in the blood are low compared to high levels of insulin, treatment focuses on getting 10 to 15 g of a fast-acting carbohydrate into the system quickly. This can be found in 4 oz of regular cola or 6 oz of ginger ale, 4 oz of apple or orange juice, four packets of table sugar, or two tablespoons of raisins.[9,10] Chocolates, which contain a high level of fat, should not be used for treating a hypoglycemic reaction, because the fat interferes with the absorption of sugar. If the person is unconscious or unable to swallow, the individual should be rolled on their side, and close attention should be given to the airway so that saliva drains out of the mouth, not into the throat. Sugar or honey should be placed under the tongue, because it is absorbed through the mucous membrane. Recovery usually is rapid.

After initial recovery, the individual should wait 15 minutes and check the blood sugar level. If the level is still less than 70 mg/dL or no meter is available and the individual still has symptoms, another 10 to 15 g of carbohydrates should be administered. Blood testing and treatment should be repeated until the BG level has normalized.[9] Even when the BG level has returned to normal, however, physical performance and judgment may still be impaired, or the individual may relapse if the quick sugar influx is rapidly depleted. After the symptoms resolve, the individual should be instructed to have a good meal as soon as possible to increase carbohydrates in the body. If the condition does not appear to improve, the emergency plan should be activated, including summoning of EMS. While waiting for EMS to arrive, the coach should monitor vital signs and treat for shock as necessary.

Diabetic Coma

Without insulin, the body is unable to metabolize glucose, leading to hyperglycemia. As the body shifts from carbohydrate metabolism to fat metabolism, an excess of ketoacids in the blood can lower the blood pH to 7.0 (i.e., normal pH is 7.35 to 7.45), leading to a condition called diabetic ketoacidosis. This is manifested by ketones in the breath, ketonemia, and ketonuria.

Signs and Symptoms

Symptoms appear gradually and often occur over several days. The individual becomes increasingly restless and confused and complains of a dry mouth and intense thirst. Abdominal cramping and vomiting are common. As the individual slips into a coma, signs include dry, red, warm skin; eyes that appear deep and sunken; deep, exaggerated respirations; a rapid, weak pulse; and a sweet, fruity acetone breath similar to nail polish remover.

Management

It is not usually possible to determine with certainty whether an individual is in a diabetic coma or insulin shock. As such, a conscious individual should be given glucose or orange juice. If recovery is not rapid, a medical emergency exists. The emergency plan should be activated, including summoning of EMS. The additional glucose will not worsen the condition, provided that the individual is transported immediately. If the person is unconscious or semiconscious, nothing should be given orally. APPLICATION STRATEGY 18.2 summarizes the management of insulin shock and diabetic coma.

Exercise Recommendations

Controlled diabetes depends on a balance of glucose levels, insulin production, nutrition, and exercise. Before any exercise program begins, a physician should be consulted about proper diet,

---

APPLICATION STRATEGY 18.2

Management Algorithm for Diabetic Emergencies

Look for a medic alert tag!
Is the person conscious?

YES
Administer 10 to 15 g of fast-acting carbohydrate:

4 oz of regular cola

6 oz of ginger ale

4 oz of apple or orange juice

Four packets of table sugar

Two tablespoons of raisins

Does the individual show signs of improvement after the initial carbohydrates?

YES
Wait 15 minutes, and check the blood sugar level.

If the BG level is still below 70 mg/dL or if symptoms persist:

Give another 10 to 15 g carbohydrates.

Repeat blood testing and treatment until BG is normalized.

After the symptoms resolve:

The individual should eat a good meal as soon as possible

NO
Activate the emergency plan, including summoning EMS.

Roll the individual on his or her side so that saliva will drain out of the mouth.

Maintain an open airway.

Place sugar or fast-acting carbohydrates under the tongue.

Do not give liquids.

NO
Activate the emergency plan, including summoning emergency medical services.

BOX 18.2	Guidelines for Safe Exercise by Physically Active Individuals with Diabetes

- Have a routine medical examination, and be cleared for activity.
- Develop a balanced program of diet and exercise under a physician's supervision.
- Wear identification (e.g., bracelet or necklace) indicating that the individual has diabetes.
- Eat at regular times throughout the day.
- Avoid exercising at the peak of insulin action and in the evening, when hypoglycemia is more apt to occur.
- Adjust carbohydrate intake and insulin dosage before physical activity.
- Check BG levels before, during (if possible), and after physical activity.
- Prevent dehydration by consuming adequate fluids before, during, and after physical activity.
- Have access to fast-acting carbohydrates during exercise to prevent hypoglycemia.
- Avoid alcoholic beverages, or drink them in moderation.
- Avoid cigarette smoking.

and normal BG levels should be documented (strenuous exercise is contraindicated for some diabetics). With the advent of BG self-monitoring, exercise is encouraged if certain precautions are followed. BG levels should be taken 30 minutes before and 1 hour after exercise to see how exercise affects BG. These measurements help to regulate food intake and insulin dosage.

Aerobic exercise can decrease the requirements of insulin and increase the body's sensitivity to it. Exercise can also help attain and maintain ideal body weight and decrease the risk for hypertensive diseases including cardiovascular and peripheral vascular disease, and slow the progression of diabetic nephropathy (kidney damage). It is recommended that all exercising diabetics should follow the guidelines listed in Box 18.2. Despite the benefits of exercise, Type 2 diabetics who have lost protective neural sensation should not participate in treadmill walking, prolonged walking, jogging, or step exercises. Recommended exercises include low-resistance walking, swimming, bicycling, rowing, chair exercises, arm exercises, and other non-weight-bearing exercises. Sports that require resistance strength training are permissible as long as there are no indications of retinopathy (noninflammatory degenerative disease of the retina) or nephropathy. Scuba diving, rock climbing, and parachuting are strongly discouraged.

SEIZURE DISORDERS AND EPILEPSY

A seizure is an abnormal electrical discharge in the brain. A seizure disorder entails recurrent episodes of sudden, excessive charges of electrical activity in the brain, whether from known or idiopathic causes. Epilepsy is a general term used to describe only recurrent (at least two) idiopathic episodes of sudden, excessive discharges of electrical activity in the brain.[11,12] The discharge may trigger altered sensation, perception, behavior, mood, level of consciousness, or convulsive movements. Seizures and epilepsy often are used interchangeably; however, it is important to understand their definitions.

Causes of Epilepsy

Epilepsy appears to be directly related to age of onset and generally is categorized as provoked or unprovoked (BOX 18.3). Seizures that begin before 5 years of age usually are associated with mental or neurologic impairment. Seizures that begin between 5 and 15 years of age are not usually associated with a known metabolic or structural cause and are called idiopathic or

> ### BOX 18.3   Causes of Epilepsy
>
> - **Unprovoked or idiopathic (no cause of the seizure is identified)**
> - **Provoked:**
>   - Post-traumatic (e.g., skull fracture, intracranial hematoma)
>   - Metabolic (e.g., hyponatremia, hypocalcemia, hypoglycemia, hypomagnesemia, dehydration)
>   - Drug and drug withdrawal (e.g., alcohol, cocaine)
>   - Infections (e.g., meningitis, encephalitis, brain abscess)
>   - Anoxia and hypoxia
>   - Cerebrovascular (e.g., stroke, intracerebral or subarachnoid hemorrhage, sinus thrombosis)
>   - Hyperthermia
>   - Sleep deprivation
>   - Febrile seizures
>   - Neoplasms (e.g., primary intracranial, carcinomatous meningitis, metastatic, lymphoma, leukemia)
>   - Perinatal or hereditary (e.g., congenital anomalies, genetic and hereditary disorders, perinatal trauma)

unprovoked seizures. These seizures respond very well to treatment, and individuals usually can participate in physical activity with little to no restrictions. Trauma and tumors are responsible for most seizures in young adults; strokes are the most frequent cause in those 40 years and older.[11,13]

Types of Seizures

Seizures can be divided into three basic types, namely partial or focal, generalized, and special epileptic syndromes. Because physical educators, exercise specialists, and coaches are not likely to encounter individual's special epileptic conditions, these conditions will be not be addressed.

Partial or Focal Seizures

Partial or focal seizures have a localized onset, are focused in one particular area of the brain, and are restricted to specific areas of the body.[12] Partial seizures may be subdivided into simple, in which consciousness is retained, and complex, in which consciousness is impaired.

Signs and Symptoms

A simple partial seizure is relatively common. It is classified according to the main clinical manifestations. The sensory manifestation includes bodily sensations and discomforts, such as tingling, numbness, "pins and needles," or loss of feeling. A motor manifestation is characterized by involuntary movements of the face, limbs, or head and may involve an inability to speak. The seizures, which can last for minutes or hours, may be followed by localized weakness or paralysis of the body part in which the seizure occurs. The individual may experience powerful emotions, such as fear, anxiety, depression, or embarrassment, for no apparent reason. In some cases, a feeling of the mind and body separating may be reported. The person also may experience visual, olfactory, and auditory hallucinations. Psychic symptoms may include disturbing memory flashbacks or frequent, disconcerting feelings of déjà vu, in which something or someone unfamiliar seems to be familiar, or jamais vu, in which something or someone familiar seems to be unfamiliar. Time distortions, out-of-body experiences, sudden nausea, or stomach pain may occur. Consciousness is not impaired; however, a partial or focal seizure may precede a generalized seizure and serve as an aura that consciousness is about to be altered.[14]

Complex partial seizures affect a larger area of the brain and, therefore, impair consciousness. They are characterized by attacks of purposeful movements or experiences followed by impairment of consciousness. In other words, although appearing to be conscious, the individual is in an altered state of consciousness, an almost trance-like state.

If engaged in activity, an individual's movements usually are disorganized, confused, and unfocused, but observers may find it hard to believe that the individual does not know of their actions. The average seizure lasts from 1 to 5 minutes. The individual is unresponsive to verbal stimuli and may exhibit disorientation or confusion. Afterward, the individual is unable to recall the actions that took place. These types of seizures usually start between 10 and 30 years of age.

Generalized Seizures

Generalized seizures can affect the entire brain. These seizures may be further subdivided into convulsive and nonconvulsive types.

The tonic–clonic, or grand mal, seizure is the most common and severe seizure of the convulsive type. It may occur in an intermittent or a continuous form. Tonic refers to prolonged contractions of skeletal muscles, whereas clonic refers to rhythmic contractions and relaxation of muscles in rapid succession.

An intermittent seizure may be tonic, clonic, or both, and it often is associated with loss of consciousness. Many individuals experience a sensory phenomenon (aura), such as a particular taste or smell, before the seizure. The average seizure lasts from 50 to 90 seconds but may extend up to 5 minutes. Because the unconscious, seizing individual is overtaken by the excessive electrical discharge during the seizure, control of bladder and bowel functions may be lost, resulting in urination or defecation. This action typically is embarrassing and unpleasant but not unexpected. When the seizure ends, the brain may shift into a sleep pattern. As such, the individual may be unarousable for a brief period of time (i.e., seconds to a few minutes). The muscles relax during this period, and the person awakens. Following the seizure, the person often is disoriented, confused, and lethargic and may not remember what happened.

A continuous tonic–clonic seizure (status epilepticus) is a medical emergency. Continuous convulsions can last 30 minutes or longer, or recurrent generalized convulsions can occur without the person regaining full consciousness between attacks. If the convulsions exceed 60 minutes, irreversible neuronal damage may occur. Any seizure that lasts longer than 5 minutes should be seen as indicating a serious problem. Accordingly, the emergency action plan, including summoning of emergency medical services (EMS), should be activated.

Myoclonic seizures are characterized by sporadic or continuous clonus of muscle groups. They are associated with progressive mental deterioration. These types of seizures are seldom seen in the physically active population.

Post-traumatic seizures are provoked by head trauma and are classified as impact, immediate, early, and late. Impact seizures occur at the time of trauma and are considered to result from electrochemical changes induced by the trauma. Immediate seizures occur within the first 24 hours of trauma. Early seizures occur within the first week after head trauma and often are associated with prolonged post-traumatic amnesia lasting more than 24 hours. A late seizure occurs after the first week of head trauma but primarily within 1 year, and it may be associated with a history of childhood epilepsy.[15]

The typical absence, or petit mal, attack is characterized by a slight loss of consciousness, or blank staring into space, for 3 to 15 seconds without loss of body tone or falling. Slight twitching of the facial muscles, lip smacking, or fluttering of the eyelids may occur. Onset of the condition usually is between 4 and 8 years of age; it tends to resolve by age 30.

Immediate Management of Seizures

It is important that the coach note the time at the onset and the end of a seizure. Seconds may seem like minutes; unless accurately timed, the actual length of the seizure may be exaggerated. Management of any seizure is directed toward protecting the individual from injury. Nearby objects should be removed or padded so that the individual does not strike them during uncontrollable muscle contractions. The individual should not be restrained, but the head should be protected at all times. Although the individual may bite the tongue during the seizure, nothing (e.g., fingers or any object) should be placed into the mouth. In an effort to avoid embarrassment to the individual, any

APPLICATION STRATEGY 18.3
Management of Seizures

DURING THE SEIZURE
- Note the time that the seizure began.
- Help the individual to a supine position; protect the head.
- Remove glasses and loosen clothing.
- Do not:
  - Stop or restrain the person.
  - Place fingers or any object in the mouth.

AFTER THE SEIZURE
- Ensure an adequate airway.
- Turn the individual to one side to allow saliva to drain from mouth.
- Protect the person from curious bystanders.
- Do not leave until the individual is fully awake.

IF THIS IS
- A first-time seizure
  - The individual should be seen by a physician
- A continuous seizure, or if another seizure occurs in rapid succession
  - Activate the emergency action plan, including summoning EMS

SEND DOCUMENTATION, INCLUDING A WRITTEN DESCRIPTION OF
- Type of seizure; localized or generalized.
- How it started.
- Length of time from onset until return of consciousness.
- Number of seizures.

observers or spectators should be removed from the area, if possible, to allow privacy. When the seizure ends, it is not unusual for the individual to fall into a sleep pattern.

It is essential to document the length of time of the seizure and the amount of time the individual sleeps. If a single, continuous seizure or a series of intermittent seizures exceeds 5 minutes, the emergency action plan, including summoning EMS, should be activated. APPLICATION STRATEGY 18.3 summarizes the management of a seizure.

Physical Activity Guidelines

In nearly all instances, seizure disorders can be controlled with proper medication. Traditionally, good seizure control has been identified as being seizure-free for 6 months or a year. Participation in physical activity and sports, particularly those sports with a danger of falling, contact sports, and water sports, should be carefully evaluated by a neurologist before such participation is allowed. Several issues must be addressed in determining participation levels; namely, what type of physical or sport activity is being performed?

- Is there a risk of death or severe injury if the individual has a seizure during activity?
- Is there a pre-existing brain injury or any neurologic dysfunction?
- Is there a risk of potential brain injury from participation in the activity (e.g., concussion or intracranial hematoma)?
- Will exercise adversely affect seizure control?
- What are the potential effects of anticonvulsive medications on performance (e.g., impaired judgment or delayed reaction time)?

Head injury during activity participation can certainly precipitate seizures. Individuals with epilepsy, however, are no more prone to seizures after a head injury than are individuals without epilepsy. In addition, epilepsy does not increase the risk of injury while participating in sports,[12] although certain activities (e.g., football, scuba diving, mountain climbing, and automobile racing) should be discouraged if they put the individual or others at risk should a seizure occur. Any individual with a history of seizures should be prohibited from boxing, regardless of seizure control. Individuals who experience frequent seizures should choose physical activities accordingly. It is highly recommended that children with seizure disorders be allowed to participate in physical activity and sports, provided that good seizure control and proper supervision are available at all times.

SUMMARY

1. Bronchial asthma is caused by a constriction of bronchial smooth muscles (bronchospasm), increased bronchial secretions, and mucosal swelling, each leading to inadequate airflow during respiration (especially during expiration). Wheezing, a common sign of asthma, results from air squeezing past the narrowed airways. The condition is classified as intermittent, seasonal, or chronic.

2. EIB affects up to 90% of those with asthma and up to 35% of those without known asthma. Key signs are a dry, regular cough within 8 to 10 minutes of the start of moderate exercise as well as stomach cramps after exercise.

3. The management of bronchial asthma and EIB involves medication, both as a prophylactic and in response to an attack.

4. Insulin is needed after carbohydrate ingestion to transfer glucose from the blood into the skeletal and cardiac muscles. It also promotes glucose storage in the muscles and liver in the form of glycogen. If little or no insulin is secreted by the pancreas, glucose bypasses the body cells and rises to abnormally high levels in the blood. The excess glucose is excreted in the urine, drawing with it large amounts of water and electrolytes and leading to weakness, fatigue, malaise, and increased thirst.

5. When glucose cannot enter the cells, the cells shift from carbohydrate metabolism to fat metabolism for energy, resulting in dehydration and ketoacidosis, which can depress cerebral function. Acetone, formed as a by-product of fat metabolism, is volatile and blown off during expiration, giving the breath a sweet or fruity odor.

6. There are four types of DM:
   - Type 1 (insulin-dependent) DM has an onset before age 30 in people who are not obese.
   - Type 2 (non-insulin-dependent) DM has an onset after age 40 and is the most common form. It is highly associated with a family history of diabetes, older age, obesity, and lack of exercise.
   - Gestational DM occurs when a pregnant woman cannot produce enough insulin to handle the higher BG level because of hormones secreted during the latter half of pregnancy. The condition usually resolves after delivery, but it places the woman at risk for developing Type 2 DM later in life.
   - Diabetes secondary to other conditions includes individuals with genetic defects of beta-cell function or with defects of insulin action and persons with pancreatic disease, hormonal disease, and drug or chemical exposure.

7. Severe hypoglycemia can lead to insulin shock. The signs and symptoms include a rapid onset with dizziness; headache; intense hunger; aggressive behavior; pale, cold, and clammy skin; profuse perspiration; salivation; drooling; and tingling in the face, tongue, and lips.

8. An individual progresses into a diabetic coma (i.e., hyperglycemia) over a long period of time. Common symptoms include dry mouth, intense thirst, abdominal pain, confusion, and fever. Severe signs include deep respirations; rapid, weak pulse; dry, red, warm skin; and a sweet, fruity acetone breath.

9. Because it may be difficult to determine which condition is present, a fast-acting carbohydrate should be given to the individual. If the individual is in insulin shock, recovery usually is rapid. If recovery does not occur, the emergency plan should be activated.

10. An individual with diabetes should have a consistent daily intake of carbohydrates at each meal and snack to minimize BG fluctuations.

11. A seizure disorder entails recurrent episodes of sudden, excessive charges of electrical activity in the brain, whether from known or unknown (idiopathic) causes. Epilepsy is a general term used to describe only recurrent idiopathic episodes (at least two) of sudden, excessive discharges of electrical activity in the brain. The discharge may trigger altered sensation, perception, behavior, mood, or level of consciousness or may lead to convulsive movements.

12. Seizures are classified as partial, generalized, or special epileptic syndromes.

13. The most serious seizure is the tonic–clonic seizure, which may occur in an intermittent or a continuous form. An intermittent seizure, which usually only lasts from 50 to 90 seconds but may extend to 5 minutes, often is preceded by a particular taste or smell (aura).

14. The typical absence (petit mal) attack is characterized by a slight loss of consciousness or blank staring into space for 3 to 15 seconds without loss of body tone or falling.

15. The simple partial seizure is characterized by involuntary movements of the face, limbs, or head, and the individual may experience tingling or numbness. The localized motor seizures may be followed by localized weakness or paralysis of the body part in which the seizure occurs.

16. Complex partial (psychomotor) seizures are characterized by purposeful movements or experiences followed by impairment in consciousness.

17. Management of any seizure is directed toward protecting the individual from injury. The area surrounding the individual should be clear of objects; immovable objects should be padded.

The individual should not be restrained, but the head should be protected at all times. Nothing should be placed in the mouth of an individual having a seizure. When the seizure ends, an adequate airway should be ensured. If the time of the seizure exceeds 5 minutes, activation of the emergency action plan is warranted.

18. In the majority of cases, individuals with a seizure disorder can be allowed to participate in certain physical activities and sports, provided that good seizure control and proper supervision are available at all times.

APPLICATION QUESTIONS

1. During a workout session, a client at a fitness club becomes very dizzy, complains of a headache, and reports being very hungry. The individual is sweating profusely, the skin appears to be pale and clammy, and movement is somewhat clumsy. In addition, the person appears to be swallowing an excessive number of times. What condition should the fitness specialist suspect? How should the fitness specialist manage the condition?

2. During tennis practice, a high school player has a seizure. How should the coach manage the condition?

3. During a physical education class, a seventh-grade student has a partial seizure between soccer drills. The physical education teacher is not aware of the student having a history of seizures. What could have caused the seizure?

4. A high school varsity basketball player has EIB. What signs and symptoms can be expected when the individual experiences EIB? How should the coach manage the condition?

5. A middle-aged individual with diabetes is a new member at an exercise facility. Explain guidelines that the individual should follow to promote safe participation in exercise.

6. 20 minutes into a physical education class involving weight training and cardiovascular activities, a 16-year-old diabetic male student suddenly feels weak and faint. How should the physical educator determine whether this individual is experiencing insulin shock?

REFERENCES

1. Rupp NT. 1996. Diagnosis and management of exercise-induced asthma. Phys Sportsmed, 24(1):77–87.
2. Tan RA, and Sheldon SL. 1998. Exercise-induced asthma. Sports Med, 25(2):1–6.
3. Disabella V, and Sherman C. 1998. Exercise for asthma patients: little risk, big rewards. Phys Sportsmed, 26(6):75–84.
4. Hermansen CL, and Kirchner JT. 2004. Identifying exercise-induced bronchospasm. Postgrad Med, 115(6):15–20.
5. 2003. Diabetes: new ways to deal with an old problem. Ebony 58(5):64–68. MAS Ultra-School Edition, EBSCO host (accessed November 9, 2010).
6. Mayfield M. 1998. Diagnosis and classification of diabetes mellitus: new criteria. Am Fam Physician, 58(6):1355–1363.
7. National Institutes of Health. Diabetes in America. Washington, DC: National Institute of Diabetes and Digestive and Kidney Diseases, 1995.
8. Whitney EN, and Rolfes SR. Understanding Nutrition. Belmont, CA: Wadsworth, 1999.
9. Jimenez CC. 1997. Diabetes and exercise: the role of the athletic trainer. J Athl Train, 32(4): 339–343.
10. Seitzman A, and Anderson C. 1998. Lower your risk for lows. Diabetes Forecast, 51(6):60–65.
11. Lang D. 1997. Seizure disorders and physical activity: convulsions, collision, and sports. Phys Sportsmed, 25(10):24e–24k.
12. Agnew CM, Nystul MS, and Conner MC. 1998. Seizure disorders: an alternative explanation for students' inattention. Prof School Coun, 2(1):54–60.
13. Jordan BD, and Sundell R. Epilepsy and the athlete. In The team physicians' handbook, edited by MB Mellion, et al. Philadelphia: Hanley & Belfus, 2002.
14. Kistner D, and DeWeaver KL. 1997. Nonconvulsive seizure disorders: importance and implications for school social workers. Social Work Educ, 19(2):73–86.
15. Robbins L, and Lang SS. Headache Help: A Complete Guide to Understanding Headaches and the Medicines that Relieve Them. MA: Houghton Mifflin, National Headache Foundation, 1998.

GLOSSARY

Acclimatization Physiologic adaptations of an individual to a different environment, especially climate or altitude.

Active inhibition A technique whereby an individual consciously relaxes a muscle before stretching.

Acute injury Injury with rapid onset caused by traumatic episode, but with short duration.

Adhesions Tissues that bind the healing tissue to adjacent structures, such as other ligaments or bone.

Alveoli Air sacs at the terminal ends of the bronchial tree where oxygen and carbon dioxide are exchanged between the lungs and surrounding capillaries.

Amenorrhea Absence or abnormal cessation of menstruation.

Analgesic Agent that produces analgesia.

Anaphylaxis An immediate, shocklike, frequently fatal, hypersensitive reaction that occurs within minutes of administration of an allergen unless appropriate first-aid measures are taken immediately.

Anatomic position Used as a universal reference to determine anatomic direction; the body is erect, facing forward, with the arms at the side of the body, palms facing forward.

Anatomic snuffbox Site directly over the scaphoid bone in the wrist; pain here indicates a possible fracture.

Angina Chest pain during physical exertion.

Angiogenesis Development of new blood vessels.

Anisotropic Having different strengths in response to loads from different directions.

Antacid Agent that neutralizes stomach acid.

Anterograde amnesia Loss of memory of events after a head injury.

Apnea Temporary cessation of breathing.

Aponeurosis A flat, expanded, tendonlike sheath that attaches a muscle to another structure.

Apophysis An outgrowth or projection on the side of a bone; usually where a tendon attaches.

Apophysitis Inflammation of an apophysis.

Appendicitis Inflammation of the appendix.

Arrhythmia Disturbance in the heart beat rhythm.

Aseptic necrosis Death or decay of tissue caused by a poor blood supply in the area.

Assumption of risk When sport participants knowingly participate in an activity with the inherent possibility of potential injury.

Asthma Disease of the lungs characterized by constriction of the bronchial muscles, increased bronchial secretions, and mucosal swelling, all leading to airway narrowing and inadequate airflow during respiration.

Atherosclerosis Condition whereby irregularly distributed lipid deposits are found in the large and medium-sized arteries.

Athletic training A discipline whereby athletic trainers work in collaboration with physicians to optimize activity and participation of their patients.

Atrophy A wasting away or deterioration of tissue because of disease, disuse, or malnutrition.

Axial force Loading directed along the long axis of a body.

Axonotmesis Damage to the axons of a nerve followed by complete degeneration of the peripheral segment, without severance of the supporting structure of the nerve.

Ballistic stretch Increasing flexibility by using repetitive bouncing motions at the end of the available range of motion.

Bankart lesion Avulsion or damage to the anterior lip of the glenoid as the humerus slides forward in an anterior dislocation.

Battery Unpermitted or intentional contact with another individual without their consent.

Battle's sign Delayed discoloration behind the ear caused by basilar skull fracture.

Bending Loading that produces tension on one side of an object and compression on the other side.

Bennett's fracture Fracture-dislocation to the proximal end of the first metacarpal at the carpal-metacarpal joint.

Bimalleolar fracture Fractures of both medial and lateral malleolus.

Blowout fracture Fracture of the floor of the eye orbit, without fracture to the rim; produced by a blow on the globe with the force being transmitted via the globe to the orbital floor.

Brachial plexus A complex web of spinal nerves (C5-T1) that innervate the upper extremity.

Bradykinin Normally present in blood; a potent vasodilator. Increases blood vessel wall permeability and stimulates nerve endings to cause pain.

Bronchitis Inflammation of the mucosal lining of the tracheobronchial tree characterized by bronchial swelling, mucus secretions, and dysfunction of the cilia.

Bronchospasm Contraction of the smooth muscles of the bronchial tubes causing narrowing of the airway.

Burner Burning or stinging sensation characteristic of a brachial plexus injury.

Bursa A fibrous sac membrane containing synovial fluid typically found between tendons and bones; acts to decrease friction during motion.

Bursitis Inflammation of a bursa.

Callus Localized thickening of skin epidermis caused by physical trauma, or fibrous tissue containing immature bone tissue that forms at fracture sites during repair and regeneration.

Calor Localized heat; one of the four classic signs of inflammation.

Cardiac asystole Cardiac standstill.

Cardiac tamponade Acute compression of the heart because of effusion of fluid or blood into the pericardium from rupture of the heart or penetrating trauma.

Carpal tunnel syndrome Compression of the median nerve as it passes through the carpal tunnel, leading to pain and tingling in the hand.

Cauda equina Lower spinal nerves that course through the lumbar spinal canal; resembles a horse's tail.

Cauliflower ear Hematoma that forms between the perichondrium and cartilage of the auricle (ear) caused by repeated blunt trauma.

Chondral fracture Fracture involving the articular cartilage at a joint.

Chondromalacia patellae Degenerative condition in the articular cartilage of the patella caused by abnormal compression or shearing forces.

Chronic injury An injury with long onset and long duration.

Circumduction Movement of a body part in a circular direction.

Clonic Movement marked by repetitive muscle contractions and relaxation in rapid succession.

Cold diuresis Excretion of urine in cold weather; caused by blood being shunted away from the skin to the core to maintain vascular volume.

Collagen protein substance found in connective tissue; it provides strength in resisting tensile forces

Collateral ligaments Major ligaments that cross the medial and lateral aspects of a hinge joint to provide stability from valgus and varus forces.

Colles fracture Fracture involving a dorsally angulated and displaced/radially angulated and displaced fracture within 1½ inches of the wrist.

Commission Committing an act that is not legally one's duty to perform.

Comparative negligence The relative degree of negligence on the part of the plaintiff and defendant, with damages awarded on a basis proportionate to each person's carelessness.

Compartment syndrome Condition in which increased intramuscular pressure brought on by activity impedes blood flow and function of tissues within that compartment.

Compression A pressure or squeezing force directed through a body that increases density.

Concussion Violent shaking or jarring action of the brain resulting in immediate or transient impairment of neurologic function.

Conjunctivitis Bacterial infection leading to itching, burning, watering, and inflamed eye; pinkeye.

Constipation Infrequent or incomplete bowel movements.

Contraindication A condition adversely affected if a particular action is taken.

Contrecoup injuries Injuries away from the actual injury site because of rotational components during acceleration.

Contusion Compression injury involving accumulation of blood and lymph within a muscle; a bruise.

Coronal plane A vertical plane at right angles to a sagittal plane that divides the body into anterior and posterior portions.

Coup injuries Injuries at the site where direct impact occurs.

Cramp Painful involuntary muscle contraction, either clonic or tonic.

Crepitus Crackling sound or sensation characteristic of a fracture when the bones ends are moved.

Cruciate ligaments Major ligaments that crisscross the knee in the anteroposterior direction, providing stability in that plane.

Cryotherapy Cold application.

Curvatures A bending, as in the spine (kyphosis, scoliosis, lordosis).

Cyanosis A dark bluish or purple skin color caused by deficient oxygen in the blood.

Cyclist's palsy Paresthesia in the ulnar nerve distribution; seen when bikers lean on the handlebar for an extended period.

Dead arm syndrome Common sensation felt with a recurrent anterior shoulder subluxation and multidirectional instability.

de Quervain's tenosynovitis An inflammatory stenosing tenosynovitis of the abductor pollicis longus and extensor pollicis brevis tendons.

Detached retina Neurosensory retina separated from the retinal epithelium by swelling.

Diabetes mellitus Metabolic disorder characterized by near or absolute lack of the hormone insulin, insulin resistance, or both.

Diabetic ketoacidosis Condition in which an excess of ketoacids in the blood can lower the blood pH to 7.0; manifested by ketones in the breath, blood, and urine.

Diagnosis Identification of an injury/ illness based on assessment of signs and symptoms

Diarrhea Loose or watery stools.

Diffuse injuries Injury over a large body area, usually caused by low velocity-high mass forces.

Diplopia Double vision.

Dislocation Traumatic injury that occurs when the bones that comprise a joint are forced beyond their normal position, resulting in the displacement of one joint surface on another.

Disposition A physical property or tendency related to an injury or illness.

Diuretics Chemicals that promote the excretion of urine.

Dural sinuses Formed by tubular separations in the inner and outer layers of the dura mater, these sinuses function as small veins for the brain.

Duty of care legal obligation to provide a professional standard of care to protect individuals under one's care or supervision from unreasonable risks that could potentially be harmful

Dyspepsia Gastric indigestion.

Dyspnea Labored or difficult breathing.

Ecchymosis Superficial tissue discoloration.

Edema Swelling resulting from a collection of exuded lymph fluid in interstitial tissues.

Elasticity The ability of a muscle to return to normal length after either lengthening or shortening.

Elastin protein substance found in connective tissue that provides added elasticity to some connective tissue structures

Emesis Vomiting.

Epicondylitis Inflammation and microrupturing of the soft tissues on the epicondyles of the distal humerus.

Epidermis The outer epithelial portion of the skin.

Epiphyseal fracture Injury to the growth plate of a long bone in children and adolescents; may lead to arrested bone growth.

Epiphyseal plate Cartilaginous disc found near the ends of the long bones.

Epistaxis Profuse bleeding from the nose; nosebleed.

Erb's point Located 2 to 3 cm above the clavicle at the level of the transverse process of the C6 vertebra; compression over the site may injure the brachial plexus.

Excitability A muscle's ability to respond to a stimulus; irritability.

Exculpatory waiver a release signed by the individual or parent of an individual under the age of 18 that releases a physician from liability of negligence.

Expressed warranty Written guarantee that states the product is safe for consumer use.

Extensibility The ability of a muscle to be stretched or to increase in length.

Extensor mechanism Complex interaction of muscles, ligaments, and tendons that stabilize and provide motion at the patellofemoral joint.

Extrinsic Origination outside of the part where something is found or upon which it acts; denoting especially a muscle.

Extruded tooth Tooth driven in an outwardly direction.

Extruded disc Condition in which the nuclear material bulges into the spinal canal and runs the risk of impinging adjacent nerve roots.

Exudate Material composed of fluid, pus, or cells that has escaped from blood vessels into surrounding tissues after injury or inflammation.

Facet joint Joint formed when the superior and inferior articular processes mate with the articular process of adjacent vertebrae.

Fasciitis Inflammation of the fascia surrounding portions of a muscle.

Fibroblast A cell present in connective tissue capable of forming collagen fibers.

Flatulence Presence of an excessive amount of gas in the stomach and intestines.

Flexibility Total range of motion at a joint dependent on normal joint mechanics, mobility of soft tissues, and muscle extensibility.

Focal injuries Injury in a small concentrated area, usually caused by high velocity-low mass forces.

Force A push or pull acting on a body.

Foreseeability of harm Condition whereby danger is apparent, or should have been apparent, resulting in an unreasonably unsafe condition.

Fracture Disruption in the continuity of a bone.

Frontal plane A longitudinal (vertical) line that divides the body or any of its parts into anterior and posterior portions. (aka coronal plane)

Gamekeeper's thumb Sprain of the metacarpophalangeal (MCP) joint of the thumb; the thumb is in near extension and is forcefully abducted away from the hand, tearing the ulnar collateral ligament at the MCP joint.

Ganglion cyst Benign tumor mass commonly seen on the dorsal aspect of the wrist.

Gastritis Inflammation, especially mucosal, of the stomach.

Gastrocolic reflex Propulsive reflex in the colon that stimulates defecation.

Gastroenteritis Inflammation of the mucous membrane of the stomach or small intestine.

Glenoid labrum Soft tissue lip around the periphery of the glenoid fossa that widens and deepens the socket to add stability to the joint.

Golgi tendon organ proprioceptors located in tendons and joint ligaments that can be stimulated during stretching; stimulus causes a reflex inhibition in the antagonist muscle.

Hallux The first, or great, toe.

Hallux rigidus Degenerative arthritis in the first MTP joint of the foot associated with pain and limited motion.

Heat cramps Painful involuntary muscle spasms caused by excessive water and electrolyte loss.

Hemarthrosis Collection of blood within a joint or cavity.

Hematoma A localized mass of blood and lymph confined within a space or tissue.

Hematuria Blood or red blood cells in the urine.

Hemothorax Condition involving the loss of blood into the pleural cavity but outside the lung.

Heparin An anticoagulant that is a component of various tissues and mast cells.

Hernia Protrusion of abdominal viscera through a weakened portion of the abdominal wall.

HIPPA Health Insurance Portability and Accountability Act, which includes laws intended to protect the privacy of patients.

Hip pointer Contusions caused by direct compression to an unprotected iliac crest that crushes soft tissue and sometimes the bone itself.

Histamine A powerful stimulant of gastric secretion, a constrictor of bronchial smooth muscle, and a vasodilator (capillaries and arterioles) that causes a fall in blood pressure.

Homeostasis The state of a balanced equilibrium in the body's various tissues and systems.

HOPS Evaluation process that involves history, observation, palpation and special tests.

Hyperglycemia Abnormally high levels of glucose in the circulating blood that can lead to diabetic coma.

Hyperhydration Overhydration; excess water consumption of the body.

Hyperthermia Elevated body temperature.

Hypertrophic cardiomyopathy Excessive hypertrophy of the heart, often of obscure or unknown origin.

Hypertrophy General increase in bulk or size of an individual tissue not caused by tumor formation.

Hyphema Hemorrhage into the anterior chamber of the eye.

Hypoglycemia Abnormally low levels of glucose in the circulating blood that can lead to insulin shock.

Hypothalamus A region of the diencephalon that forms the floor of the third ventricle of the brain; responsible for thermoregulation and other autonomic nervous mechanisms underlying moods and motivational states.

Hypothenar The fleshy mass of muscle and tissue on the medial side of the palm.

Hypothermia Decreased body temperature.

Hypovolemic shock Shock caused by a reduction in volume of blood, as from hemorrhage or dehydration.

Hypoxia A reduced concentration of oxygen in air, blood, or tissue, short of anoxia.

Idiopathic Of unknown origin or cause.

Impingement syndrome Chronic condition caused by repetitive overhead activity that damages the supraspinatus tendon, glenoid labrum, long head of the biceps brachii, and subacromial bursa.

Implied warranty Unwritten guarantee that the product is reasonably safe when used for its intended purpose.

Indication A condition that could benefit from a specific action.

Individuality When individuals have different responses to a conditioning program due to age, gender, body type, heredity, lifestyle, fitness level, illness/chronic conditions, and previous experience.

Infectious mononucleosis An acute illness associated with the Epstein-Barr herpetovirus; characterized by fever, sore throat, enlargement of lymph nodes and spleen, and leukopenia that changes to lymphocytosis.

Inflammation Pain, swelling, redness, heat, and loss of function that accompany musculoskeletal injuries.

Influenza Acute infectious respiratory tract condition characterized by malaise, headache, dry cough, and general muscle aches.

Informed consent Consent given by a person of legal age who understands the nature and extent of any treatment and available alternative treatments before agreeing to receiving treatment.

Innominate Without a name; used to describe anatomic structures.

Intrinsic In anatomy, denoting those muscles of the limbs whose origin and insertion are both in the same limb.

Intruded tooth Tooth driven deep into the socket in an inwardly direction.

Irritability Ability of muscle to respond to a stimulus.

Ischemia Local anemia caused by decreased blood supply.

Ischemic necrosis Death of a tissue caused by decreased blood supply.

Jersey finger Rupture of the flexor digitorum profundus tendon from the distal phalanx caused by rapid extension of the finger while actively flexed.

Jones fracture A transverse stress fracture of the proximal shaft of the fifth metatarsal.

Kehr's sign Referred pain down the left shoulder indicative of a ruptured spleen.

Ketoacidosis Condition caused by excess accumulation of acid or loss of base in the body; characteristic of diabetes mellitus.

Ketonuria Enhanced urinary excretion of ketone bodies.

Kyphosis Excessive curve in the thoracic region of the spine.

Legg-Calvé-Perthes disease Avascular necrosis of the proximal femoral epiphysis seen especially in young males ages 3 to 8 years.

Little leaguer elbow Tension stress injury of the medial epicondyle commonly seen in adolescents.

Little league shoulder Fracture of the proximal humeral growth plate in adolescents caused by repetitive rotational stresses during pitching.

Lordosis Excessive convex curve in the lumbar region of the spine.

Lumbar plexus Interconnected roots of the first four lumbar spinal nerves.

Malaise Lethargic feeling of general discomfort; out-of-sorts feeling.

Malfeasance Committing an act that is not one's responsibility to perform

Mallet finger Rupture of the extensor tendon from the distal phalanx caused by forceful flexion of the phalanx.

Malocclusion Inability to bring the teeth together in a normal bite.

Marfan syndrome Inherited connective tissue disorder affecting many organs, but commonly resulting in the dilation and weakening of the thoracic aorta.

Mast cells Connective tissue cells that carry heparin, which prolongs clotting, and histamine.

McBurney's point A site one-third the distance between the anterior superior iliac spine and umbilicus that, with deep palpation, produces rebound tenderness indicating appendicitis.

Mechanism of injury The manner in which an injury occurred.

Meninges Three protective membranes that surround the brain and spinal cord.

Meningitis Inflammation of the meninges of the brain and spinal column.

Menisci Fibrocartilaginous discs found within a joint that reduce joint stress.

Misfeasance While committing an act that is one's responsibility to perform, following the wrong procedure or performing the right procedure in an improper manner.

Mitral valve prolapse A condition in which redundant tissue is found on one or both leaflets of the mitral valve. During a ventricular contraction, a portion of the redundant tissue on the mitral valve pushes back beyond the normal limit and, as a result, produces an abnormal sound followed by a systolic murmur as blood is regurgitated back through the mitral valve into the left atrium; often called a click-murmur syndrome.

Muscle cramp A painful, involuntary contraction that is either clonic (alternating contraction and relaxation) or tonic (continued contraction over time).

Muscle spasm A short, involuntary contraction caused by reflex action biochemically derived or initiated by a mechanical blow to a nerve or muscle.

Muscle spindle proprioceptors located in muscle fibers that can be stimulated during stretching; stimulus causes a reflex contraction which inhibits the stretch

Musculotendinous unit Composed of both muscle and tendon.

Myocardial infarction Heart attack.

Myositis Inflammation of connective tissue within a muscle.

Myositis ossificans Accumulation of mineral deposits within muscle tissue.

Necrosis The death of areas of tissue or bone surrounded by healthy parts.

Negligence Breach of one's duty of care that causes harm to another individual.

Neoplasm A new or abnormal formation of tissue, as a tumor or growth.

Nephropathy Any disease of the kidney.

Neurapraxia Injury to a nerve that results in temporary neurologic deficits followed by complete recovery of function.

Neurotmesis Complete severance of a nerve.

Nociceptor A receptor that is sensitive to potentially damaging stimuli that result in pain.

Nonfeasance Failing to perform one's legal duty of care.

Nonunion fracture Failure of normal healing of a fractured bone.

Nystagmus Abnormal jerking or involuntary eye movement.

Oligomenorrhea Infrequent menstrual cycles or menstruation that involves scant blood flow.

Omission Failing to perform a legal duty of care.

Osgood-Schlatter disease Inflammation or partial avulsion of the tibial apophysis due to traction forces.

Osteitis pubis Stress fracture to the pubic symphysis caused by repeated overload of the adductor muscles or repetitive stress activities.

Osteoarthritis Type of arthritis attributed to degeneration of the articular cartilage in a joint.

Osteochondral fracture Fracture involving the articular cartilage and underlying bone.

Osteochondritis dissecans Localized area of avascular necrosis that results in complete or incomplete separation of joint cartilage and subchondral bone.

Osteochondrosis Any condition characterized by degeneration or aseptic necrosis of the articular cartilage because of limited blood supply.

Osteopenia Condition of reduced bone mineral density that predisposes the individual to fractures.

Otitis externa Bacterial infection involving the lining of the auditory canal; swimmer's ear.

Otitis media Localized infection in the middle ear secondary to upper respiratory infections.

Overload principle that physiologic improvements occur only when an individual physically demands more of the body than is normally required

Paresthesia Abnormal sensations, such as tingling, burning, itching, or prickling.

Paronychia A fungal or bacterial infection in the folds of skin surrounding a fingernail or toenail.

Patellofemoral joint Gliding joint between the patella and patellar groove of the femur.

Patellofemoral stress syndrome Condition whereby the lateral retinaculum is tight, or the vastus medialis oblique is weak, leading to lateral excursion and pressure on the lateral facet of the patella; causes a painful condition.

Pericardial tamponade Compression of venous return to the heart caused by increased volume of fluid in the pericardium; usually caused by direct trauma to the chest.

Periorbital ecchymosis Swelling and hemorrhage into the surrounding eyelids; black eye.

Periostitis Inflammation of the periosteum (outer membrane covering the bone).

Peritonitis Irritation of the peritoneum that lines the abdominal cavity.

Pes cavus High arch.

Pes planus Flat feet.

Phagocytosis Process by which white blood cells surround and digest foreign particles, such as bacteria and necrotic tissue.

Pharyngitis Viral, bacterial, or fungal infection of the pharynx that causes a sore throat.

Phonophoresis The introduction of anti-inflammatory drugs through the skin with the use of ultrasound.

Photophobia Abnormal sensitivity to light.

Plantar fascia Specialized band of fascia that covers the plantar surface of the foot and helps support the longitudinal arch.

Pneumothorax Condition whereby air is trapped in the pleural space, causing a portion of a lung to collapse.

Polyphagia Excessive hunger and food consumption; gluttony

Polyuria Excessive excretion of urine that causes a huge urine output of water and electrolytes and leads to decreased blood volume and further dehydration.

Postconcussion syndrome Delayed condition characterized by persistent headaches, blurred vision, irritability, and inability to concentrate.

Primary Survey Assesment of responsiveness, airway, breathing, and circulation to identify and initiate management of any life-threatening condition

Prolapsed disc Condition in which the eccentric nucleus produces a definite deformity as it works its way through the fibers of the annulus fibrosus.

Pronation Inward rotation of the forearm; palms face posteriorly. At the foot, combined motions of calcaneal eversion, foot abduction, and dorsiflexion.

Proprioceptor A sensory receptor, commonly found in muscles, tendons, joints, and the inner ear, that detects the motion or position of the body or a limb by responding to stimuli within the organism.

Prostaglandins Active substances found in many tissues, with effects such as vasodilation, vasoconstriction, and stimulation of intestinal or bronchial smooth muscle.

Purulent Containing, consisting of, or forming pus.

Q-angle Angle between the line of quadriceps force and the patellar tendon.

Raccoon eyes Delayed discoloration around the eyes from anterior cranial fossa fracture.

Raynaud's syndrome A condition characterized by intermittent bilateral attacks of ischemia of the fingers or toes and marked by severe pallor, numbness, and pain.

Reciprocal inhibition uses active agonist contractions to relax a tight antagonist muscle

Referred pain Pain perceived at a location remote from the site of the tissues actually causing the pain.

Reflex Action involving stimulation of a motor neuron by a sensory neuron in the spinal cord without involvement of the brain.

Relative humidity The ratio of the amount of water vapor present in an air sample to the amount that could be present if the sample were saturated with water vapor.

Retinopathy Noninflammatory degenerative disease of the retina.

Retrograde amnesia Forgetting events before an injury.

Rhinitis Inflammation of the nasal membranes with excessive mucus production resulting in nasal congestion and postnasal drip.

Rhinorrhea Clear nasal discharge.

Rotator cuff The SITS muscles (supraspinatus, infraspinatus, teres minor, and subscapularis) hold the head of the humerus in the glenoid fossa and produce humeral rotation.

Rubor Redness; one of the four classic signs of inflammation.

Sacral plexus Interconnected roots of the L4-S4 spinal nerves that innervate the lower extremities.

Saddle joint A biaxial-like condyloid joint with both concave and convex areas, but with freer movement, like the carpometacarpal joints of the thumbs.

Sagittal plane A longitudinal (vertical) line that divides the body or any of it parts into right and left portions.

SAID principle states that the body responds to a given demand with a specific and predictable adaptation.

Sciatica Compression of a spinal nerve caused by a herniated disc, annular tear, myogenic or muscle-related disease, spinal stenosis, facet joint arthropathy, or compression from the piriformis muscle.

Scoliosis Lateral rotational spinal curvature.

Screwing-home mechanism Rotation of the tibia on the femur at the end of extension to produce a "locking" of the knee in a closed packed position.

Secondary survey Assessment performed following a primary survey to determine the type and extent of any injury and the immediate disposition of the condition.

Sesamoid bone An oval nodule of bone or fibrocartilage in a tendon playing over a bony surface.

Shear force A force directed parallel to a surface.

Shock Collapse of the cardiovascular system when insufficient blood cannot provide circulation for the entire body.

Sign Objective measurable physical findings that you can hear, feel, see, or smell during the assessment.

Sinusitis Inflammation of the paranasal sinuses.

Smith's fracture Volar displacement of the distal fragment of the radius; sometimes called a reversed Colles fracture.

Snapping hip syndrome A snapping sensation either heard or felt during motion at the hip.

Solar plexus punch A blow to the abdomen with the muscles relaxed resulting in an immediate inability to catch one's breath.

Somatic pain Pain arising from the skin, ligaments, muscles, bones, and joints.

Spasm Transitory muscle contractions.

Spondylolisthesis Anterior slippage of a vertebra resulting from complete bilateral fracture of the pars interarticularis.

Spondylolysis A stress fracture of the pars interarticularis.

Sports medicine Area of health and special services that applies medical and scientific knowledge to prevent, recognize, manage, and rehabilitate injuries related to sport, exercise, or recreational activity.

Sprain Injury to ligamentous tissue.

Standard of care Minimum standard that requires an individual to act as a reasonably prudent person; in a professional setting, use of the knowledge, skills, and abilities that conform to the standard of care for a particular specialization.

Static stretch Increasing flexibility by using movement that is slow and deliberate

Stenosing Narrowing of an opening or stricture of a canal; stenosis.

Stitch in the side A sharp pain or spasm in the chest wall, usually on the lower right side, during exertion.

Strain Amount of deformation with respect to the original dimensions of the structure; injury to the musculotendinous unit.

Stress The distribution of force within a body; quantified as force divided by the area over which the force acts.

Stress fracture Fracture resulting from repeated loading with relatively low magnitude forces.

Subconjunctival hemorrhage Minor capillary ruptures in the eye globe.

Subluxation A partial or incomplete dislocation.

Subungual hematoma Hematoma beneath a fingernail or toenail.

Sudden death A nontraumatic, unexpected death that occurs instantaneously or within a few minutes of an abrupt change in an individual's previous clinical state.

Supination Outward rotation of the forearm; palms facing forward. At the foot, combined motions of calcaneal inversion, foot adduction, and plantar flexion.

Symptom Subjective information provided by an individual regarding his or her perception of the problem.

Syncope Fainting or lightheadedness.

Tachycardia Rapid beating of the heart, usually applied to rates over 100 beats per minute.

Tendinitis Inflammation of a tendon.

Tenosynovitis Inflammation of a tendon sheath.

Tensile force A pulling or stretching force directed axially through a body or body part.

Tension pneumothorax Condition in which air continuously leaks into the pleural space, causing the mediastinum to displace to the opposite side and compressing the uninjured lung and thoracic aorta.

Thenar The fleshy mass of muscle and tissue on the lateral palm; the ball of the thumb.

Thermoregulation The process by which the body maintains body temperature; primarily controlled by the hypothalamus.

Thermotherapy Heat application.

Thoracic outlet syndrome Condition whereby nerves or vessels become compressed in the root of the neck or axilla, leading to numbness in the arm.

Tibiofemoral joint Dual condyloid joints between the tibial and femoral condyles that function primarily as a modified hinge joint.

Tinnitus Ringing or other noises in the ear caused by trauma or disease.

Torsion force Twisting around an object's longitudinal axis in response to an applied torque.

Tort A wrong done to an individual whereby the injured party seeks a remedy for damages suffered.

Transverse plane A horizontal line that divides the body into superior and inferior portions.

Triage Assessing all injured individuals to determine priority of care.

Turf toe A sprain of the plantar capsular ligament of the first MTP joint, which results from forced hyperextension or hyperflexion of the great toe.

Unconsciousness Impairment of brain function wherein the individual lacks conscious awareness and is unable to respond to superficial .sensory stimuli.

Urticaria Hives; an eruption of itching wheals, usually of systemic origin; may result from a state of hypersensitivity to foods or drugs, infection, physical agents, or psychic stimuli.

Valgus An opening on the medial side of a joint caused by the distal segment moving laterally.

Valsalva maneuver Holding one's breath against a closed glottis, resulting in sharp increases in blood pressure.

Varus An opening on the lateral side of a joint caused by the distal segment moving medially.

Vasoconstriction Narrowing of the blood vessels; opposite of vasodilation.

Vasodilation Enlarging of the blood vessels; opposite of vasoconstriction.

Visceral pain Pain resulting from disease or injury to an organ in the thoracic or abdominal cavity.

Volkmann's contracture Ischemic necrosis of the forearm muscles and tissues caused by damage to the blood flow.

Wedge fracture A crushing compression fracture that leaves a vertebra narrowed anteriorly.

Yield point (elastic limit) The maximum load that a material can sustain without permanent deformation.

Zone of primary injury Region of injured tissue before vasodilation.

Zone of secondary injury Region of damaged tissue after vasodilation.

Note: Page numbers followed by b, f, s, and t indicates box, figure, application strategy, and table respectively.